BULLETS
AND BRAINS

BY ANDREW NATHAN WILNER MD

A COLLECTION OF ESSAYS
ORIGINALLY PUBLISHED ON
MEDSCAPE.COM

Other Books by the Author

Epilepsy:199 Answers, 3rd Edition

Epilepsy in Clinical Practice

ISBN: 1490396926
ISBN-13: 9781490396927
Library of Congress Control Number: 2013910965
CreateSpace Independent Publishing Platform
North Charleston, South Carolina

DEDICATION

To my grandfather, Jack Leonard,
who always wrote me letters.

TABLE OF CONTENTS

FOREWORD

Distilling complex medical and scientific information into easy-to-understand, informative, and, ultimately, enjoyable prose is not easy. Jargon and daunting chemical names can get in the way, as can the reams of data that accompany most advances - which is why I would like to thank Dr. Andrew N. Wilner for making my job a little easier.

Dr. Wilner is a neurologist, fellowship-trained epileptologist, and prolific author. He has published two prior books on epilepsy, *Epilepsy: 199 Answers, 3rd Edition,* and *Epilepsy in Clinical Practice.* As the Editorial Director for Medscape Neurology News, I've had the pleasure of editing and publishing Dr. Wilner's work for the previous four years. "Editing" might actually be too strong a word given the negligible polishing his contributions require. Dr. Wilner's approach to medical journalism consistently conveys high-level concepts through an approachable, engaging voice. His writing is thoughtful, evocative, informative.

Bullets and Brains is a collection of over 100 of Dr. Wilner's essays about people and their brains. These articles all originally appeared on Medscape.com, a division of WebMD geared toward healthcare professionals, primarily as part of the prolific author's two recurring columns: "Wilner on Neurology" and "Epilepsy Notes." Although written for a medical audience, most of these essays address the impact of neurological topics on society and culture, and are easily accessible to the curious reader.

Dr. Wilner's writings span neurology. In *Bullets and Brains,* Alzheimer's disease, multiple sclerosis, Parkinson's disease, traumatic brain injury, stroke, and the intersection of neurology and psychiatry are all explored. Epilepsy, Dr. Wilner's area of interest, is addressed in more depth given his expertise on the subject and his monthly column dedicated to the disorder. The final section highlights recent guidelines on the prevention and treatment of diseases of the brain; though primarily directed toward clinicians, anyone with a personal connection or interest to the respective diseases may find this information worthwhile.

I think you will greatly enjoy the neurologic musings and insights in *Bullets and Brains.* For more from Dr. Wilner, follow his work on Medscape.com/neurology.

Bret S. Stetka, MD
Editorial Director
Medscape Neurology News
http://www.medscape.com/neurology
June 25, 2013

AUTHOR'S NOTE

Writing these essays has provided an outlet for observations regarding the rapid evolution of neurology practice in the United States and how it affects physicians, other healthcare providers, patients and caregivers. All of us have been drawn into a 21st century whirling tornado of scientific advances, complicated insurance plans, government initiatives of the Health Insurance Portability and Accountability Act (HIPAA) and Affordable Care Act, electronic medical records that save everything and obfuscate nearly all of it, Byzantine local politics, hospital mergers and bankruptcies, a challenging economy and many more variables that affect what is arguably our most important and intimate asset, our health. As a practicing neurologist and sometimes patient and caregiver, I have also been sucked inside this relentless vortex, but the knowledge that a column is due almost every week has forced me to extricate myself, at least for a few hours at a time, to crawl outside for a better view.

Bullets and Brains begins with a section on brain injury. Sports-related traumatic brain injury has recently been recognized as an important public health issue and is discussed along with bullet and blast injury. A host of topics that concern our brain's relationship with modern society follow, including mass hysteria, microgravity, nanotechnology, the effect of an earthquake on epilepsy care in Haiti, the ethics of "neuroenhancement," romance, social media and health care, stigma of epilepsy, video games, and wartime memories. Topics regarding treatment decisions are also investigated such as anti-venom for scorpion stings, "Cheesecake Factory" medicine, chronic cerebrospinal venous insufficiency (CCSVI) procedures for multiple sclerosis, dance therapy for Parkinson's disease, marijuana for epilepsy, medical evacuation from Antarctica for stroke, merits of vaccines for children, stents or surgery for carotid artery disease, and vaccines for rabies.

In the large section about epilepsy, recently approved drugs, such as clobazam (Onfi), ezogabine (Potiga) and vigabatrin (Sabril), novel treatments of deep brain stimulation and trigeminal nerve stimulation, and a watch-like epilepsy monitoring device are presented, as well as newly recognized drug side effects. Progress in epilepsy research is detailed, including advances in genetic testing, newly defined causes for epilepsy, up-to-date knowledge about medication-related birth defects and developmental delay, as well as an historical overview regarding the evolution of epilepsy care by leaders in the field.

Important physician practice issues are analyzed, such as the increasing subspecialization of neurologists into those who work in their offices or outpatient clinics and those who care for acutely ill hospitalized patients (neurohospitalists), the burgeoning use of "mid-level" providers in addition to (or instead of) physicians, government rules regarding the interaction between physicians and pharmaceutical companies, the responsibilities of the physician/passenger during in-flight medical emergencies, and the appeal of volunteer medical mission work in a foreign country.

The last section, "Prevention and Treatment Guidelines," summarizes official guidelines from various societies regarding the assessment and/or treatment of a number of conditions, such as brain death, Bell's Palsy, cerebral aneurysms, delirium, epilepsy and pregnancy, HIV and epilepsy, Huntington's Chorea, infantile spasms, intracerebral hemorrhage, microcephaly, Parkinson's disease, transverse myelitis, and traumatic brain injury. This section is intended primarily for clinicians, and offers commentary on the usefulness of these guidelines.

Writing these columns over the last four years has provided an opportunity to reflect on my own role in this rapidly evolving health care system. While there is value in remembering and extolling the merits of "the way it used to be," an improved appreciation for where we are and where we are going might allow us to anticipate and meet the future head on, rather than spend our days reeling from its effects. This strategy may support efforts to continue to provide high quality patient care as well as insist on a healthy professional practice environment, two ambitious but necessary goals.

Finally, I hope my observations shed some light on the importance of our central nervous system and the discipline of neurology in our day to day lives, provoke thought and discussion, and at least in some cases, help to navigate a complex health care system buffeted by the turbulent winds of change.

Andrew Wilner, MD, FACP, FAAN
August 20, 2013

ACKNOWLEDGEMENTS

My editor, Bret Stetka, MD, offered me the opportunity to begin writing these columns over four years ago. Since then Bret has been a dependable ally, consistent motivator, and constant source of encouragement. My literate parents also deserve mention as they recognized early on my passion for writing and remain my best critics and cheerleaders. Sarah Block and Vanessa Cancino provided helpful feedback on the manuscript. A large group of colleagues and friends, too many to name here, have been on the receiving end of these columns over the years, and I thank all of them for their continued interest and feedback. A number of people participated in interviews for these columns, including Anthony Alessi, MD, Selim Benbadis, MD, Martin Brodie, MD, Julian Cautherley, Lionel Carmant, MD, James Cloyd, PharmD, Jill Diamond, Robert Fisher, MD, PhD, Patricia Gibson, Gary Gronseth, MD, Anoo Nathan, Tom Panayiotopoulos, MD, Brett Petersen, MD, MPH, Randall Shapiro, MD, and Sherry Wulkan, MD. I appreciate the generosity of their time and willingness to share their knowledge and experience. Sally McMillan, my long-time agent, and Diana Schneider, PhD, publisher of my first two books, helped direct the development of *Bullets and Brains*.

I would also like to thank the readers of Medscape. com. Their enthusiastic reception of these essays has been much appreciated and prompted the development of this collection.

Section 1.

Traumatic Brain Injury

Chapter 1.

BULLETS AND BRAINS

January 11, 2011

Bullets and brains, despite the alliteration, don't belong together. Anyone can tell you that. Except Arizona Congresswoman Gabrielle Giffords, who may never be able to speak again after a would-be assassin's bullet traversed the left side of her brain three days ago.

Early reports suggest that at least some parts of Wernicke's area were spared by the 9 mm bullet, as Giffords was able to comprehend a question and respond by raising up two fingers. At this writing, her vocal cords remain separated by a plastic endotracheal tube attached to a ventilator preventing any possibility of speech. When the tube is removed, we'll have more information on the integrity of her Broca's area.

The first time I was up close to a "living brain" was about 20 years ago during surgery in a young man with intractable epilepsy. I was amazed when I touched its surface with my finger-so soft! I don't know why I was surprised, but somehow I expected something so important to be more substantial than what looked and felt like a big chunk of pulsating, grey Jello.

I think that memory of the brain's velvet vulnerability motivated me to write about boxing and other contact sports. When observing a roundhouse blow, I imagine that precious glob of tissue shuddering in its pool of cerebrospinal fluid, veins and arteries stretched to the point of tearing, axons shearing, and just a bit of a twist on the brainstem, maybe enough for a knockout. While boxing may have other merits, protecting the brain isn't one of them. (The high speed collision of two NFL helmets also makes me wince.)

The care of acute penetrating head injury remains the neurosurgeon's domain. According to news reports, Michael Lemole, Jr., MD, Chief of Neurosurgery at the University of Arizona Department of Surgery, Tucson, AZ, and Martin Weinand, MD, Professor of Neurosurgery, University Medical Center, Tucson, AZ, were in the operating room 38 minutes after the shooting to remove "gunshot debris, dead brain tissue, and part of her skull."

Given that the bullet entered the back of her head and exited just above her left eye, the area of brain injury included at least parts of the left occipital, parietal, temporal, and frontal lobes. The bullet's shockwave widened the swath of destruction to more than its 9 mm diameter.

According to Nina Zeldis, PhD, a rehabilitation expert who taught at Tel Aviv University for more than 20 years, deficits from this type of injury may include difficulty speaking and understanding, reading, problem solving, planning, hand/eye coordination, as well as behavior problems like impulsivity and emotional lability. In addition, Congresswoman Giffords has a high risk of developing post-traumatic epilepsy. Other than state of the art wound care, we have no medications to impede the process of epileptogenesis and prevent her from developing a lifelong seizure disorder. While we do have a host of medications to successfully treat seizures, side effects may include sedation and adverse behavioral effects adding to the morbidity of her injury.

James Eklung, MD, Chairman of Neurosciences at Inova Fairfax Hospital, Falls Church, VA, and Geoffrey Ling, MD, PhD, Colonel, Medical Corps, US Army, both experts in treating combat injuries, have been sent to Tucson to assist in Congresswoman Giffords' care. I had the privilege of listening to Dr. Ling speak during last December's American Epilepsy Society meeting in San Antonio, Texas. In the context of a discussion of blast injury, Dr. Ling showed a video of an American convoy under attack in Afghanistan. It was not for the faint of heart. Perhaps lessons learned in war will benefit Congresswoman Giffords. She has already received the worst we have to offer as a free democratic society (an attack from a mentally ill individual with a *legal* Glock 19 loaded with more than 30 rounds), at least she will receive the best we have to offer in medical care.

As a neurologist, I admire the amazing complexity of the brain, but I worry about its vulnerability to dementia, seizures, strokes, trauma, and multiple other ills. The rapid demise of Senator Ted Kennedy from an aggressive glioma and the relentless deterioration of President Ronald Reagan from Alzheimer's disease highlight our therapeutic impotence.

Those of us who work with neurologically injured patients, including neurosurgeons, neurologists, neuropsychologists, physical medicine and rehabilitation specialists, and occupational, physical, and speech therapists, cannot help but be humbled by the limitations of our therapies. While the brain *can* heal from traumatic injury, circuits reorganize, and functional recovery occur, it is a slow, incomplete, and imperfect process. Opportunities for brain research abound, and the need has never been greater as tens of thousands of our young soldiers return from foreign countries with traumatic brain injury and the increasing elderly population succumbs to strokes and dementia.

Barring a miracle (and I do not hesitate to pray for one), Congresswoman Gabrielle Giffords will never return to her work in Washington, DC. Statistically, she is lucky to be alive, as the vast majority of people with bullets to the brain do not survive. Whether she is lucky or not, only Congresswoman Giffords and her family can decide.

Update May 14, 2013

Analysis by military doctors suggested that the 9 mm bullet entered Gabrielle Giffords' head front to back, not back to front. She had a cranioplasty on May 18, 2011, to replace part of her skull with plastic. She was discharged from the rehabilitation hospital June 15, 2011, more than five months after the shooting. Although her recovery was considered to be in the top 5% for someone with her degree of injury, she has persistent speech difficulties, lost about 50% of her vision, her right arm is paralyzed, and she has trouble walking. She continues with outpatient speech and physical therapy. Gabrielle Giffords resigned from Congress on January 25, 2012. In January, 2013, Gabrielle Giffords and her astronaut husband, Mark Kelly, started "Americans for Responsible Solutions," an advocacy group for responsible gun control.

Chapter 2

BULLETS, BOMBS, AND FISTS

May 2, 2009

Today's my last day at the American Academy of Neurology meeting, but I managed to catch half of the Traumatic Brain Injury session this afternoon. One of the reasons for this symposium was painfully evident. A quick look around the room revealed several men in military uniforms. (Not being a military man myself, I learned that the green ones are Army and the blue ones, Air Force.)

According to one of the speakers, Captain Brett Theeler, MD, a PGY 4 neurology resident, 15-25% of soldiers returning from Iraq and Afghanistan have suffered mild traumatic brain injury. Dr. Theeler screened more than 5,000 soldiers and identified 1,033 who had a head injury, concussion, or blast exposure. A headache questionnaire was administered to 978/1,033 (95%) (954 males and 24 females) to determine the types of headache. Headaches requiring medication occurred about 7 times/month and often had migraine-like features. Usually the soldiers treated the headaches with over the counter medications such as nonsteroidal anti-inflammatory drugs (NSAIDs) and acetaminophen. The soldiers were usually not disabled by the headaches.

During the same session, Anthony Alessi, MD, a neurologist from Norwich, CT, presented a paper on the value of electroencephalography (EEG) as a screening tool for brain injury in boxers.

I have to admit that it seemed kind of bizarre that, on the one hand, we were talking about traumatic brain injury due to the horrors of war, and, on the other hand, we were talking about brain injury due to a sport played for entertainment. As Dr. Alessi pointed out, "The only way to score a point in boxing is to neurologically impair your opponent."

Dr. Alessi explained that EEG had traditionally been used to screen boxers for neurologic abnormalities. However, his review of 98 EEGs performed in 86 boxers who had fought in 5,809 fights failed to find a significant abnormality, and no boxer was disqualified from fighting on the basis of an EEG. Consequently, he recommended to the local boxing authorities that they drop the EEG requirement and replace it with a neurologic history and examination, and neuroimaging (CT or MRI), neuropsychological testing, and EEG when indicated. The boxing authorities accepted his recommendation. Since then, more contestants have been denied licensing based on abnormal neurologic exams and imaging. Dr. Alessi was gratified, "We were able to put together data that changed behavior."

Dr. Alessi explained that a neurological examination that reveals persistent lateralized nystagmus, fourth nerve palsy, slow response, or coordination problems suggests that the boxer has sustained cumulative head injury and should not be allowed to fight.

While a ban on boxing would eliminate the problem of boxing related head injury, the sport has many avid supporters. Consequently, Dr. Alessi recommended that neurologists become more involved in boxing in order to help safeguard those who choose to box.

Chapter 3

BOXING: ROUND TWO

September 23, 2009

I wanted to follow up on the May 2nd, 2009, post about traumatic brain injury from the American Academy of Neurology meeting, particularly the section about boxing. Although there weren't many responses to the poll, the voting was 4:1 that boxing should be banned.

In an effort to learn more about boxing and neurology, I called Tony Alessi, MD, who presented the paper on boxing and EEG. Dr. Alessi is a private practice neurologist in Norwich, CT, and has been treating boxers for 13 years. He is also the host of a ReachMD neurology radio show.

Dr. Alessi attends a fight about once a month as a ringside physician. I figured he liked boxing, but Dr. Alessi set me straight, "I am not a boxing fan. I don't recommend boxing. I hate it. The neurologist's role at ringside is to advocate for the fighter; that's a duty to these athletes who are really our patients. In Connecticut, the physician can end the fight. There are three physicians at every fight in Connecticut, a primary care doctor, neurologist, and typically a plastic surgeon or emergency doctor, and any one of them can cancel the fight. In many situations, the fighter wants to quit, but there is no honorable way to end the fight. If I do it, I may have just saved his life."

Jill Diamond, an avid boxer and chairwoman of the North American Boxing Federation's (NABF) women's division, taught me a little bit more about why boxers box.

According to Ms. Diamond, "Boxers do it because it is a job, and a job they can be proud of if they are good."

For Ms. Diamond, boxing offers many rewards, "I box as a workout. There are tangible results. It's raw, imaginative, creative, primal, structured, traditional, and has a sense of community. It's a very natural form of human expression, and thankfully it's regulated by the government."

Ms. Diamond observed that boxing is a growing sport for women, "Women find the competition and the confidence exhilarating. Essentially, boxing is legalized assault."

Woman and boxing is especially popular outside the US, in countries such as Germany, Argentina, and Japan.

"In the US there is a cultural problem; men 50 and over usually don't want to see women box. Men under 35 are fine with it. Men are still your basic audience for boxing," said Ms. Diamond.

Ms. Diamond explained that part of her mission is to make boxing, an intrinsically unsafe sport, safer. "At my fights, there is drug testing, a ringside physician, and a fight supervisor to check the weights and dressing rooms. Medical standards vary from state to state and country to country. When we saw deaths in the Philippines, we sent doctors there to teach when to stop fights and how to treat someone with a knockout."

Ms. Diamond added, "I would like to see standardized rules for all states and countries, standardized medical testing, and a computerized system for sharing boxers' medical information."

Sherry Wulkan, MD, a board certified internist, is a commissioned ringside physician for the New York and New Jersey State Athletic Control Boards. Dr. Wulkan provided me with information and a number of articles regarding boxing and neurologic injury. For example, there appear to be at least 3 different mechanisms for a knockout.

1. Stimulation of the trigeminal nerve, vagus nerve, or carotid sinus causes a reflex drop in heart rate, cerebral blood vessel constriction, and peripheral blood vessel dilatation, a "neurovascular knockout."

2. Strikes to the side of the head or the angle of the jaw from a punch known as a "hook" result in rotational forces that can disrupt brain function by one of four hypothetical mechanisms: a) twisting of the brainstem with disturbance of the reticular activating system, b) stimulation of the trigeminal nerve, c) activation of the carotid sinus, and d) diffuse axonal injury.

3. The "pummeling knockout," which occurs without loss of consciousness, but with dissociation and confusion. This type of knockout is believed to be caused by traumatic disruption of neuronal activity.

Of course, knockouts may present concomitantly with cerebral contusions, subdural hematomas, and concussions. To see what happens to neurons and astroglia after a fight, check out the paper by Zetterberg et al. (2006). For some historical context, see Martland (1928) regarding the "punch drunk" syndrome.

Dr. Wulkan observed, "The only two legal areas of contact between participants are the body above the belt line and the head. We know that the number of ring-years (number of rounds sparred x the number of years as a participant), age, quantity of "wars," knockouts, concussions, and lifestyle habits when not in training are some of the more important variables that play a role in the development of chronic traumatic brain injury. "

Dr. Wulkan added, "There are many renowned neurologists, neurosurgeons, sports medicine physicians, and physiologists who have dedicated their careers to either clinical or basic science research in this field. They are attempting to develop diagnostic tools that could more readily pinpoint risk factors for head injury, improve the efficiency and rapidity of diagnosis and treatment of brain injury through technological advances, and help discover better treatment for those showing early signs of neurologic dysfunction."

Dr. Wulkan concluded, "Above all, I have tremendous respect for the dedication, drive, and conditioning of these athletes, and have come to view boxing and mixed martial arts as highly competitive, fast, chess games. As a medical community, it is our job to make the sport as safe as possible and to continue to do research about the short and long term effects of combat sports on participants. Perhaps some of what we learn may cross over to other disciplines, or can be of some benefit to patients who sustain neurologic damage from other types of trauma."

Given the rising enthusiasm of women for boxing, I asked Dr. Alessi if he would allow his daughter, now a medical student, to box. He replied without hesitation, "Absolutely not."

References

Martland HS. Punch Drunk. JAMA 1928;91(15):1103-1107.

Zetterberg H, Hietala MA, Jonsson M et al. Neurochemical aftermath of amateur boxing. Arch Neurol 2006;63:1277-1280.

Chapter 4

BOXING AND ME

February 2, 2013

Introduction

I've addressed boxing in several blogs, focusing on its intrinsic potential to harm the brain. The American Academy of Pediatrics recommends that pediatricians "vigorously oppose boxing for any child or adolescent." The deleterious effect of repetitive mild traumatic brain injury on amateur and professional boxers and other athletes, as well as the effects of blast injury on soldiers, have become important research topics and public health issues (Stern et al. 2011). The diagnosis of chronic traumatic encephalopathy (CTE) has been associated with football, hockey, soccer and wrestling and linked to suicides in professional athletes (Omalu et al. 2010).

While boxing's popularity has declined in the US, it remains prominent internationally. Nonetheless, three countries have banned boxing (Cuba, North Korea, and Norway). Given the overwhelming evidence that boxing is bad for the brain, I have struggled to comprehend its appeal. Who would want to stand in a confined space while someone tries to hit you as hard as they can, doing their best to knock you out? If it's for exercise, there are many other strategies to increase one's heartbeat without putting one's head in the way of a flying fist. Like Boxer Duk Koo Kim, one could even die from a subdural hematoma. In the long term (never mind the short term), getting knocked out cannot be healthy for the brain. Yet, boxing has persisted as a popular sport, at least since the ancient Greeks included it in their Olympic games.

An Unexpected Invitation

A few days ago, I complained to my friend Dan*, a semi-retired martial arts expert, that my regular workouts had become a little dull. He responded by inviting me to join him at his gym and box. There would be three of us and the trainer. Each one would box 1 minute, then rotate to the next. We would do 10 rounds, a grand total of 10 minutes each. Dan told me it was totally safe, as the trainer would just catch my punches in his gloves and not hit back. My knee-jerk response was a categorical "No way!" But upon further reflection, his invitation seemed like an excellent opportunity to gain some personal insight into this incredibly popular and mystifying sport.

The Club

The boxing club appeared to have been modeled after the neighborhood gym in the first Rocky Balboa movie. Half a dozen very fit guys in their twenties were punching each other and pounding big sausage-shaped bags like there was no tomorrow. There wasn't much chit-chat, just some intermittent grunting and the sound of leather gloves colliding. Although three of the boxers had Mohawk haircuts, I was told it wasn't a club requirement.

My First Lesson

Dan instructed me to keep my hands up by my face, "like you're on the telephone," and how to step forward, backward and to the side. There were two basic punches that I would do, the left jab and the right cross. He carefully told Manny, the trainer, that it was my first time.

Dan was the first to start. On each of Manny's gloves was painted a white circle, about 4 inches wide. Apparently, this was the target. Manny barked out instructions, "jab, jab, cross, 4, 6, 4, 8," and Dan struck as quickly and powerfully as he could. As I watched the ferocity of Dan's punches, perfected after decades of martial arts training, I made a mental note to steer clear of any arguments with him.

Dan's buddy Floyd was next, with more of the same.

Into the Ring

Then it was my turn. I followed Dan's instructions and held the gloves up near my face. I ducked my head a little bit like I had seen on TV. Even though I knew the trainer was only there to receive my punches, feeble as they might be, it seemed prudent to protect my head. I watched Manny hold up his right glove and say "cross," so I aimed for his glove and gave it a good, solid punch. Then jab, then cross, then a combination. But while engaged in this simulated "fight," an extraordinary thing happened. I sensed that what I really wanted to do was punch Manny right in his smiling face, which kept bobbing between his two gloves. We had been briefly introduced before the session, and he seemed like a pretty nice guy. But it took a lot of self-control to keep hitting that round circle in his glove and not clock him right in those shining teeth. I didn't have the nerve to actually hit him, and he just did his job absorbing my punches in his gloves. At the end of our session, he congratulated me on my hard punches, impressed at my first-time effort.

Most people would consider me rather mild mannered. I haven't been in a fistfight since elementary school (although I don't think Dan can say the same). I don't know why I wanted to knock Manny out. It also worried me to think that maybe he had the same feeling, especially since he was in great shape and 30 years younger. Obviously, discipline is a big part of boxing.

As Dan predicted, 10 minutes of boxing felt like more than an hour on a Stairmaster. At the end of the workout, we were all a sweaty mess. While waiting for my heart rate to drop below 100, I told Dan about my unexpected aggressive feelings while in the ring. I asked him whether he ever wanted to hit the trainer. "Sure," he said, "It's instinct."

That sounded right. One could argue that I've seen too many "Rocky" movies, but my new emotion did not feel like a learned response. Even for a pacifist neurologist, it appears that there's some hard wiring in the brain that responds to a potentially violent confrontation, rivets attention on your adversary, and makes you want to knock the other guy's lights out. Maybe it's self-preservation, an excess of epinephrine or testosterone, or some hormone that we haven't discovered yet.

Conclusions

Boxing is a challenge for the mind and body, a tactical chess game and test of physical endurance. But there's more to it than that. There's unbridled passion-something inside just wants to wallop your opponent. Perhaps that's not the only reason why boxing is so popular, but I suspect it's a large part of the explanation.

My first boxing experience was a little unsettling and yielded unexpected insight into the visceral nature of this sport. Maybe I've inadvertently discovered why we spend hundreds of billions of dollars a year on our defense budget.

If only we could just keep it in the ring.

*All names have been changed for my own protection.

References

Omalu BI, Bailes J, Hammers JL, Fitzsimmons RP. Chronic traumatic encephalopathy, suicides and parasuicides in professional American athletes: the role of the forensic pathologist. Am J Forensic Med Pathol 2010;31(2):130-132.

Purcell LK, Leblanc CMA and the American Academy of Pediatrics. Policy Statement. Boxing participation by children and adolescents. Pediatrics 2011;128(3):617-623.

Stern RA, Riley DO, Daneshvar DH et al. Long-term consequences of repetitive brain trauma: chronic traumatic encephalopathy. PM&R 2011;3:S460-467.

Chapter 5

NEW HOPE FOR PEOPLE WITH TRAUMATIC BRAIN INJURY

March 15, 2012

Introduction

There is no Food and Drug Administration (FDA) approved medication that alters the natural history of traumatic brain injury. Although much attention was paid to the high quality care that Arizona Congresswoman Gabrielle Giffords received after her gunshot wound to the head last year, in reality, her treatment probably amounted to what might be called "advanced first aid;" debridement, hemostasis, and possibly a prophylactic anticonvulsant. Apart from some minor neurosurgical refinements gleaned from the Vietnam and Iraq wars, her treatment was little different than it would have been decades ago. Neurologic recovery was left to rehabilitation and "tincture of time." More than a year later, despite considerable improvement and the best medical care in the world, she resigned from her job in Congress. According to her video statement, "I have more work to do on my recovery, so to do what is best for Arizona I will step down this week." Her halting words are testimony to the devastating impact of the single bullet that pierced her skull and brain.

High Human and Dollar Cost

Traumatic brain injury is a serious public health problem. Approximately 1.7 million people suffer a traumatic brain injury per year in the US. While most injuries are mild, traumatic brain injury results in 275,000 hospitalizations and 52,000 fatalities each year. Approximately 5.3 million Americans live with a disability secondary to traumatic brain injury. In addition to the human cost, the estimated direct and indirect economic cost of traumatic brain injury was $76.5 billion in 2010.

Amantadine in Traumatic Brain Injury

A recent multicenter study published in the *New England Journal of Medicine* suggests that a bright new therapeutic era for patients with traumatic brain injury may have begun (Giacino et al. 2012). The authors report a randomized, double blind, placebo controlled trial of 184 patients with severe traumatic brain injury that demonstrated accelerated recovery in the treatment group. At study onset, patients were in vegetative or minimally conscious states. Unlike Congresswoman Giffords, they all had nonpenetrating head injuries. Based on the encouraging results of prior studies, the treatment group received amantadine (100-200 mg BID), a dopamine receptor agonist and weak noncompetitive N-methyl D-aspartate receptor antagonist for 4 weeks. Outcomes included rate of improvement on a Disability Rating Scale (DRS) and the Coma Recovery Scale-Revised (CRS-R). After a 2 week washout period, the assessments were repeated at 6 weeks.

The study did *not* demonstrate that the amantadine group had better final outcomes, only that they improved more rapidly at 4 weeks. At the end of the study, there was no significant functional difference between the amantadine and placebo groups.

Amantadine is an interesting drug, having received FDA approval for prophylaxis and treatment of uncomplicated influenza A infections, parkinsonism, and drug-induced extrapyramidal reactions (PDR). Already in generic form, it would be available to traumatic brain injury patients at relatively low cost.

More New Indications for Old Drugs?

The fact that amantadine is an "old" drug makes one wonder how many other FDA approved medications already sitting on pharmacy shelves might be effective for traumatic brain injury. Perhaps there should be a concerted effort to test drugs already proven "safe and effective" for new indications? As a financial incentive, could there be a special category of market protection for old drugs that demonstrate effectiveness for new indications such as traumatic brain injury? If this scenario is not embraced by the pharmaceutical industry, could the National Institutes of Health step up to the plate? (Of note, the study by Giacino et al. was funded by the National Institute on Disability and Rehabilitation Research, not a pharmaceutical company.)

Future Treatment of Traumatic Brain Injury

If ever there was an "unmet medical need," traumatic brain injury is it. The positive results of this study inspire a flurry of questions: Would amantadine be more effective if administered immediately after injury? If so, it could be carried by Medics for blast injuries in the battlefield and by Emergency Medical Services who arrive at the scene of motor vehicle accidents. Is it helpful for those with concussions and postconcussive syndromes? Is it useful for penetrating as well as nonpenetrating head injuries? Could it be used prophylactically for those at risk of significant head injury (e.g., soldiers, boxers and hockey players)?

Methodology and Results-Some Concerns

1. Accurate randomization of patients with traumatic brain injury would seem very problematic as even focal lesions might be accompanied by diffuse axonal injury that would be difficult to quantify.

2. The median time from injury to amantadine treatment was 48 days, but the range was very wide; 28-112 days. Although this was partially controlled for by separating the patients into 2 groups (28-70 and 71-112 days), one could imagine that treatment at day 28 might have different effects than treatment at day 70.

3. Approximately 1/3 of patients received potentially confounding medications, such as anticonvulsants (more common in the amantadine group) and narcotics (more common in the placebo group).

Adverse Events

While there were no significant side effects from amantadine in this study, multiple potential adverse reactions such as anxiety, ataxia, depression, dizziness, orthostatic hypotension, nausea, seizures and others could add to the morbidity of traumatic brain injury. One patient in the amantadine group died from cardiac arrest, a "possible" complication of the drug.

Unanswered Questions

The long term effects of accelerated recovery are unknown. Is there a price to pay for more rapid recovery? For example, are patients more likely to develop posttraumatic epilepsy? Or does more rapid improvement decrease the risk of posttraumatic epilepsy? What about cognitive ability and emotional lability? How are these affected in the long term? What happens if the drug is continued indefinitely? What is the drug's effect on neurotransmitter levels, their receptors, and brain metabolism? Many important questions need to be addressed before a treatment that changes the natural history of brain healing is widely adopted.

Conclusions

This paper casts a glimmer of light into the bleak world of medical therapy for traumatic brain injury. Patients treated with amantadine had a statistically significant benefit in their rate of recovery after 4 weeks without an increase in adverse effects. In particular, seizures were not more frequent. However, when the drug was discontinued for 2 weeks, the functional scores of the amantadine and placebo groups no longer differed. While more rapid improvement is likely beneficial, perhaps limiting days in the hospital and complications, the value of this treatment is questionable if the end result is the same as placebo.

Nonetheless, these encouraging results should spark enthusiasm for increased traumatic brain injury research. If amantadine really works, other drugs may work as well or even better. As a first step, other dopamine agonists could be tested. Electrical and magnetic stimulation therapies should also be examined. Armed with improved understanding of traumatic brain injury pathophysiology as well as the development of increasingly detailed anatomical and functional imaging, researchers are better positioned than ever before to identify successful therapeutic strategies.

For the last year, Gabrielle Giffords has worked diligently with her physicians and therapists to achieve functional recovery. If vigorous research efforts continue, someday soon we may be able to accelerate and enhance recovery for those whose lives have been tragically altered by traumatic brain injury. If amantadine really improves brain healing, it represents an opportunity to help millions of people.

References

Giacino JT, Whyte J, Bagiella E et al. Placebo-controlled trial of amantadine for severe traumatic brain injury. NEJM 2012;366:819-826.

Chapter 6

AMERICAN ACADEMY OF PEDIATRICS-NO MORE MANNY PACQUIAOS, PLEASE

October 3, 2011

Introduction

I was first exposed to boxing several years ago when I visited the Philippines and watched Manny Pacquiao fight Juan Manuel Marquez on pay-per-view. It was pretty amazing.

But if the American Academy of Pediatrics has its way, there will be no more boxing success stories like Manny Pacquiao's:

Emmanuel Dapidran Pacquiao was born in Bukidnon, Philippines, the 4th of 6 children. After his parents separated, his mother could not support the family, and Manny went to Manila to look for work at the age of 14. He lived on the streets, started boxing, and the rest, as they say, is history. Manny Pacquiao is the first eight-division world boxing champion, "Fighter of the Decade," and the world's greatest "pound-for-pound" boxer. Boxing also opened up a career for Pacquiao in acting, singing, and politics. He is a member of the House of Representatives of the Philippine Congress. In the Philippines, his fan base is so large that it is said that the crime rate goes down during a Pacquiao fight...

For many young people, boxing offers the opportunity to engage in regular exercise, develop discipline, self-confidence, and character, and a respectable way to earn a living. There's even a remote chance to become a superstar. It's all good.

Other contact sports, such as football or hockey, may be even more dangerous. Boxing, however, is unique. Unlike other sports, as the American Academy of Pediatrics (AAP) points out, "boxing encourages and rewards direct blows to the head and face" (AAP 2011). This is not so good.

Pacquiao would be the first to agree that boxing is a violent sport. His childhood friend Eugene Barutag fell unconscious in the ring in 1995...and never woke up. Pacquiao was the only one who attended Barutag's wake.

Parallel Universe

One could imagine a parallel universe, with slightly different rules of biophysics, where boxing would be good for your brain. It could be that a sudden left hook to the jaw, with jarring rotational forces, clears out the cobwebs and improves intracerebral circulation, leading to a longer and happier life (as opposed to axonal injury). In this same parallel universe, smoking would be good for you. In that universe, nicotine is a vitamin, and all that smoke in your lungs purifies the body and even kills germs that cause tuberculosis (as opposed to causing lung cancer).

But in our universe, smoking is unhealthy, and blows to the head are bad for the brain. This has been well documented in boxing since the description of the "punch drunk" syndrome many years ago (Martland 1928), later termed dementia pugilistica. Martland wrote, "For some time fight fans and promoters have recognized a peculiar condition occurring among prize fighters which, in ring parlance, they speak of as 'punch drunk.' Fighters in whom the early symptoms are well recognized are said by the fans to be 'cuckoo,' 'goofy,' 'cutting paper dolls,' or 'slug nutty.'"

Martland astutely observed that symptoms were more likely in those "who take considerable head punishment," making an intuitive leap from repetitive traumatic head injury to the development of what we now refer to as chronic traumatic encephalopathy (CTE). CTE is associated with memory impairment, behavior and personality changes, Parkinsonian symptoms, and speech and gait abnormalities (McKee et al. 2009).

In addition, boxers face the risk of subdural hematomas (SDH). In a review, the authors state, "Boxing is a violent sport in which athletes accept the risk of brain damage or death. The most common life-threatening injury encountered by its participants is SDH, and the most feared consequence of chronic insult to the nervous system is dementia pugilistica or punch drunkenness" (Miele et al. 2007).

Repetitive head injuries in sports may cause neurologic symptoms. For example, after 9 concussions, the star soccer player Taylor Twellman had to prematurely retire from the game due to postconcussion syndrome (Cantu 2010). CTE has been associated with football, hockey, soccer, and wrestling, but most often with boxing (McKee et al. 2009, 2010). Repetitive head trauma related to collision sports has also recently been linked to motor neuron disease (McKee et al. 2010).

American Academy of Pediatrics Policy Statement
The AAP recommends that pediatricians:

- Vigorously oppose boxing for any child or adolescent

- Educate patients who may be engaged in or considering engaging in boxing, as well as parents/caregivers/teachers/coaches, regarding the medical risks of boxing

- Encourage young athletes to participate in alternative sports in which intentional blows to the head are not central to the sport such as swimming, tennis, basketball, and volleyball

- Advocate that boxing organizations ensure that appropriate medical care is provided for children and adolescents who choose to participate in boxing, ideally including medical coverage at events, preparticipation medical examinations, and regular neurocognitive testing and ophthalmologic examinations

These new AAP guidelines are co-sponsored by the Canadian Paediatric Society and are consistent with positions from the American, Australian, British, Canadian, and World Medical Associations (AAP 2011).

Treatment?

Neurons are precious. Neurologists are constantly reminded how little we can do to repair brain injury caused by degenerative neurologic diseases such as Alzheimer's, Parkinson's, or multiple sclerosis. There is an epidemic of mild traumatic brain injury in soldiers returning from Iraq and Afghanistan, and we have pitifully few tools to help these young men and women. Our complete impotence in doing anything more than "supportive care" for penetrating traumatic brain injury, like Katherine Giffords', is a source of continual despair and motivation for more research.

However, neurologists and other healthcare providers can discourage a sport that focuses on inflicting blows to the head.

Conclusions

I'm writing this blog from Manila, and I confess to feeling like a heretic. There are at least 2 boxing gyms within a couple blocks of my office. Manny Pacquiao's true-life rags-to-riches story has no doubt inspired thousands if not millions of would-be boxing champions. But with all due respect to Manny, I have to agree with the American Academy of Pediatrics. The prevention of traumatic brain injury trumps the many virtues of boxing, at least for this neurologist. Those who insist on boxing should master the art of ducking, and most importantly, don't fight Manny Pacquiao.

References

American Academy of Pediatrics. Policy Statement-Boxing participation by children and adolescents. Pediatrics 2011;128(3):617-623.

Cantu RC. World Cup Soccer: a major league soccer superstar's career-ending injury, concussion; and World Neurosurgery: A common thread. World Neurosurgery 2010;74:224-225.

Martland HS: Punch Drunk. JAMA 1928;91(15):1103-1107.

McKee AC, Gavet BE, Stern RA et al. TDP-43 proteinopathy and motor neuron disease in chronic traumatic encephalopathy. J Neuropathol Exp Neurol 2010;69:918-929.

McKee AC, Cantu R, Nowinski C et al. Chronic traumatic encephalopathy in athletes: Progressive tauopathy after repetitive head injury. J Neuropathol Exp Neurol 2009;68:709-735.

Miele VJ, Bailes JE, Cantu RC, Rabb CH. Subdural hematomas in Boxing: The spectrum of consequences. http://www.medscape.com/viewarticle/5539654/3/2007.

Chapter 7

AMERICAN ACADEMY OF NEUROLOGY FILM FESTIVAL FOCUSES ON BRAIN DISORDERS

March 24, 2013

Introduction

Last night I attended the 4th Annual American Academy of Neurology Film Festival at the American Academy of Neurology (AAN) meeting in San Diego, CA. There were over 80 entries, which had to include the phrase, "Let's put our brains together to cure brain disease." The grand prize went to "Hope for HumaNS," by Suzanne Gazda, MD, a neurologist from San Antonio, TX. Dr. Gazda's film was a technically superb documentary about "Nodding Syndrome," an endemic disease in Northern Uganda and South Sudan that causes intellectual decline, seizures, and death. Dr. Gazda founded an organization, Hope for Humans, to encourage research on the diagnosis and treatment of Nodding Syndrome, as well as to provide care for children afflicted with this mysterious disorder.

The first runner up was "Epillepsy," by Ingrid Pfau, Bozeman, MT, a moving self-portrait of a thoughtful young woman with cerebral palsy and intractable epilepsy. The film features her grim story of living with a disorder that can present without warning, alter consciousness, and requires constant treatment with pill after pill in order to control seizures. Ingrid, who is also a Master of Fine Arts student in the Science and Natural History Filmmaking program at Montana State University, narrated the film, which included many special effects.

"The Crash Reel"-A Snowboarder's Nightmare
The film festival concluded with a new feature-length documentary, "The Crash Reel," directed by Lucy Walker, the award winning British Film Director. "The Crash Reel" premiered at the Sundance Film Festival and will appear later this year on HBO. One of the producers, Julian Cautherley, was on hand to answer questions. "The Crash Reel" tells the heartbreaking story of Kevin Pearce, an immensely talented snowboarder who crashed and sustained a traumatic brain injury while training for the 2010 Olympics. Using archival footage of Kevin's youth, snowboarding competitions, hospital footage, interviews with his family, friends, fellow competitors, and doctors, the film intimately depicts this young man's life before and after the accident. Home videos and interviews reveal Kevin's gregarious personality, impressive talent, relentless drive, and boundless enthusiasm for snowboarding. The film provides insights into the competitive world of snowboarding, including Kevin's friendship with Olympic champion snowboarder Shaun White, which fractured when he started to beat Shaun at events.

The Fall
A miscalculation during a training run landed Kevin flat on his face and into a coma. He required helicopter evacuation, 26 days in the neurologic intensive care unit with several tubes including an intraventricular drain, and several months at the Craig Rehabilitation Hospital in Denver,

Colorado. During his protracted recovery he experienced focal seizures treated with lamotrigine and levetiracetam. His course was further complicated by depression, requiring medication and counseling. Kevin's lack of insight regarding his new physical and cognitive limitations caused further stress for him and his family. Alan Weintraub, MD, Medical Director of the Brain Injury Program at Denver's Craig Hospital, appears briefly in the film.

"The Crash Reel" offers a realistic view of the devastating, life changing effects of traumatic brain injury to an ambitious and talented teenager and his family. The film ends about 2 years after the injury. By this time, Kevin has returned to living independently, but reluctantly reached the inescapable conclusion that he can never return to competitive snowboarding. He still has double vision, impaired memory, and sometimes says socially inappropriate things. He says that he must adapt to a new life as a "brain injured" person. He spends his time giving motivational speeches, working as a commentator at snowboarding events, and searching for a goal that could replace his passion for snowboarding. The movie's treatment of disabilities is further textured because Kevin's brother David has Down's Syndrome. David is high functioning enough to know that he has a severe, irreversible disability. He is able to articulate that his disability makes him so depressed that he often returns to his room to cry. The story ends with both Kevin and his brother struggling to adapt their dreams to the reality of their disabilities.

Kevin's family is amazingly supportive. One of his brothers quits his job in order to be by Kevin's side and help motivate him during his prolonged rehabilitation. Kevin's brain injury prevents him from remembering and appreciating much of his family's attention, adding to the extreme pathos of the situation. Every patient with a chronic disorder should be so lucky to have a family like Kevin's.

The film highlights several issues:

1. Traumatic brain injury can result in loss of judgment and insight, which can further endanger the victim and create stress for caregivers and the healthcare team. For example, upon his release from rehab, Kevin was determined to resume his competitive snowboarding career, even though it was clear to everyone but him that he had lost the quick reflexes and cognitive and physical agility required for this extreme sport. Further, his history of a traumatic brain injury meant that he faced an even greater risk of another head injury upon resuming snowboarding, which might result in more severe impairment or death.

2. Olympic class athletes are incredibly motivated. The qualities of determination, persistence, and discipline that enable them to excel in their sport are the same ones that facilitate recovery from traumatic brain injury.

3. Athletes may need to be protected from themselves. The current height of the snowboarding "half-pipe," 22.5 feet, sets the stage not only for dramatic cinematography but also potentially crippling and lethal falls. Athletes know that they have to "push the

limits" to succeed and will continue to attempt ever more complicated and dangerous tricks. Sponsors and others involved in extreme sports need to control the competitive environment in order to limit the participants' risks.

4. Many competitive snowboarders lack health insurance. Although insurance is provided for sanctioned events, private sponsored events may leave snowboarders without coverage. A particularly poignant example was provided in the story of Sarah Burke, a competitive skier who suffered a traumatic brain injury on the same course as Kevin. She died 9 days later, but not before incurring a $500,000 hospital bill.

5. Snowboarding and competitive skiing are dangerous. Many of Kevin's friends told stories of broken bones and multiple concussions. The new American Academy of Neurology Concussion Guidelines may help this group of athletes.

Conclusions

These films provide valuable patient perspectives on neurologic illness, and I hope the AAN continues its film festival next year. The inclusion of a feature film and the visit from the producer made the evening that much more interesting. "The Crash Reel" is well done and inspirational. Snowboarders will enjoy this film, as it contains many exciting excerpts from snowboarding competitions. This deeply personal film highlights the risks of traumatic brain injury from snowboarding and its potential cognitive, physical, and social consequences. This film doesn't pull any punches. It includes an interview with an athlete who became quadriplegic after a fall who states, "I didn't even know what 'quadriplegic' meant. Kevin also has a painful discussion with another brain injured boy who clings to a fantasy that he might return to snowboarding despite the fact that he is hemiplegic and so cognitively impaired he can't even tell his elbow from his foot. Although we do get to glimpse Kevin's MRI, I would have liked to learn more details about his injury (e.g., basilar skull fracture? why persistent diplopia?) and his resultant epilepsy.

The producers plan to make "The Crash Reel" available at ski resorts to increase awareness of the potential for brain injury from snowboarding and skiing. They have also developed a "loveyourbrain" educational initiative that partners with nonprofit organizations to highlight the need to prevent traumatic brain injury. Healthcare professionals and others who experience the world of traumatic brain injury will appreciate this honest documentary and want to share it with their patients. After seeing this film, parents with active teenagers will spend more money on helmets.

Section 2.

Assorted Neurology Topics

Chapter 8

NEUROLOGY-THE LAST 200 YEARS, AN UPDATE...

September 10, 2012

Introduction

If you have been too busy in your clinic or research laboratory to review the last 200 years' worth of developments in clinical neurology, a recent article in the *New England Journal of Medicine* (NEJM) may help you out (Ropper 2012).

200 years in 8 pages

Allan Ropper, MD, expertly attacked this formidable topic and managed to keep it to 8 pages, including 95 references. An Associate Editor of the NEJM, Dr. Ropper is also Executive Vice Chair of Neurology, Brigham and Women's Hospital, Boston, MA, author of four editions of Adams and Victor's *Principles of Neurology*, and one of the founders of neurological intensive care, credentials that eminently qualify him for this daunting task. Of course, Dr. Ropper stood on the shoulders of giants, as his review was facilitated by a paper in 1962, which had already reviewed the past 150 years, leaving him to address merely the last 50 years...

Clinical Trials Rule

Dr. Ropper stressed the importance of properly performed clinical trials, many of which were published in the *NEJM*, to the transformation of neurology from an "elegant diagnostic specialty" to a therapeutic specialty. Examples of clinical trials that have become cornerstones to the modern neurologic treatment of stroke include the use of tissue plasminogen activator for acute stroke (tPA), carotid endarterectomy for prevention of transient ischemic attack and stroke, calcium channel blockers to reduce the risk of ischemic stroke after subarachnoid hemorrhage, low dose warfarin for nonrheumatic atrial fibrillation, and more recently, dabigatran for stroke prevention in atrial fibrillation. Pivotal therapeutic articles have also been published in the *NEJM* for brain tumors, coma, central nervous system infections, headache, epilepsy, multiple sclerosis, neuromuscular disease, Parkinson's, and spinal and traumatic brain injury. Landmark articles regarding normal pressure hydrocephalus, subclavian steal, aortic-arch atherosclerosis, lumbar disk sciatica, progressive multifocal leukoencephalopathy, prion disease, and many others have appeared in the *NEJM*. The *NEJM* also addressed the evolution of medical treatment in psychiatry with publications on dementia, depression, and psychosis. Even with the proliferation of journals dedicated to neurology, such as the *Annals of Neurology, Archives of Neurology, Brain, Neurology, Frontiers in Neurology, Practical Neurology,* and subspecialty journals such as *Epilepsia, Epilepsy & Behavior, Headache, Movement Disorders, Multiple Sclerosis Journal, Stroke* and others, the *NEJM* has remained a key source of relevant clinical information.

One Step Forward, One Step Back
The *NEJM* has not been immune from publishing research that ultimately turned out to be unfounded, such as articles on magnetism. (I personally gave up on the *NEJM* after I spent a rare free Saturday afternoon in medical school

reading that "A strong association between coffee consumption and pancreatic cancer was evident in both sexes" (MacMahon et al. 1981). This revelation, even in those pre-Starbuck days, provoked much discussion at the hospital, primarily at coffee breaks. But I was disheartened to find that my afternoon dutifully spent reading the *NEJM* had been wasted when I read a few years later that further research by the *same group of investigators* in *the same esteemed journal* that "none of the estimates reached statistical significance" (Hsieh et al. 1986). Ever since those conflicting reports about the importance of coffee left a bitter taste in my mouth, I view epidemiologic research on common exposures (e.g., chocolate, electricity, food, sunlight) with hefty skepticism. However, after this initial phase of disillusionment with the *NEJM*, the many challenging and informative neurological cases featured in the "Case Records of the Massachusetts General Hospital" section lured me back when I prepared for my neurology boards. These case studies feature discussions that are a *tour de force* of differential diagnosis and are a pleasure to read and reread.

Conclusions

This paper celebrates the 200th anniversary of the *NEJM*. It is economically written and provides an important historical context for the clinical endeavors of 21st century neurologists. The quality, quantity, and durability of the *NEJM* over the last 200 years are certainly impressive. One cannot dispute Dr. Ropper's assertion that "Neurology has been transformed by these articles." For neurology residents, his review provides an outline of major topics that should be mastered when preparing for a comprehensive neurology examination. For clinical neurologists, the topics listed are bread and butter for a day at the office or hospital. As clinical research continues to remodel neurology from a diagnostic to a therapeutic specialty, the next generation of articles should be even more helpful for people who suffer from neurologic disorders. I'm not sure who will write the progress report for the *NEJM's* 250th Anniversary Edition, but it should make for a fascinating read.

References
Hsieh CC, MacMahon B, Yen S et al. Coffee and pancreatic cancer (Chapter 2). NEJM 1986;315:587-589.

MacMahon B, Yen S, Trichopoulos D et al. Coffee and cancer of the pancreas. NEJM 1981;304:630-633.

Ropper AH. Two centuries of neurology and psychiatry in the Journal. NEJM 2012;367:58-65.

Chapter 9.

DELIRIUM-THE ELEPHANT IN THE ROOM

July 28, 2012

Introduction
Imagine if there was a common medical disorder associated with a one year mortality of 40% and a cost of $7 billion per year. It often escapes recognition and is associated with poor outcomes such as falls, pressure ulcers, prolonged hospitalization, need for long term care, and increased mortality. In addition, current knowledge, if properly applied, could prevent approximately 1/3 of cases. Despite these grave statistics and potential for remedies, it receives relatively little attention.

Delirium is such a disorder.

A Common Clinical Problem
At my community hospital, delirium was the third most common complaint requiring a neurology consult, after cerebrovascular disease (transient ischemic attack and stroke) and seizures. Delirium is present at the time of hospital admission in 14-24% of patients, 6-56% of hospitalized patients, 15-53% of patients postoperatively, 70-87% of intensive care patients, 60% of patients in nursing homes, and up to 83% of patients at end of life. The importance of delirium was recognized in a recent Clinical Guideline from the National Institute for Health and Clinical Excellence. The Guideline contained 13 specific recommendations to limit the occurrence of

delirium in people at risk (O'Mahony et al. 2011). (A brief review of the Guidelines appears in Chapter 94.)

Postoperative Delirium

An article by Saczynski et al. addressed the particular circumstance of delirium post cardiac surgery, which included coronary artery bypass graft (CABG) or valve replacement in patients 60 years or older (mean age 73). Of the 461 eligible patients, 200 declined. Of the 261 who consented, 26 were not enrolled for a variety of reasons, including 6 who developed delirium preoperatively. Ten patients were lost to follow-up. Two hundred and twenty-five were included in the final analysis.

Patients were tested preoperatively with the Mini-Mental State Examination (MMSE) and postoperatively with the MMSE, digit span, Confusion Assessment Method (CAM), and the Delirium Symptom Interview. The Katz Index of Independence in Activities of Daily Living assessed functional ability.

Study Results

Patients who developed delirium were significantly older, more likely to be female, nonwhite or Hispanic, had a higher Charlson Comorbidity Index score, history of stroke or transient ischemic attack, less education, and lower baseline MMSE scores. Patients had a drop of MMSE immediately after surgery, but those without delirium returned to baseline within 5 days. Those with a longer duration of delirium (3 or more days) had a greater postoperative drop in the MMSE score and a slower recovery. At 12 months, 31% of patients with delirium had still not returned to their cognitive baseline compared to

20% of those without delirium, which was nearly statistically significant (p=0.055). However, after adjustment for differences in baseline MMSE, there was no significant difference in mean MMSE scores at 6 and 12 months after surgery. Of interest, the 10 patients who died during the follow-up period had significantly lower preoperative MMSE status scores.

Study Limitations

1. Two hundred patients, nearly half of the 461 who were eligible, declined participation, possibly creating enrollment bias.

2. Details of the surgeries were not provided. (Did those who developed delirium have longer surgeries, trouble with anesthesia, hypotension, infection, or a greater incidence of other intraoperative complications?)

3. Although the MMSE is a well accepted measure, more detailed neuropsychological testing would have been informative with respect to particular domains of intellectual function that might be more vulnerable to changes related to cardiac surgery.

4. There is no discussion of electroencephalogram (EEG), MRI or other laboratory results that might have contributed to understanding the pathogenesis of delirium.

More Questions Than Answers

The authors present a thorough study of elderly patients pre and post cardiac surgery. But why did nearly half of them develop delirium? And why did it take so long for it to go away? Did those who developed delirium already have an underlying dementing process as suggested by their lower MMSE scores, or were they more susceptible to some new, unidentified insult because of their lower preoperative cognitive function? If so, is that insult completely reversible? Did their higher Charlson Comorbidity Index predispose them to complications during surgery that may have been subtle, but significant enough to cause brain injury? What is it about aging that predisposes older people to develop delirium? Conversely, what protects younger individuals from delirium? Why is delirium so common in the intensive care unit that it is almost surprising if a patient doesn't get it?

Therapeutic Opportunity

One might think that a whole army of neurologists and others would have already pounced on the opportunity to prevent and treat this common, devastating, and expensive disorder. One could even imagine a fellowship devoted to understanding the pathophysiology of delirium, its clinical manifestations, and methods of prevention and treatment. A wide variety of fellowship training is available for neurologists, including ACGME (Accreditation Council for Graduate Medical Education) fellowships in clinical neurophysiology, endovascular surgical neuroradiology, neurodevelopment disabilities, neuromuscular medicine, neuroradiology, pain management/pain medicine, sleep medicine and vascular neurology, as well as non-accredited fellowships. Not one of these focuses primarily on the problem of delirium.

According to a recent review article, "The pathophysiological mechanisms of delirium remain unclear (Martins and Fernandez 2012). Really? After all these years of consulting on countless patients with "altered mental status" the cause is still unclear?

Another review article states, "Current treatment paradigms typically focus on supportive care and management of the underlying etiology. Directed therapies that target neurochemical and neurotransmitter pathways that mediate encephalopathy are not currently available and represent an important area for future research" (Frontera 2012). In other words, when it comes to specific therapy for delirium, we have nothing to offer. Zilch. If ever there was an "unmet medical need" that should attract the attention of investigators, pharmaceutical companies, and investors, this is a big one.

Why is there not more emphasis on the prevention and treatment of delirium? Is delirium trapped in a Catch-22 that limits progress? Would there be more academic interest in delirium if the research appeared more promising? Would there be more promising research if there was more academic interest?

Conclusions

Delirium is a cause of much human misery and dollar expenditure. The problem is confronted daily by geriatricians, internists, intensivists, neurologists, rehabilitation specialists, and others. Perhaps because of its multiple etiologies, delirium does not fall neatly into any one subspecialty.

Indeed, the multidisciplinary nature of delirium is well illustrated by the diverse home institutions of the authors of the Saczynski paper, which include the Division of Geriatric Medicine and Meyers Primary Care Institute, the Aging Brain Center, Institute for Aging Research, Divisions of General Medicine and Primary Care and Gerontology, and a Neurology department.

Perhaps because delirium is so ubiquitous, it is often fatalistically accepted as a natural consequence of illness, rather than a potentially preventable, treatable disorder. According to estimates from the NICE Guidelines, approximately 1/3 of cases could be prevented using current therapies. But the implementation of these preventive strategies has yet to become standard of care, (in part because their evidence base is limited). The advent of specific therapies, such as medications that target the underlying pathophysiologic impairments, seems woefully distant.

The elephant in the room is not invisible, but the herds of elephants that roam unfettered in our hospitals have mostly been ignored. The important observations by Saczynski et al. call attention to the magnitude of this problem, its potential for prevention, need for extended care after surgery for patients who develop delirium, and the necessity for continued research that could result in effective therapy.

References

FitzGerald DB, Mitchell AL. Career choices: the fellowship search. Neurology 2008;70:e5-e8.

Frontera JA. Metabolic encephalopathies in the critical care unit. Continuum (Minneapolis Minn) 2012;18(3 Critical Care Neurology):611-639.

Inouye SK. Delirium in older persons. NEJM 2006;354:1157-1165.

Martins S, Fernandes L. Delirium in elderly people: a review. Frontiers in Neurology 2012;3(101):1-12.

O'Mahony R, Murthy L, Akunne A et al. Synopsis of the National Institute for Health and Clinical Excellence Guideline for Prevention of Delirium. Ann Intern Med 2011;154:746-751.

Saczynski JS, Marcantonio ER, Quach L et al. Cognitive trajectories after postoperative delirium. NEJM 2012;367: 30-39.

Chapter 10

MICROGRAVITY: A NEW RISK FACTOR FOR IDIOPATHIC INTRACRANIAL HYPERTENSION?

July 22, 2012

Introduction

Physicians routinely ask a laundry list of questions to identify possible etiologies for a patient's symptoms. For example, the question, "Any foreign travel?" has always been a mainstay when investigating a fever of unknown origin. A recent trip to Southeast Asia might be a tip-off to otherwise unsuspected dengue, malaria or tuberculosis.

A fascinating paper by Kramer et al. suggests that physicians exploring possible etiologies of decreased vision need to extend the concept of "foreign travel" to include, "Any exposure to microgravity?" Their investigation was triggered by reports of visual degradation by ~60% of astronauts on long-duration space missions. Two cases of optic disc edema have also been documented in-flight. According to the authors, "Exposure to microgravity can result in a spectrum of intraorbital and intracranial findings similar to those in idiopathic intracranial hypertension."

Using a 3-Tesla MRI, the authors examined 27 consecutive astronauts who had significant microgravity exposure. MRI examination included thin section, 3-dimensional, axial T2-weighted images of their brains and orbits. Nineteen of the astronauts (mean age 48.4) had spent an average of

108 days in microgravity and 8 (mean age 47.8) had averaged 130 days.

Results

The MRI images provide impressive *in vivo* anatomical detail of the globe, optic nerve, and neighboring structures. Nearly all (96%) of the astronauts had a central area of T2 hyperintensity in their optic nerves. Seven (26%) astronauts had posterior globe flattening, 4 (15%) optic nerve protrusion, 4 (15%) optic nerve sheath diameter distension in association with optic nerve sheath kinking, and 3 (11%) moderate concavity of the pituitary dome with posterior stalk deviation. None of the astronauts had evidence of central venous thrombosis, hydrocephalus, mass lesions, or vasogenic edema to account for the above abnormalities. Three of the astronauts who had posterior globe flattening and optic disc protrusion had a lumbar puncture that revealed elevated cerebrospinal fluid (CSF) pressures of 23, 28, and 29 cm H_2O, performed at 12, 453, and 57 days after return to earth, respectively.

Discussion

There are those who question the suitability of man for flight-after all, if man were meant to fly, wouldn't he have wings? With respect to distancing one's self from the earth's gravitational field, there may be significant medical considerations that lend some substance to this argument. Prolonged exposure to microgravity is known to cause adverse health effects, such as bone mineral loss and muscle atrophy. Other physiologic systems, such as cardiovascular, neurovestibular and psychological may also be affected.

With respect to visual symptoms and anatomical changes in the globe and optic nerve, Kramer et al. hypothesize that the microgravity environment may result in cephalad fluid shifts, manifesting as facial congestion and possibly increased intracranial pressure. Some of the findings note above, such as posterior globe flattening (N=3), optic nerve sheath kinking (N=1), optic nerve protrusion (N=1), and increased concavity of the pituitary gland with posterior stalk displacement (N=1) were observed more than 100 days after a mission, suggesting that anatomical distortions may be persistent or potentially permanent.

Limitations

The paper suffers from numerous limitations. The astronauts were not imaged pre-flight, eliminating a baseline comparison regarding any of the MRI findings. Imaging was also done irrespective to specific symptoms or interval from the most recent mission. Perhaps because this paper focuses on imaging, no clinical summary of the 27 astronauts was provided. It would have been interesting to learn how many had visual disturbance, the nature and duration of the disturbance, the relationship to other disorders, such as migraine, and whether symptoms of possible idiopathic intracranial hypertension included headache. Perhaps these details will appear in a future publication.

Conclusions

The era of commercial space flight is fast approaching with the promise of permitting more and more people the opportunity to leave the surface of the earth for extended periods of time. In recognition of the medical ramifications of prolonged space flight and microgravity, a one day conference, Emerging Opportunities in Space Life Sciences Research, Johns Hopkins School of Medicine, Baltimore, MD, August 13, 2012, will address the effects of long-duration space flights on the human body. The research is supported by the Discovery Program at Johns Hopkins University and the National Space Biomedical Research Institute. Research into the physiologic implications for prolonged space flight is still in its infancy. Neurologists and others dedicated to understanding the brain and visual system have much to learn and offer regarding the care of current and future astronauts. While astronauts must pay careful attention to their spacecraft's flight path, they should orbit the earth more comfortably knowing that their health, including the anatomy and physiology of their own orbits, will be under close observation upon their return.

References

Kramer LA, Sargsyan AE, Hasan KM et al. Orbital and intracranial effects of microgravity: Findings at 3-T MR imaging. Radiology 2012;2263(3):819-827.

Chapter 11

ROMANCE AND THE BRAIN-A NEUROLOGIST'S GUIDE FOR A BETTER VALENTINE'S DAY

February 13, 2012

Introduction

Four presentations about the brain, love and sex appear on the Forum Network, a collection of free online lectures from the Public Broadcasting Service (PBS) and National Public Radio (NPR). These lectures address the topics from vastly different perspectives and are thought provoking:

1. Rebecca M. Jordan Young, November 19, 2010 (58 minutes)
Brainstorm: Flaws in the Science of Sex Differences (a lecture based on her book of the same title)
Ms. Jordan takes a "walk on the wild side" and challenges the concept of prenatal "hardwiring" of sexual identity based on her analysis of >400 research papers and interviews of 21 scientists. She questions the validity of much sex and gender research and suggests that behavioral flexibility regarding sexual activity is more common than we realize.

2. Helen Fisher, February 4, 2009 (1:18 minutes)
This is Your Brain on Love
Ms. Fisher, a biological anthropologist and excellent speaker, describes the neurotransmitter systems responsible for sex drive, romantic love, and attachment, and how these 3

systems may all work together to solidify relationships...or not! She categorizes personality into four biological types and associates them with specific brain neurochemistry; the "Explorer" (dopamine), "Builder" (serotonin), "Director" (testosterone), and the "Negotiator" (estrogen and oxytocin). Based on the responses to thousands of questionnaires she developed for a dating site, Chemistry.com, Ms. Fisher goes on to suggest the personality types that match well together. While she admits that this classification is oversimplified, she feels it nonetheless has value.

Ms. Fisher warns that a drug such as fluoxetine (Prozac), a selective serotonin reuptake inhibitor (SSRI) that elevates serotonin, also decreases dopamine, and may impair emotions of love and attachment. Despite her extensive scientific research on the subject, Ms. Fisher concedes, "There will always be magic to love."

Lynn Margulis, September 18, 2008 (01:30:02–audio only) Tales of Science and Love

An evolutionary biologist, Ms. Margulis discusses the spread of syphilis throughout Europe and its effect on the writings and ultimate madness of the philosopher Friedrich Nietzsche. (Although a fascinating historical tale, this lecture might not do much to set the desired mood for Valentine's Day!) She also proposes that Lyme disease and syphilis are chronic infections and never eradicated in the human body despite appropriate antibiotics. Along these contrarian lines, she is unwilling to accept that the HIV virus is responsible for AIDS and that antiretroviral drugs are effective treatment. Of interest to women students, she cautions against striving for the "superwoman" role of successful marriage, children and a stellar scientific career, lamenting that it is simply not feasible. Given her two failed marriages, she does not consider herself a "role model" and "refuses to offer any recipe for personal fulfillment."

4. Tal Ben-Shahar, October 4, 2006 (01:57:58)
Positive Psychology: The Science of Happiness
Tal Ben-Shahar is a popular Harvard professor who teaches a course that focuses on relationships, self-esteem, passion and the science of "positive psychology," which he insists differs from "pop psychology." Ben-Shahar points out that happiness is not merely the negative of unhappiness. He claims that focusing on optimism and hope, for example, can decrease the frequency and severity of mental illness, improve relationships, and lead to greater happiness. While achieving a state of persistent "happiness" may be beyond human possibility, positive psychology addresses the practical question, "How can I become happier?" In this lecture, Ben Shahar articulates 6 principles that lead towards that elusive goal.

Conclusion
While the lay literature regarding romance is extensive, the science of romance appears wanting. Yet these novel presentations shed some light into the age-old mysteries of the central nervous system, love and sex.

For more on this topic, listen to Frank Sinatra croon, "How Little We Know."

Chapter 12

VIDEO GAMES-SHOULD PARENTS WORRY?

December 16, 2011

Introduction

If you are a pediatrician or family physician, chances are that parents have asked you whether video games are good or bad for their child's brain. According to a recent article that featured a discussion by 6 experts in the field, the answers are quite complex (Bavelier et al. 2011).

Their conclusions? In short, it depends upon the video game and the child. More detail below:

The Video Screen, A 21st Century Distraction

Video games are immensely popular. Sales of video games are expected to grow from $66 billion worldwide in 2010 to $81 billion in 2016 (Takahashi 2011). As a point of reference, video game sales are now greater than those of the music industry.

There's no debate that too much time playing video games may distract children from required studying, socializing, practicing a musical instrument or participating in sports. Displacement of "real world" activities by video games has been associated with decline in school performance, obesity, and repetitive strain disorders.

In a past generation, teenage boys were often accused of spending too much time away from their studies tinkering with cars and motorcycles. But it was the invention of the television that heralded the invasion of the home by "screens" (computers, video games, cell phones, iPads, Nooks, and others) that would compete with traditional childhood activities (e.g., eating, sleeping, going to school, playing outside). Arguments between parents and children over watching "too much TV" now seem rather prosaic in light of the enhanced distractions of the Internet, (which includes free TV). Fussing with cellphones, software, social networking, hacking, and video games, along with the computerization of automobile engines, seem to have largely replaced motor repair and conventional TV as teenage time sinks.

Addiction

Infrequently, video games may become an obsession that can be added to the long list of potentially addictive activities (e.g., alcohol, drugs, eating, gambling, work) in susceptible individuals. Depression, anxiety, social phobia, and poor school performance have been associated with excessive video game use, but a clear cause and effect relationship has not been determined. These symptoms may improve with reduction in video game play.

Type of Video Game

There are literally millions of different video games. One of the most popular is the "action" video game, where the objective usually requires killing opponents in various ways.

Parents may be justifiably concerned about the level of violence in these games.

According to one discussant, "Violent video games alone are unlikely to turn a child with no other risk factors into a maniacal killer. However, in children with many risk factors, the size of the effect may be sufficient to have practical negative consequences."

Another discussant pointed out that violent content, per se, was not necessarily bad. For example, one could imagine that the goal of a violent game was to rescue teammates, thereby teaching teamwork and social coordination skills. In this example, both content and context are important.

The structure and mechanics of video games may lead to improved visual attention skills, including the "ability to acquire three dimensional information from flat screens" and "mental rotation skills." These properties may be useful in general education and rehabilitation medicine as well.

Photosensitive Epilepsy

Seizures associated with the flashing display of video games were first reported in a teenager who played the space wars game "Astro Fighter" (Rushton 1981). Children with photosensitive epilepsy may have their seizures triggered by the rapid flashes of light and changes in color and patterns in some video games (Bureau et al. 2004). Exposure to such games may even trigger a child's first seizure and lead to the diagnosis of photosensitive epilepsy. Obviously, these children should avoid the offending games. Sitting further away from the screen (at least 2 meters) so that the flashing image does not fill the entire field of vision may be helpful for children who insist on playing. Sleep deprivation associated with prolonged video game playing may increase the risk of seizures.

Conclusions

Children who enjoy video games should not pursue them to the extent of excluding other important activities such as homework, socialization, practicing a musical instrument and sports. When video game use interferes with normal life, or when associated with anxiety, depression, or social phobia, parents should refer their children for treatment. Certain skills, such as hand/eye coordination, may be improved by participating in video games, although it is not clear to what extent these skills carry over into the "real world." The degree to which violent content in video games influences psychosocial functioning probably depends upon the type of game, hours played, the child's personality and other factors. The video game format lends itself to educational instruction and may also have an important role in rehabilitation for those with neurologic injury. For the moment, educational and rehabilitation applications lag behind those available for entertainment, but neuroscience research into attention, cognition, learning, memory, perception, personality and processing may eventually harness the video game as a powerful and educational clinical tool.

References
Bavelier D, Green CS, Han DH et al. Brains on video games. Nature Reviews Neuroscience 2011;12:763-768.

Bureau M, Hirsch E, Vigevano F. Epilepsy and videogames. Epilepsia 2004;45(Suppl. 1):24-26.

Rushton DN. The Lancet 1981;317(8218):501 (letter).

Takahashi D. With online sales growing, video game market to hit $81B by 2016. http://venturebeat. com/2011/09/07/with-online-sales-growing-video-game-market-to-hit-81b-by-2016-exclusive/, September 7, 2011.

Chapter 13

VAMPIRE BAT CAUSES FATAL RABIES ENCEPHALITIS IN USA

September 1, 2011

Introduction
A flurry of fictional vampires has recently invaded American television, movie screens and bookstores. While the Centers for Disease Control and Prevention (CDC) offers no statistics on vampire attacks, the CDC did report the first case of fatal rabies in the US from a vampire bat (August 12, 2011).

Clinical History
According to the patient's mother, the 19 year old boy had been bitten by a bat on the left foot while sleeping in Michoacan, Mexico, before coming to Louisiana to work as a laborer on a sugar cane plantation. After one week of work, he developed generalized fatigue, left shoulder pain, and left hand numbness. Initially, his symptoms were attributed to overexertion. He then experienced hyperesthesia of his left shoulder, left hand weakness, generalized areflexia and drooping of the left upper eyelid. A presumptive diagnosis of the Miller-Fisher variant of acute inflammatory demyelinating polyneuropathy (Guillain Barre) syndrome was made. He became febrile, had respiratory distress, and lapsed into a coma. A lumbar puncture revealed 87 white blood cells (97% lymphocytes) and a protein of 233 mg/dl. Rabies virus specific immunoglobulin G and immunoglobulin M

were present in the cerebrospinal fluid. Rabies virus antigen was detected in postmortem brain tissue, and antigenic typing isolated the vampire bat rabies variant.

I chatted with Brett Petersen, MD, MPH, Medical Officer, Poxvirus and Rabies Branch, CDC, who was kind enough to answer my many questions. He told me that this case is unusual because vampire bats are only found in Latin America, not in the US. (Other bat species have caused rabies in the US, however.) Dr. Petersen explained that patients may develop hypersalivation and hydrophobia due to painful laryngeal spasms. "Even the sight of water can create pain," he stated.

According to Dr. Petersen, bat rabies is uniformly fatal, even for infected bats. However, the long incubation period of the virus allows it to be transmitted from bat to bat. In human cases, the median incubation period is 85 days. In general, for a person to be infected with bat rabies, the virus must be inoculated under the skin from the bat's saliva. This requires a bite or a scratch (Hooper et al. 2011), although infection by aerosolized virus has been proposed.

Rabies is caused by a Lyssavirus and has the highest case fatality of any infectious disease (Blanton et al. 2010). With rare exceptions, every patient dies.

Vampire Bats
Characterized by big ears and razor sharp teeth, vampire bats feed at night, quietly landing or jumping onto their prey. However, because of the bat's padded feet and wrists, the victim may be unaware of the bat's presence. Heat sensors in the bat's nose detect accessible blood vessels close to the skin's surface. The bat has an anticoagulant in its saliva

that allows it to lap up blood with its tongue. After feeding for approximately 30 minutes, the bat may have ingested so much blood that it is barely able to fly. Victims may not realize they have been bitten. Bat teeth are very fine and may leave only pinpoint puncture marks ≤1 mm that may be nearly undetectable (De Serres et al. 2008). In the past 20 years, most of the people infected with bat rabies did not report a bat bite (De Serres et al. 2008).

The number of rabies cases in the US has decreased dramatically due to the elimination of canine rabies by vaccination programs for dogs. Rabies now comes from wildlife such as bats, foxes, skunks and raccoons (Blanton et al. 2010). This is in contrast to the global situation, where rabies kills approximately 55,000 people per year, mostly due to rabid dogs (De Serres et al. 2008). Humans are not natural reservoirs for rabies virus (Hooper et al. 2011).

Since the elimination of dogs as a rabies reservoir in the US, bat rabies has become the most common cause of human rabies. In 2009, only 4 cases of rabies were identified in the US. Of these, 3 were due to bats. A fourth case of rabies was in a physician who had been bitten by a rabid dog while traveling in India.

Vampire bats are the leading cause of human rabies in Latin America. One concern about global warming is that it could possibly affect the range of vampire bats, introducing them into the Southern USA, resulting in an increase in bat rabies.

Post-Exposure Prophylaxis
Over 20,000 people receive rabies post-exposure prophylaxis in the US each year, and there are no reported failures

(Hooper et al. 2011). The purpose of post-exposure prophylaxis is to prevent the virus from reaching the central nervous system. While the neurotropic virus travels through peripheral nerve axons to the central nervous system, there is no clinical evidence of infection. Post-exposure prophylaxis is 100% effective if administered before symptoms develop. However, once the rabies virus has entered the central nervous system and caused symptoms, the outcome is nearly always fatal.

The current recommendations for post-exposure prophylaxis are 4 doses of rabies vaccine and 1 dose of rabies immunoglobulin. The wound should be vigorously cleaned and infiltrated with rabies immunoglobulin. The immunoglobulin provides immediate protection while the vaccination induces endogenous antibodies. While the older rabies vaccine was made from nervous tissue and was painful, the current vaccine is made from human diploid cell culture or purified chick embryo cells and is no more painful than other vaccines. In 2008, the CDC revised its vaccination guidelines from 5 shots down to 4, administered on days 0 (right away), 3, 7, and 14. Allergic reactions are infrequent (1/1000), but patients should be closely supervised (De Serres et al. 2009). Persons with altered immunocompetence should receive the older 5 dose regimen. If work or travel predispose individuals to rabies exposure, they can be vaccinated prophylactically. There is also research on an intranasal vaccine (Cruz et al. 2008).

Conclusions

For those who have received excessive exposure to vampires from TV, cinema and other media, their suffering may continue, as a vaccine is still unavailable. However, if one is bitten by a bat, the CDC recommends the following:

1. If the bat is available, test it for rabies. If the test is negative, no anti-rabies prophylaxis is needed.

2. If the bat flies away, assume it was rabid and administer post-exposure prophylaxis according to the CDC guidelines.

3. Treat as soon as possible after the bite.

Rabies, although rare in the US, should be considered in the differential diagnosis of unexplained acute, progressive encephalomyelitis. Because of the relatively long incubation period of the rabies virus, a travel history should be obtained from the patient because of the possibility of infection outside the US. Prompt post-exposure treatment is critical-once a patient has developed symptoms, there is no established therapy (Jackson 2011).

More information can be found on the CDC rabies web page.

References
Blanton JD, Palmer D, Rupprecht CE. Rabies surveillance in the United States during 2009. JAVMA 2010;237(6):646-657.

Cruz ET, Romero IAF, Mendoza JGL et al. Efficient post-exposure prophylaxis against rabies by applying a four-dose DNA vaccine intranasally. Vaccine 2008;36:6936-6944.

De Serres G, Skowronski DM, Mimault P et al. Bats in the bedroom, bats in the belfry: Reanalysis of the rationale for rabies postexposure prophylaxis. Clinical Infectious Diseases 2009;48:1493-1499.

De Serres G, Dallaire F, Cote M, Skowronski DM. Bat rabies in the United States and Canada from 1950 through 2007: Human cases with and without bat contact. Clinical Infectious Diseases 2008;46:1329-1337.

Hooper DC, Roy A, Barkhouse DA et al. Rabies virus clearance from the central nervous system. Chapter 4 Advances in Virus Research 2011;79:55-71.

Jackson AC. Therapy of human rabies. Chapter 17 Advances in Virus Research;79:365-372.

Chapter 14

ANTI-VENOM NEUTRALIZES SCORPION TOXIN

August 15, 2011

Introduction

A new anti-venom relieves neurologic and other symptoms caused by the sting of the Arizona Bark scorpion, *Centruroides sculpturatus* (FDA 2011a). The anti-venom, Anascorp, Centruroides (Scorpion) Immune F (ab')$_2$ (Equine) Injection was approved under the Food and Drug Administration's (FDA) orphan drug program on August 3, 2011. This is good news especially for children, who are the ones most commonly stung and who experience the most severe reactions, including death (FDA 2011a). Anascorp is manufactured by Instituto Bioclon, S.A. de C.V., in Tlalpan, Mexico.

Neurotoxic Scorpion Forges International Ties

The Arizona Bark Scorpion, *Centruroides sculpturatus*, also known as the Deadly Sculptured Scorpion, is the only neurotoxic scorpion in the United States. Approximately 11,000 people are stung each year in Arizona, the scorpion's preferred US residence and the site of the venom clinical research (FDA 2011b). The Arizona Bark Scorpion also frequents California, New Mexico, Nevada, Texas, and northern Mexico (Berg and Tarantino 1991). In Mexico, neurotoxic scorpions constitute a much larger public health problem than in the US, stinging more than 250,000 people per year (Boyer et al. 2009). Collaboration between investigators at the University of Arizona Health Sciences Center, Tucson, AZ, Children's Hospital of Philadelphia, Philadelphia, PA, the Instituto de Biotecnologia, Universidad Nacional Autonoma de Mexico, Cuernavaca, Morelos, and the Instituto Bioclon, Mexico Distrito Federal, Mexico, culminated in the recent FDA anti-venom approval. Previously, a goat-derived whole-IgG anti-venom had been available, which risked serum reactions. Manufacture of that product, which was not FDA approved, ceased in 1999, leaving no treatment option other than supportive care.

Double-Blind Study

Anascorp anti-venom was approved after a prospective, randomized, double-blind study that compared scorpion specific $F(ab')_2$ anti-venom to placebo in 15 children (6 months-18 years) with severe scorpion stings (Boyer et al. 2009). All patients required admission to pediatric intensive care and had systemic toxic effects that included at least one of the following 3 symptoms: neuromotor agitation with wild flailing of the extremities, oculomotor manifestations, and respiratory compromise. Other symptoms due to scorpion toxin may include agitation, blurred vision, dysarthria, hyperpyrexia, hypersalivation, hypertension, local pain, noncardiogenic pulmonary edema, paresthesias, perioral numbness, restlessness, stridor, tachycardia, tachypnea and wheezing. Elevated creatine phosphokinase (CPK), cerebrospinal fluid pleocytosis, and renal failure have been reported (Berg and Tarantino 1991). Eight children received the anti-venom and 7 received placebo. Within 4 hours of intravenous treatment, all 8 patients who received anti-venom were free of neurotoxic symptoms compared to only 1/7 (14%) placebo treated patients (p=0.001). In addition, at 4 hours, none of the anti-venom treated patients had detectable venom in their blood compared to 4/6 (67%) placebo treated patients (p=0.02). Further, the need for sedation was greatly reduced in the anti-venom group, which required a cumulative midazolam dose of only 0.07 mg/kg at 4 hours compared to 1.77 mg/kg in the placebo group (p=0.01).

Anascorp venom was remarkably free of side effects. All adverse effects were mild. One patient had vomiting and diarrhea several days after treatment and another had vomiting 6 days after treatment.

The new intravenous anti-venom is produced from horses immunized with venom from southern Mexican scorpions (C. limpidus, C.l. tecomanus, C. noxious, and C. suffusus suffusus) related to the Arizona Bark scorpion. Due to the horse serum, acute serum reactions or delayed serum sickness are potential complications of treatment, although they did not occur during this study. Such reactions were common, however, with the prior, unregulated goat-derived anti-venom (Banner 1991).

Unusual Oculomotor Abnormalities

Roving eye movements are an unusual symptom that should trigger consideration of an Arizona Bark scorpion sting if the clinical history is in doubt. These oculomotor abnormalities are visible on a short video that accompanies the NEJM article. (Although the video describes these movements as "nystagmus," they look more like opsoclonus to my eye.)

Toxic Venom

The venom appears to activate Na+ channels, with variants that preferentially affect insects or vertebrates. The *Centruroides sculpturatus* venom causes excessive neuronal firing, similar to the venom of the potentially lethal *Buthus quinquestriatus* scorpion found in Israel and North Africa (Berg and Tarantino 1991). Sixteen different genes have been cloned from the venomous glands of *Centruroides sculpturatus* (Corona et al. 2001).

Conclusions

The FDA approval of Anascorp anti-venom represents a dramatic advance in the treatment of scorpion stings by *Centruroides sculpturatus* that will decrease morbidity and mortality, especially in children. The combination of flailing limb movements and roving eye movements are highly suggestive of envenomation with this species. Many envenomations are probably due to accidental physical contact between people and unseen scorpions in clothing or bedclothes. Vigorous shaking of clothing and shoes as a precaution prior to getting dressed is probably worthwhile for those who live in endemic areas. Further investigation into the pathophysiology of scorpion toxin, particularly with respect to the hyperkinetic motor and unusual eye movements it can produce, may reveal new insights into human nervous system physiology.

References

Banner W Jr. A scorpion by any other name is still a scorpion. Ann Emerg Med 1999;34:669-670.

Berg RA, Tarantino MD. Envenomation by the scorpion *Centruroides exilicauda* (*C sculpturatus*): Severe and unusual manifestations. Pediatrics 1991;87:930-933.

Boyer LV, Theodorou AA, Berg RA et al. Antivenom for critically ill children with neurotoxicity from scorpion stings. NEJM 2009;360:2090-2098.

Corona M, Valdez-Cruz NA, Merino E et al. Genes and peptides from the scorpion *Centruroides sculpturatus* Ewing, that recognize Na+ channels. Toxicon 2001;39:1893-1898.

FDA Press Release: FDA approves the first specific treatment for scorpion stings. http://www.fda.gov/NewsEvents/Newsroom/PressAnnouncements/ucm266611.htm, August 3, 2011(a).

FDA Press Release (For Consumers): FDA approves first scorpion sting antidote. http://www.fda.gov/ForConsumers/ConsumerUpdates/ucm266515.htm, August3, 2011 (b).

Chapter 15

DOES THE LESION FIT THE CRIME?

July 27, 2011

The type of crime committed by a patient may assist neurologists in localizing the brain lesion underlying that patient's dementia according to a recent retrospective review from two dementia clinics at the University of California at Los Angeles and the VA Greater Los Angeles Healthcare Center, Los Angeles, CA (Mendez et al. 2011). The authors identified 33 (27 males, 6 females) patients with dementia who had gotten into trouble with the law. The patients had committed the following sociopathic acts; physical assaults (7), unsolicited sexual approach or touching of adults (5), theft, especially shoplifting (5), excessively disruptive behavior (4), indecent exposure in public (3), assault with a weapon due to delusional beliefs (2), moving traffic violations, including hit and run accidents (2), unsolicited sexual approach or touching of children (1), stalking with homicidal behavior (1), breaking and entering into others' homes (1), destruction of others' property (1), kidnapping her child (1). None of the crimes were committed during an acute delirium.

When divided into "impulsive" (N=22) crimes (i.e., shoplifting, grabbing and fondling both men and women, disruptive public behavior) versus "nonimpulsive" (N=11) (i.e., attempting to punch or choke family members, stalking and premeditated threats at ex-wife), those in the "impulsive" group were more than twice as likely to have greater frontal-caudate involvement than temporal and parieto-occipital on neuroimaging than those in the "nonimpulsive" group (p<0.05). "Impulsive" patients were younger (62.36 vs. 73.60 years, p<0.001) and scored higher on the Mini-Mental State Examination (MMSE) (24.12 vs. 19.72, p<0.01). Several behavioral variables were also better in the "impulsive" group; Consortium to Establish a Registry in Alzheimer's Disease (CERAD) Savings Score (6.86 vs. 4.55, p=0.001), CERAD Recognition (7.64 vs. 5.55, p=0.001), and Constructions Score (8.68 vs. 6.64, p=0.001).

Violent "nonimpulsive" crimes were only committed by those with agitation-paranoia as part of their dementia. These patients had more cognitive impairment, especially in the domains of memory and visual spatial construction. (Given their dementia, none of the patients were tried or imprisoned for their antisocial behavior.)

Comment

Since people with dementia have lost cognitive ability in multiple domains, it is not surprising that they may fail to conform to social norms and break the law. Multiple variables, including the person's premorbid personality and social conduct, extent of dementia, quality of care and supervision, as well as opportunity likely influence the incidence and prevalence of sociopathic behavior in this population. The authors observed that people who committed "impulsive" crimes tended to be younger, less severely demented, and were more likely to have frontal than temporal lesions than those who committed "nonimpulsive" crimes.

This paper does not tell us how often sociopathic behavior is associated with dementia. Probably the authors have examined hundreds if not thousands of patients with dementia, but have chosen to present only 33 cases. What was the denominator? The premorbid legal history of these patients is also not provided; criminal activity may have been a "pre-existing condition" in some. It would also be of interest to learn how often dementia *presents* with criminal activity.

There is some inconsistency in the scheme of frontal vs. temporal localization regarding "impulsive" and "nonimpulsive" behavior as portrayed in the paper. For example, one patient with "impulsive" behavior (shoplifting) was diagnosed with frontal temporal dementia, but her SPECT scan showed hypoperfusion in both anterior temporal lobes. Another patient who had "Wernicke's aphasia as a result of strokes" and "nonimpulsive" aggressive behavior had left subfrontal hypometabolism on PET scan, as well as other areas (not described). It appears there remains much to be learned about localization and cerebral networks regarding complex illegal behaviors.

If sociopathic behavior is more common in demented individuals than generally appreciated, caregivers and law enforcement personnel may benefit from additional education on this topic. Strategies to prevent criminal behavior are inherent in custodial care, but may need special emphasis for certain patients.

Perhaps neurologists should add an additional question to the social history, "Have you ever broken the law?" The answers may provide additional information regarding lesion localization and underlying pathophysiology. They may also spice up the dictations in the neurobehavior clinic.

References

Mendez MF, Shapira JS, Saul RE. The spectrum of sociopathy in dementia. The Journal of Neuropsychiatry and Clinical Neurosciences 2011;23:132-140.

Chapter 16

OMG! VACCINES WORK!

June 19, 2011

Introduction

A recent, retrospective study revealed that the incidence of bacterial meningitis decreased by 31% over 10 years, likely the result of vaccinations (Thigpen et al. 2011). In addition, the median age of those infected increased from 30.3 to 41.9 years, evidence that vaccinating the young has protected them from infections while leaving older, unvaccinated people more vulnerable.

The authors analyzed data on bacterial meningitis from 1998-1999 to 2006-2007 in 8 surveillance areas of the Emerging Infections Programs Network, which includes 17.4 million people. The 5 most common pathogens for bacterial meningitis were *Haemophilus influenza type b (Hib)*, *Streptococcus pneumonia, group B streptococcus (GBS), Listeria monocytogenes, and Neisseria meningitides*. Cerebrospinal fluid confirmation of the clinical diagnosis was required.

The beneficial effect of vaccines during the surveillance period is striking. The incidence of bacterial meningitis from *Haemophilus influenza* decreased by 25%. For strains of bacterial meningitis from *Streptococcus pneumonia* included in the PCV7 vaccine, infections decreased by 92%. Conversely, rates of meningitis from *group B streptococcus*, for which there is no vaccine, did not change.

Deadly Choices

In a recent Medscape One-on-One video interview, Eli Adashi, MD, discussed the dangers of the anti-vaccine movement with Paul Offit, MD, Chief of Infectious Disease at Children's Hospital, Philadelphia, PA. Dr. Offit is a pediatrician and author of *Deadly Choices: How the Anti-Vaccine Movement Threatens Us all*, Basic Books, 2011.

It's a Conspiracy

According to the Centers for Disease Control and Prevention (CDC), "Unfounded claims can cause harm to children if they result in less protection for them against potentially serious diseases."

However, judging from some of the online comments to Dr. Adashi's program, not all health care workers are convinced of the value and safety of vaccines. Their uncertainty may be contributing to the 40% of parents who refuse or delay vaccination of their children, a factor that appears related to the increase in measles, mumps, and other outbreaks.

A recent blog by Steven Salzberg published in *Forbes* regarding the importance of measles vaccination was attacked by Robert Schecter of "The Vaccine Machine," a website that "fights the misinformation and propaganda disseminated by the Machine and its unwitting media allies and stands firmly in opposition to the forced vaccination of America's children." Schecter argues that the health risk from measles is exaggerated, "but more importantly we must begin to dismantle the hidden police [state] which already exists and has as its foundation mandatory vaccination."

Yikes! If there's a "hidden police state," I guess it's well hidden, because I haven't found it yet. But I'll keep looking...

While those who choose not to vaccinate themselves or their children may consider this their "right," their refusal not only puts themselves at risk, but others as well, particularly those who are immunocompromised or with chronic medical conditions (Thigpen et al. 2011). Unvaccinated newborns, who have yet to have a say in the matter, are the most vulnerable (Thigpen et al. 2011).

A Global Concern

The problem of bacterial meningitis may be better appreciated when examined from a global perspective. Data from the CDC are enlightening:

Haemophilus influenzae type b (Hib) is a bacterial disease that each year causes pneumonia and meningitis in young children, resulting in three million illnesses and 400,000 deaths. Bacterial meningitis alone kills more than 65,000 young children in the developing world each year. The United States has been able to virtually eliminate pediatric bacterial meningitis through several interventions including the introduction of Hib vaccines.

Your Son is Going to Die

Here is an excerpt from the Introduction of *Deadly Choices: How the Anti-Vaccine Movement Threatens Us All.*

On February 17, 2009, Robert Bazell, a science correspondent for NBC Nightly News, told the story of an unusual outbreak in Minnesota: a handful of children had contracted meningitis caused by the bacterium Haemophilus influenzae type b, or Hib. What made this outbreak so unusual was that it didn't have to happen;

a vaccine to prevent Hib had been around for twenty years. But most of the Minnesota children-including one who died from the disease-weren't vaccinated. The problem wasn't that their parents couldn't afford vaccines, or that they didn't have access to medical care, or that they didn't know about the value of vaccines. The problem was that they were afraid: afraid that vaccines contained dangerous additives; or that children received too many vaccines too soon; or that vaccines caused autism, diabetes, multiple sclerosis, attention deficit disorder, learning disabilities, and hyperactivity. And despite scientific studies that should have been reassuring, many weren't reassured. When the outbreak was over, one mother reconsidered her decision: "The doctor looked at me and said, 'Your son is going to die. He doesn't have much time.' Honestly, I never really understood how severe the risk [was] that we put our son at."

Infants Don't Get to Choose

While working as an emergency room (ER) physician several decades ago, I vividly remember treating one febrile 7 month old boy. Unlike most of the children I saw in the ER, this one wasn't cranky, crying or screaming. He just lay there, limp and quiet on his mother's shoulder. I had never done a lumbar puncture on a 7 month old, but meningitis seemed likely. A spurt of green pus that shot though the needle and splattered onto my white coat confirmed the diagnosis. A helicopter ride to a tertiary medical center and vials of antibiotics saved the child's life.

It would be nice if no one ever needed to participate in that scenario again, not doctor, parent, or patient. I hope that little boy never developed any neurological sequelae such as cognitive and behavioral dysfunction, deafness, seizures, speech and language deficits, spasticity or vision loss.

Moderate to severe sequelae of bacterial meningitis occur in approximately 25% of survivors (Chandran et al. 2011).

Less Vaccinations, More Epilepsy

As an epileptologist, I have treated people suffering from intractable epilepsy due to meningitis. Of course, they were "lucky," since they survived. The overall mortality rate of meningitis is 15%, which did not change during the 10 year surveillance period (Thigpen et al. 2011).

Conclusions

It is ironic that modern science provides the power to eradicate epidemic infections (like measles), but irrational human behavior limits our ability to apply these tools, resulting in unnecessary morbidity and mortality for individuals and a costly societal burden. The educational efforts of the CDC, Dr. Offit, and others, as well as the observations presented by Thigpen and colleagues may convince some of those who doubt the value of vaccines to change their minds. Given the ongoing "debate" about the merits of vaccination, this *New England Journal of Medicine* study should be front-page news.

Adverse events may occur with any treatment, but the rigorous approval process of vaccinations by the Food and Drug Administration (FDA) as well as the excellent safety track record of current vaccines should reassure those who hesitate to vaccinate themselves or their children. Expanded coverage of the new PCV13 pneumococcal vaccine promises to be even more beneficial than the older PCV7 vaccine. However for those who contract meningitis, case fatality rates remain at a stubborn 15%. Our limited ability to improve fatal outcomes further emphasizes the importance of vaccination for meningitis prevention.

Believe it.

References

Chandran A, Herbert H, Misurski D, Santosham M. Long-term sequelae of childhood bacterial meningitis: An under appreciated problem. Posted 1/6/2011, http://www.medscape.com/viewarticle/734981.

Thigpen MC, Whitney CG, Messonnier NE et al. Bacterial meningitis in the United States, 1998-2007. NEJM 2011;364:2016-25.

Chapter 17

A NEUROLOGIST ON A MISSION

March 4, 2011

Introduction

What can a neurologist do on a medical mission? That was my first thought when I was invited to join "Lingkod Timog," a volunteer medical mission group 5 years ago. Since then, I've become the group's medical director. The name of the organization, Lingkod Timog, translates from Tagalog (Filipino) to "Service to the South." It refers to the Southern Philippines, the location of most of our missions. Lingkod Timog was established 7 years ago by Irene Covarrubias-Sabban and Cecilia Heredia, wives of Philippine military officers. Unlike some medical mission groups, Lingkod Timog has no religious or political affiliation.

Medical Missions-Overview

Medical missions can take many forms. Some are primarily concerned with disaster relief, such as after a tsunami or earthquake. Perhaps the best known of these groups are Medecins sans Frontieres (Doctors without Borders) and Project Hope. Others focus on quick "in and out" surgery that can dramatically improve people's lives, such as cataract removal (e.g., Himalayan Cataract Project) or facial cleft repair (e.g., Operation Smile). Some missions emphasize the development of local infrastructure or training villagers to become health care providers, following the "Give a man a fish, and you feed him for a day. Teach a man to fish, and you feed him for a lifetime," paradigm. At least one group serves rural areas in the USA (Remote Area Medical). A "Physicians Guide" to medical missions published in *Medical Economics* provides an overview regarding the pros and cons of participating in medical missions with links to a variety of organizations.

The Tagbanua

Lingkod Timog just returned from a medical mission to care for the Tagbanua, a tribe of indigenous people who live on the island of Palawan, Philippines. The Tagbanua live in the hills, earn a subsistence living farming, and obtain no regular medical care. They have a rich tribal culture, but their population has decreased to only about 150 families. Upon arrival in Puerto Princessa, we met with the Governor, Baham Mitra, as well as the Public Health Director to square away our itinerary and goals. By their very nature, medical missions are "ad hoc" projects, requiring extensive planning and local cooperation.

Partners

In order to leverage its effectiveness, Lingkod Timog partners with other organizations. During this mission, physicians, dentists, and nurses joined our group from the Philippine Marines, Army and Navy. The marines, under the direction of General Juancho Sabban, also provided logistic support, such as crowd control, security, and transportation. Security can be a bit dicey in the Philippines, but the marines had matters well in hand. Teresa Wycoco, MD, from the Puerto Princessa City Health Office, supervised a family planning tent to help counter the high infant mortality associated with large families. We set up a medical clinic for adults, pediatrics, a minor surgery center, and a dental extraction clinic. An optometrist refracted patients and provided free reading glasses. Medicines and supplies came from a variety of sources, including donations from the Lions Club of the Philippines, residents of Newport, RI, (Lingkod Timog's USA home base), and others. Shell Philippines supplied mosquito nets coated with insect repellant, as malaria is still endemic in Palawan. Malaria education was also provided.

Tables and Chairs
Our "clinic" consisted of tables and chairs in the Cabayugan Elementary School, a 1.5 hour drive on a mostly paved road from the main city of Puerto Princessa. A "feeding tent" provided at least one nutritious meal to patients and their family members. Food was contributed by a local restaurant owner, Butch Chase. We wrote prescriptions for medications, which were dispensed by our "pharmacy" in an adjacent building. Music was provided for entertainment, and some enterprising food vendors set up shop on the school grounds.

Neurology Office
I worked with a civilian nurse who doubled as a translator. It's a given that nearly all my neurology consultations at the hospital in the USA require some type of imaging, usually an MRI. Yet on these medical missions, I rely on the time-honored contents of my Black Bag; a flashlight, ophthalmoscope, reflex hammer, stethoscope, and tuning fork. There

is no Internet for "Googling." Consequently, I depend entirely upon that portable cognitive processor between my shoulders. (During the mission, I felt better about my status as the lone neurologist when I discovered that the Army physician at the next table was a radiologist!)

5 Interesting Cases

1. An 8 year old girl previously treated for malaria complained of persistent fevers. I couldn't help but notice her facial rash, which had never been addressed. She had no seizures or developmental delay. It appeared she was asymptomatic. She did not suffer any stigma in her community from the port-wine stain that covered just the left half of her face. While we arranged for a repeat malaria smear, I engaged in some neurology teaching about Sturge-Weber syndrome.

2. A 40 year old farmer had atrophy of his right quadriceps muscle and an absent knee jerk, suggestive of a femoral neuropathy. He was referred to the 50 bed military hospital for spine xrays and a more thorough evaluation. (The marines will provide transportation for him at a later date.)

3. A 60 year old woman complained of chronic head pain after a thorn pricked her scalp a year ago. After running through my usual differential of migraine, tension headache, temporal arteritis, and brain tumor, I asked to examine her head. She had a 1 cm sebaceous cyst on the crown of her head, which we later removed in the minor surgery clinic.

4. A 69 year old man complained of decreased vision, both near and far for the last several years. Ophthalmologic examination revealed dense bilateral cataracts, and he was referred to the local hospital for extraction.

5. An otherwise healthy 30 year old woman complained of excessive blinking of both eyes. She had no eye pain or visual complaints. She was mostly distressed because other people noticed it, and she was embarrassed. I think she had benign essential blepharospasm, and I reassured her that it was nothing serious, "Hindi malubha."

Conclusions

A medical mission is an opportunity for a neurologist to help people, but it can be much more than that. It is a team effort of like-minded volunteers who choose to devote their free time to a humanitarian effort. From a doctor's point of view, there is no paperwork, no medical-legal concerns (could the patients even spell my name?), and an opportunity to escape from the narrow confines of subspecialization and face the challenges of a broad spectrum of familiar (diabetes, hypertension) and unfamiliar (malaria, tuberculosis) illnesses. It was a relief to be reminded that all headaches are not migraine or due to medication overuse. The patients with neurologic syndromes such as Sturge-Weber, benign essential blepharospasm, and femoral neuropathy had the benefit of a diagnosis and appropriate referral, which they may not have received had they not been seen by a neurologist.

Medical missions are not the optimal approach to health care, but represent desperate attempts to fill gaps in local health care systems. A successful mission requires months of planning and expectations tailored to the available time and resources available. To compensate for the frustration that stems from the inevitable insufficient supplies and technology, one can dispense guidance, large doses of compassion, reassurance, and referral to local healthcare facilities. The Tagbanua were invariable appreciative, regardless of how much relief they actually received from their chief complaints. While medical care in remote areas may be more suited to the skill sets of emergency and family physicians, ophthalmologists, and plastic surgeons, even a neurologist can provide valuable service on a medical mission. In addition, each medical mission has been a priceless learning experience for me, about medicine and humanity. I can't wait for the next one!

Chapter 18

A NEUROLOGIST ON A MISSION-II

March 26, 2012

Introduction

This past February, my medical mission group, Lingkod Timog, traveled to the island of Palawan, Philippines, for its 8th annual medical mission. Lingkod Timog is a non-profit nongovernmental organization (NGO), founded by Cecilia Heredia and Irene Covarrubias-Sabban, wives of Filipino military officers. During our annual missions to rural areas of the Philippines, our group receives considerable logistical support from the Philippine Armed Forces, especially the Marines, led by Irene's husband, General Juancho Sabban. This informal but essential military connection enables us to travel and work safely in remote areas that are rarely visited by outsiders for reasons of accessibility and security. While there are many limitations to what our small group can accomplish, each year Lingkod Timog treats more than a thousand patients. With the cooperation of local government and public health officials, we focus on indigenous people who would otherwise not receive any modern medical care.

Tagbanua and Tao't Bato

Like last year (see Chapter 17), we provided medical services and food for the Tagbanua. We set up a makeshift clinic in Barangay Simpucan, about an hour and half drive northwest from Palawan's main city of Puerto Princessa near picturesque Sabang Beach.

In addition, we held a clinic for the Tao't Bato (Cave Dwellers). We drove south in a convoy to Barangay Ransaan, Municipality of Rizal, a 6 hour ride over mostly unpaved roads with world-class potholes. This bone-jarring drive was punctuated by a minor car accident precipitated by a pothole that almost swallowed the van in front of us. Upon arrival at the designated area, we learned that the Tao't Bato actually live yet another 8 hours away by foot via a jungle trail, a journey we were not prepared (physically or mentally) to make. Consequently, we treated those Tao't Bato who hiked from their homes and were shuttled the rest of the way in trucks driven by Philippine Marines. We also treated people from different tribes and other residents of Barangay Ransaan.

Medical Care

Most patients complained of aches and pains, coughs, colds, headaches, skin rashes and urinary tract infections. We diagnosed and distributed medicines for these common ailments. We also screened for diabetes, gastrointestinal parasites, hypertension, malaria, malnutrition, and tuberculosis and triaged for more serious illness that required hospitalization. (Because none of the patients could actually afford hospital admission, which requires up-front cash payment, those that need it can go for free to the Armed Forces of the Philippines Hospital in Puerto Princessa.) Our dental team extracted teeth and provided dental hygiene instruction. The surgical team removed lipomas, cysts, performed circumcisions and other minor surgeries. We also introduced the concept of family planning, as families are large and infant mortality high.

Participants and Sponsors
Our doctors come from diverse specialties, including anesthesiologists, radiologists, and public health. All participants are volunteers. Various sponsors, including Shell, which has a vigorous anti-malaria program, and local businessmen, such as Butch Chase and Ramon Mitra, supported the mission as well. During the medical missions, we try and emphasize to local government officials the importance of improving the existing health care infrastructure of these rural locations with the ultimate goal of eliminating the need for Lingkod Timog and the many other medical mission groups that routinely visit the Philippines.

An Interesting Case
As a board certified internist as well as a neurologist, I work with the other doctors to see general medical cases, but I am always on the lookout for neurologic ones. Here is a particularly unusual case:

This 50 year old man presented with generalized weakness and new onset of right foot drop. Through an interpreter, he said that he became sick when he was about 10 years old and had always been weak. Lately, he developed foot drop and had trouble walking. He had no sensory loss. On examination, he had diffuse muscle wasting. The intrinsic muscles of both hands were severely atrophied, as were the gastrocnemius and soleus muscles bilaterally. Reflexes were diffusely depressed, but present. There was no Babinski sign. He had no fasciculations.

Differential Diagnosis

Because the patient had muscle weakness since childhood, amyotrophic lateral sclerosis seemed out of the picture. The most likely explanation for his diffuse muscle atrophy was childhood polio. His increasing diffuse weakness and foot drop were probably caused by post polio syndrome. A superimposed peroneal neuropathy, L5 radiculopathy, lumbar plexopathy, or other cause, might also be responsible for the foot drop.

Post Polio Syndrome

Post polio syndrome is a fascinating entity. It first became well known during the time of my residency training. Publications about it peaked in the late nineties (Halstead 2011). Despite decades of research, it remains a diagnosis of exclusion based on clinical characteristics. There are still 10-20 million polio survivors worldwide, but the exact number with post polio syndrome is unknown. There is no definitive treatment, which relies on rehabilitation. Due to the ubiquitous implementation of the polio vaccine, polio and post polio syndrome are now in dramatic decline. The last cases of polio infection occurred in the USA in 1979 and in 1993 in the Philippines. Only 452 new cases of polio were reported in 2010, most from Africa and India (Halstead 2011). The Philippines has an active child immunization program and 3 doses of oral polio vaccine are routinely administered to Filipino children beginning at 6 weeks of age. The Philippines was certified polio-free in 2000. Because this Filipino man lives on the fringes of civilization, he probably never received the polio vaccine and likely had a severe case of polio as a child. Now in his 50s, the effects of aging are taxing his remaining motor units, and his weakness is increasing. Because polio has been eradicated in the Philippines, this gentleman will be one of the last cases of post polio syndrome in the country. Given the limited resources available, I recommended mild exercise to try and maximize his remaining muscle function.

The Unexpected

Participating in a medical mission always delivers satisfaction from helping other people. In addition, sometimes interacting with another culture allows one to see something that one has never seen before. I was reminded of this rewarding aspect of the medical mission by working with Tiago Villanueva, a Portuguese-Filipino physician. Tiago had traveled from Portugal to participate in his first medical mission in the Philippines, and he assisted with boundless enthusiasm. Seeing patients without the benefit of a computer terminal was a new experience for him, but he adapted quickly. He was fascinated by the rural culture, which included children riding water buffalo (carabao) and jeepneys stuffed to overflowing with fearless passengers perched on the roof. While parts of the bustling capital of Manila could easily be confused with major cities in other parts of the world, life in the Philippine provinces remains barely tinged with modernity. Satellite dishes mounted on pedestals in front of a few rustic dwellings spoke to the haphazard infiltration of modern conveniences in communities without hot water, reliable electricity, or sewage systems.

Although I have visited many rural communities, I did see something I had never seen before. A native girl had accessorized her earlobe with her own hand-rolled cigarettes, a resourceful meld of fashion and practicality!

We noticed that hand-rolled cigarettes were quite popular in Barangay Ransaan and counseled against the dangers of tobacco. Luckily, the time, trouble, and expense of rolling one's own cigarettes suggests that even amongst those who smoke, quantitative tobacco use is low.

Next Year

The location and logistics for next year's mission will take months to plan. If we return to Palawan, perhaps we can tackle that jungle trek to reach the caves of the Tao't Bato?

I'll bring my medical kit, my camera, and an open mind.

References
Halstead LS. A brief history of postpolio syndrome in the United States. Arch Phys Med Rehabil 2011;92:1344-1349.

Chapter 19

AN EPIC ADVENTURE

January 20, 2013

Introduction

A few months ago, I accepted an invitation to work over Christmas and New Year's as a locum tenens neurohospitalist. As the starting date approached, I began to have misgivings. Although the neurology service included a team of residents and nurse practitioners, all of them would take vacation for the better part of the week, leaving me to manage on my own. How long would it take to learn my way around? If it was like most hospitals, constructed over the years in fits and starts with renovations and additions, navigating a cluster of buildings with lengthy corridors wouldn't be easy. Would the staff be helpful to a newcomer, indifferent, or worse? I've often worked during Christmas, and sometimes there is a "we're all in this together" attitude that softens the reality that nearly everyone else is on vacation. What would the mood be at this hospital? I would be the only neurologist on call 24/7 in this 500 bed academic hospital, opening up a real possibility for multiple consults from the emergency room, intensive care units, medical and surgical floors, obstetrics, as well as telephone calls from outpatients and outlying hospitals. How many stroke patients would come to the emergency room requiring urgent assessment for thrombolysis with tPA in the middle of the night? Other questions lingered. For example, if this was such a good hospital, why had they been unable to recruit a full staff of neurohospitalists? Could I get the work done and still get enough sleep? Would physical exhaustion impair my ability to maintain an engaging professional demeanor at all times, as the locum tenens agency advised?

My Big Worry

But one concern trumped all the others-could I figure out the electronic medical record (EMR)*? The hospital had attained the Health Information and Management Systems Society's (HIMSS) much vaunted "Stage 7" status-patient care without paper charts. This seemed a dubious digital accomplishment. I use several computers, and when they stop working, my productivity approaches zero. I wouldn't want to put my health care in their hands. This hospital relied on the EpiCare Inpatient Clinical System (hereafter referred to as Epic) for its medical charting. Although I consider myself reasonably computer literate, I had never cared for patients using a fully electronic chart. Despite what it may say on the Epic website, it seemed unlikely that this monstrous program was "user-friendly." In order to arrive as well prepared as possible, I requested a tutorial on Epic, but it never arrived. (There may have been some Catch-22 in play; since I didn't yet have staff privileges, I couldn't use the medical record...) I insisted on a full day of on-site computer training prior to assuming my clinical responsibilities-at least whatever inadequacies I might manifest as a neurologist would not be compounded by ineptitude with the EMR.

Man vs. Machine

After an intense day of training with several knowledgeable and supportive IT personnel, I learned that the computer could reveal all the information traditionally contained in a paper chart, if only one knew where to click. I could copy and paste, reorder medications that had been "reconciled" by someone else, write notes, send messages, even view xrays. The system accomplished its mission of getting all the information in one place. However, data entry was tedious and accessing lab reports required jumping from screen to screen. When I requested advice from other clinicians, it was like asking for directions to a local restaurant-everyone had a different way of getting there. From a workflow point of view, it also seemed that somehow physicians had never been consulted regarding the system's basic design. With each click, I became convinced that the engineers who created Epic had been influenced far more by the principles of Rube Goldberg than Steve Jobs.

Woops!

Putting what I had learned about Epic into practice was not without a few stumbles. Before interviewing a young man with possible nonepileptic seizures, I noticed that "HIV positive" was listed in his past medical history. When I asked him about this, his skin paled and he adamantly denied it. (I thought he would have a seizure right then and there, which would have been a good thing from a diagnostic point of view.) He not only agreed to repeat the blood test, but insisted on it. I had not completed his social history, but it appeared that he had 7 children, most by different mothers, and he might well be in a high risk group for HIV. This little flurry of inquiry took time away from our main goal, that of sorting out his unexplained seizures, but the blood test was done and we put it behind us.

After I finished his history and neurological exam, I formulated a mental plan. Whereas in "the old days," I could have dictated a comprehensive note in about 3 minutes, I spent more than half an hour trying to enter data in the EMR. Dictation is an option for Epic, but only in some fields, which means switching back and forth from a telephone or Dictaphone to the keyboard. That particular technical ballet proved too challenging for me, so I limited myself to the cumbersome keyboard entry.

The next day, when I reviewed his record again, I saw that "HIV positive" was one of many diagnoses in his past medical history on a "pick list," but that it was only an option, not an entry. This subtlety in presentation had unfortunately escaped me the first time around. A paper chart would not have lent itself to this kind of mistake. Happily, the man's test came back negative.

The next night I lapsed into despair as consults piled up in the emergency room and I sat paralyzed in front of the computer screen, desperately trying to electronically admit a patient. I could not figure out how to enter the patient's medications into the admission orders. It initially seemed odd that the emergency room staff had no idea how to do this either until it was pointed out that they are not the ones who admit patients. Finally, I telephoned the "on call" IT person. Like a surgeon summoned at home to perform a life-saving procedure, the IT tech drove to the hospital, located me in the vast maze of the emergency room, and patiently helped enter the patient's orders.

Potential for Improvement

The ease of use of the computer-clinician interface clearly has significant potential for improvement. Clicking checkboxes is tedious and inordinately prone to error. (How many of us have mistakenly selected "Uruguay" instead of the "United States" on a credit card application or other online form?) If voice recognition could replace check boxes, the EMR would be much more clinician friendly. Physician workflow patterns should be recognized and facilitated. For example, after checking an xray report, the obvious subsequent option should be to see the xray. This next step should be made easy rather than complex (e.g., hidden link, necessity to reenter password, long delay for xray to appear) in order to encourage physicians to actually look at the images rather than ignore them out of frustration. The clinical summary, arguably the most important part of the medical chart, should be elevated to prominence, rather than lost among a myriad of scattered data fields.

Why EMR?

The U.S. government has implemented a program to financially reward physicians who are able to extract "meaningful use" out of their EMRs, and will soon financially penalize those who don't (Kern et al. 2013). More than half of office-based physicians use EMRs, including approximately 2/3 of family physicians. The benefits to patient care are expected to counterbalance the expense and intrusion of the EMR system.

One of the potential values of EMR is to save money. A RAND 2005 report estimated that "widespread use of electronic records could save the United States health care system at least $81 billion a year" (Abelson and Creswell 2013). The potential for savings seems evident. For example, there would be no need to repeat diagnostic tests, as the results would be easily searchable in the record. However, RAND admits to overstating the savings potential (Abelson and Creswell 2013).

Presumably, patient care would benefit as well. Reminders regarding vaccinations or mammograms could pop up on a patient's electronic chart, virtually insuring that all preventive medical interventions would be enacted.

Another intended use of EMR is electronic performance measurement. Initial audits of the EMR to demonstrate clinical effectiveness have met problems of accuracy (Kern et al. 2013). Whereas check box responses can be easily tallied, "free text" entries may not be recognized. Kern et al. have gone so far as to suggest, "physicians need to recognize EHRs not as electronic versions of paper records but as tools that enable transformation in the way care is delivered, documented, measured, and improved." In other words, physicians should change their workflow to accommodate the EMR-a monumental case of the "tail wagging the dog" if ever there was one.

A Few Positives

By the end of the week, with the kind assistance of numerous IT consultants and directions from friendly doctors who passed by my workstation, I achieved a passable competence with Epic. I even liked some of its features. The best part was being able to log-on and write orders on patients I had seen earlier who were many corridors and stairways away. I could also check patient labs throughout the day from any computer terminal. I could even see xrays without walking to the radiology department. The other EMR feature I liked was that all of the notes were legible. In the past, I have often had to guess at what some of my erudite colleagues had written due to the highly evolved nature of their penmanship. I was stunned to realize that the time-honored tradition of searching for a patient's chart at the nursing station, the bedside, in the radiology suite, on the medication cart or a thousand other places had disappeared. This achievement joins other momentous world events such as the collapse of the Berlin Wall, the adoption of the Euro, and Man's First Step on the Moon.

Conclusion

The EMR is a fact of life. As a modern tool for patient care and research, its use (and foibles) should be taught in first year medical school along with the operation of the blood pressure cuff and ophthalmoscope. (Perhaps the next generation of medical students, raised with smartphones in their cribs, may not require such instruction?) Physicians currently in practice must somehow find time to master this massively intrusive contrivance for the benefit of their patients and their own self preservation. For my part, I'm glad to have had my first Epic experience in such a sympathetic environment. When I return for another assignment, my efficiency ought to be much improved. I just hope I can upgrade my computer skills as fast as they upgrade the software.

*Also referred to as electronic health record (EHR).

References

Abelson R, Creswell J. In 2nd look, few savings from digital health records. The New York Times, January 10, 2013.

Chapter 20

"CRASHING THROUGH" -A MUST READ FOR THOSE WHO WOULD UNDERSTAND VISION AND THE SELF

September 12, 2010

A well-read colleague at the hospital lent me a copy of this nonfiction book, *Crashing Through*. It tells a powerful story about the trials and tribulations of a blind man who regains his sight. Physicians, particularly neurologists and psychiatrists, as well as other health care professionals, will find it interesting.

The book is really 4 stories in one, and it's worth reading for any one of these.

The first story is that of an amazing individual, Michael May, who was blinded in an accident at age 3. Through his incredible curiosity, determination, and physical stamina, with the support of an extraordinary mother, he succeeded as an entrepreneur, inventor, intrepid traveler, athlete, husband, father, Gold Medalist skier in the Paralympics and in many other endeavors. The title "Crashing Through" refers to the main character's *modus operandi*. If there were barriers, he would "crash through" them, either figuratively or literally. For those of us who ever felt that life was too hard, Michael May's story is humbling and inspiring.

The second story is a medical one. What happens when new technology, a stem cell transplant, offers a blind man the chance to see? What are the chances of success? How does one weigh the risks of immunosuppression versus the cataclysm of rejection? The writer, Robert Kurson, does an excellent job of explaining the surgery and post-op care in terms a layperson can understand.

The third story has to do with the physiology of our 5 senses: sight, sound, smell, taste, and touch. If you have relied on only 4 senses since you were 3 years old, what happens in your brain when the fifth sense is suddenly restored? How does the brain process these new images? If for nearly all your life you have imagined the world by reaching out and touching objects or listening for the subtlest of sounds to judge distances, how do you integrate vision into your life? Do the images make sense? Can you identify letters? Can you read words? Can you determine distances by using perspective? What do colors mean? Can you interpret facial expressions? Are you seeing what you imagined reality to be all these years? Is your wife really as beautiful as you thought? How do you know what is beautiful? What is ugly? Is this new sense too overwhelming to use?

And the last story has to do with one's self image. What happens to a man's identity when he has lived all his adult life as a blind man, never felt sorry for himself for lack of vision, become a leader in the "blind community," and enjoyed the attention received as a successful blind man when he abandons the realm of the blind and joins the world of the "sighted?" And what happens if that restored vision isn't perfect? It is this story that is the most unpredictable and intriguing.

Disclaimer: I have no financial interest in the book and have never met Michael May, but I sure would like to!

References

Kurson, R. Crashing Through. The extraordinary true story of the man who dared to see. Random House Trade Paperbacks, New York, 2008.

Chapter 21

FILM CONTEST DEBUTS AT AMERICAN ACADEMY OF NEUROLOGY

February 1, 2010

For the first time, the American Academy of Neurology (AAN) Foundation is sponsoring a contest for the best short, original movie that highlights the need to support research to prevent, treat, and cure brain disorders. Videos must be 3-7 minutes in duration and include the tagline, "Let's put our heads together to support brain research." The submission deadline is February 16th, 2010. Films will be judged on creativity (originality, appeal, inspirational) and technical composition. Two winners will be chosen, one for the $500 Storyteller Prize and one for the $1000 Filmmaker Prize. The latter prize is for films that demonstrate greater technical expertise. Films will be screened on Sunday, April 11, 2010, at the American Academy of Neurology's 62nd annual meeting in Toronto, Canada. Both prizes include a free trip to the Neuro Film Fest at the AAN meeting.

The winning videos, along with others selected by the committee, will also be available on the AAN's YouTube Channel where the public can vote on the best video. The most popular video on the YouTube Channel will receive the $500 Fan Favorite prize. Contest instructions are available at the AAN Neuro Film Festival webpage.

While a large public education effort has brought stroke into the lexicon of the average American, many neurologic diseases remain mysterious to the layperson. People commonly ask what my medical specialty is, and when I respond "neurologist," I often feel that I must explain further. Usually, I start with "headaches" and "migraine" to find familiar ground, before I advance to "Lou Gehrig's disease" or "multiple sclerosis." The level of ignorance regarding most neurologic disorders is matched only by the degree of fear surrounding these diagnoses. Publicity around the H1N1 virus has recently highlighted Guillain Barre syndrome for the public, although unfortunately the media has focused on drama rather than information regarding both the virus and the rare occurrence of Guillain Barre due to the H1N1 vaccine.

The ready availability of inexpensive and easy to use high quality movie cameras and editing software makes this new contest a timely and worthwhile addition to the AAN's activities. Any neurologic disorder is fair game for the contest. I wonder whether the making of such a film might be therapeutic for patients and their caregivers, especially if it chronicles a neurologic disorder such as Alzheimer's disease or multiple sclerosis, where caregivers and the patient must deal with the effect of the disease over many years. The film could explore day to day challenges and issues regarding dependency, treatment, the lack of a cure, and hope. Neurologists involved in such a project might keep note of how it affects their therapeutic alliance with the patient and family.

I hope there are many high quality entries to this year's festival and that the AAN makes it an annual event. A contest such as this provides a venue for documentary medical films that could be months in the making, providing a longitudinal look at the human experience of neurologic disorders. Films focused on people living with these illnesses will promote awareness and decrease stigma. Insights derived from such films may directly benefit patients in interactions with their own families, friends, physicians, and other health care providers, as well as generate support for research intended to alleviate suffering from neurologic disorders.

Update May 17, 2013

The AAN film festival has proven successful and continues as an annual meeting event (See Chapter 7).

Chapter 22

GENERIC DRUGS: UPCOMING MEETING AND A CALL FOR PAPERS

November 16, 2009

Introduction

As health care costs increase and more brand name drugs go off patent, the pressure on physicians to prescribe generic drugs continues to mount. Whether generic substitution is prudent for patients with epilepsy or other diseases remains a matter of intense debate. While generic drugs are similar to the innovator drug, they are not identical, and small differences in bioavailability may be important for individual patients regarding efficacy and side effects (Liow et al. 2007). Recognition of this problem is not new-a review published in *Neurology* warned against "uncontrolled generic substitution" (Nuwer et al. 1990). Recent research suggests that problems encountered with generic substitution are not limited to older antiepileptic drugs, but occur with newer antiepileptic drugs as well (Bazil 2009). Use of generic antiepileptic drugs may also paradoxically increase the costs of health care due to an increase of other prescription medications, emergency care, hospitalizations, and other health care utilization (Bazil 2009).

The American Academy of Neurology opposes mandatory and arbitrary generic substitution in the treatment of epilepsy (Liow et al. 2007). Several other organizations oppose generic substitution for epilepsy (Steinhoff et al. 2009).

For the manufacturers of brand name drugs, the impact of generic drugs on profitability may be significant. The long-term consequences of competition by generic products on new drug development are unknown. To compete in the marketplace, manufacturers of brand name drugs are even buying generic drug manufacturers!

As evidence of the worldwide interest in generic drug use, a number of conferences have been devoted to this topic. It has even been proposed that generic prescribing be taught in medical school in an effort to increase the availability of drugs to economically disadvantaged patients.

Upcoming Meeting

The World Generic Medicines Congress Europe 2010, London, UK, February 23-26, 2010, testifies to the importance of generic drugs for pharmaceutical companies, physicians, and last, but hopefully not least, patients. This will be the 4th annual conference. More than 130 representatives from generic pharmaceutical manufacturers attended last year's meeting.

Call for Papers

An open-source journal, *Pharmaceuticals*, has devoted a special upcoming issue to generic drugs. *Pharmaceuticals* is an international, peer-reviewed, quarterly open access journal published by Molecular Diversity Preservation International. At their invitation, I have volunteered as Guest Editor. Submissions may address any aspect of generic drugs for patients with epilepsy, other neurologic diseases, or other disorders. Original research and thoughtful reviews will be considered. Papers must not have been previously published. Simultaneous submissions are discouraged. Manuscripts will be rapidly vetted, and if accepted, published online in a matter of days to weeks.

Please contribute to this special issue of *Pharmaceuticals*. Additional research on generic drugs will help guide physicians in the best choice of medications for their patients.

I look forward to some interesting reading!

References

Bazil CW. Generic substitution: Are antiepileptic drugs different? Nature Reviews Neurology 2009;5:587-588.

Liow K, Barkley GL, Pollard JR et al. Position statement on the coverage of anticonvulsant drugs for the treatment of epilepsy. Neurology 2007;68:1249-1250.

Nuwer MR, Browne TR, Dodson WE et al. Generic substitutions for antiepileptic drugs. Neurology 1990;40:1647-1651.

Steinhoff BJ, Runge U, Witte OW et al. Substitution of anticonvulsant drugs. Ther Clin Risk Manag 2009;5(3):3449-3457.

Update May 17, 2013

The World Generic Medicines Congress Europe had its most recent meeting February 26-March 1, 2013, in London, England.

Chapter 23

BARIATRIC NEUROLOGY: THE NEXT SUBSPECIALTY?

October 5, 2009

Thou art so fat-witted, with drinking of old sack, and unbuttoning three after supper and sleeping upon benches after noon, that thou has forgotten to demand that truly which thou wouldst truly know.

Shakespeare
King Henry IV
Act I, Scene II

Introduction

Two papers published in *Neurology* suggest new associations between obesity and the brain. Whitmer et al. (2008) report that central obesity increases the risk of dementia more than three decades later, while Daniels et al. (2009) found an association between obesity and new-onset epilepsy in children.

Well recognized adverse health effects of obesity (body mass index (BMI) ≥30) include coronary artery heart disease, type 2 diabetes, cancers (endometrial, breast, and colon), hypertension, dyslipidemia, stroke, liver and gallbladder disease, sleep apnea and respiratory problems, osteoarthritis, gynecological problems and increased congenital heart defects in the offspring of obese women. Obesity can also decrease longevity, quality of life, economic productivity and results in billions of dollars in excess health care costs. The case for aggressive treatment of obesity is apparent, and family practitioners, pediatricians, internists, endocrinologists, bariatric surgeons, and others are assiduously trying to decrease the incidence and prevalence of obesity in their patients.

Central Obesity and Increased Risk of Dementia More than Three Decades Later (Whitmer et al. 2008)

A longitudinal analysis examined the relationship of sagittal abdominal diameter (midlife central obesity) of 6,583 patients to the diagnosis of dementia an average of 36 years later. The results were adjusted for age, sex, race, education, marital status, diabetes, hypertension, hyperlipidemia, stroke, heart disease, and medical utilization. Participants who had increased sagittal abdominal diameter and a normal BMI had an increased risk of dementia (1.89 HR, 95% CI (0.98-3.81)), while participants who had increased sagittal abdominal diameter and obesity had the highest risk of dementia (3.60 HR, 95% CI (2.85-4.55)). Dementia diagnoses included dementia, Alzheimer's disease, vascular dementia, and dementia not otherwise specified.

Obesity is a Common Comorbidity for Pediatric Patients with Untreated, Newly Diagnosed Epilepsy (Daniels et al. 2009)

A comparison of BMI Z-scores (indexed for age) of 251 children (aged 2-18 years) with newly diagnosed epilepsy to the standard CDC growth curve revealed that 18.7% were overweight, 19.9% were obese, and 38.6% were overweight or obese (p<0.0001). A group of 597 regional controls had a lower percentage of overweight (14.7%) and obese (13.7%)

children, and significantly lower BMI-Z scores than the epilepsy group (p=0.0009). Because the study was performed on new onset patients, common causes for increased weight in children with epilepsy such as decreased levels of physical activity and side effects of antiepileptic drugs could not be held responsible. Socioeconomic factors were not closely examined. Whether there is a common mechanism for the development of obesity and epilepsy in children could not be determined.

Assessment

In my neurology training, I remember little emphasis on the diagnosis and treatment of obesity. A search of the current *Adams and Victor's Principles of Neurology* revealed only 20 citations for obesity, addressing such conditions as hypothalamic syndromes, obstructive sleep apnea, pseudotumor cerebri, side effects of antiepileptic and psychotropic medications and stroke. With the advent of statin therapy, stroke neurologists have taken an interest in treating dyslipidemias as well as obesity. The importance of diagnosing (not too hard) and treating obesity (very hard) to neurologists appears to be increasing.

These two papers suggest an intrinsic link between obesity and the development of central nervous system disease, specifically epilepsy and dementia. More studies are needed to confirm this tantalizing hypothesis. If, indeed, visceral adipocyte-derived factors are neurotoxic, as Whitmer et al. suggest, or obesity attacks the central nervous system in other ways, this new understanding of the pathophysiology of epilepsy and dementia will force the recognition and management of obesity into the realm of the neurologist. The magnitude of the problem is enormous because of the high prevalence of obesity in children and adults.

We know little of the brain's physiologic response to obesity. It may be that Shakespeare was on to something when he had the Prince of Wales call the corpulent Falstaff "fat-witted." More than 400 years later, it's up to us to find out.

References

Daniels ZS, Nick TG, Liu C et al. Obesity is a common co-comorbidity for pediatric patients with untreated, newly diagnosed epilepsy. Neurology 2009;73:658-664.

Chapter 24

PFO-PATHOLOGICAL OR A NORMAL VARIANT?

July 31, 2009

As a teenager, I first learned about the importance of a "hole in the heart" (patent foramen ovale) in reference to scuba diving. (A patent foramen ovale (PFO) is a remnant of the fetal circulation, a hole between the two atria, necessary for life in utero. After birth, the PFO closes...in most people.)

A PFO is important for scuba divers because nitrogen bubbles that might form in the blood due to changes in pressure while diving may pass from the venous system (where they would normally be filtered out by the lungs), into the arterial system, where they may act as "air emboli" and block blood vessels in the brain, spinal cord or elsewhere.

But even this straightforward argument suffers from "holes," as injuries of this type are extremely rare despite the common occurrence of circulating nitrogen bubbles in recreational divers and the high percentage of divers (and everyone else) with PFO. Nonetheless, some professional divers have had their PFOs closed by occluder devices to prevent a possible stroke.

According to the authors of an article published by Divers Alert Network: "Associating a common finding (PFO) with an uncommon disease (decompression illness) is a common mistake, and this often mistaken relationship is likely to be involved in the data regarding decompression illness and PFO" (Moon R, Bove A 2004).

PFOs are also on the list of causes of "cryptogenic stroke in the young." Just ask Tedy Bruschi of the New England Patriots who at age 31 got his PFO repaired after an acute stroke, just weeks after winning the Super Bowl for the 3rd time.

So, did Tedy do the right thing? Does the data support a role of PFO in stroke recurrence?

Data from a prospective Spanish multicenter study assessed 486 patients with cryptogenic stroke with contrast transcranial Doppler and echocardiography. The authors concluded, "Neither massive RLSh (right to left shunt) nor massive RLSh with concurrent atrial septal aneurysm is an independent risk factor for recurrent stroke, in either the general or younger stroke population" (Serena et al. 2008).

To further the case against PFO repair, a systematic review and meta-analysis of 15 clinical studies of patients with TIA or cryptogenic stroke just published in *Neurology* (July 14) "...does not support an increased relative risk of recurrent ischemic events in those with vs without a patient foramen ovale" (Almekhlafi et al. 2009).

Is this heresy-or science?

The American Heart Association/American Stroke Association and the American College of Cardiology Foundation Science Advisory (2009) recommended enrollment of patients with cryptogenic stroke and PFO into clinical trials to establish whether PFO closure decreases the risk of recurrent stroke (O'Gara et al. 2009). Three US trials are in progress; RESPECT, CLOSURE-1, and REDUCE. More information is available at: www.strokecenter.org/trials and www.clinicaltrials.gov.

In the meantime, what do you do in patients with acute stroke?

Do you look for PFO with a bubble study?

Do you use transcranial Doppler or transesophageal echocardiogram (TEE)?

Do you perform PFO closure to reduce the risk of acute stroke?

Do you treat a PFO with antiplatelet agents or anticoagulation with warfarin (Coumadin)?

Do you attach any importance to the presence of a concurrent atrial septal aneurysm?

Have you referred any patients to the ongoing PFO clinical trials?

If you have a patient who scuba dives and had a PFO discovered incidentally (no history of stroke), would you recommend another sport?

I appreciate your input.

For more on PFO:
Medscape video: Mark J Alberts, MD, Patient Foramen Ovale and Risk for Recurrent Stroke: www.medscape.com/viewarticle/586709

References
Almekhlafi MA, Wilton SB, Rabi DM et al. Recurrent cerebral ischemia in medically treated patent foramen ovale. A meta-analysis. Neurology 2009;73:89-97.

Moon R, Bove A, Divers Accident Network, October 2004.

O'Gara PT, Messe SR, Tuzcu EM et al. Percutaneous device closure of patient foramen ovale for secondary stroke prevention. Circulation 2009;119:2743-2747.

Serena J, Marti-Fabregas J, Santamarina E et al. CODICIA, Right-to-Left Shunt in Cryptogenic Stroke Study; Stroke Project of the Cerebrovascular Diseases Study Group, Spanish Society of Neurology. Recurrent stroke and massive right-to-left shunt: results from the prospective Spanish multicenter (CODICIA) study. Stroke 2008;39:3131-3136.

Update May 18, 2013

In the RESPECT trial, there was no significant benefit in the primary intention-to-treat analysis for adults with cryptogenic stroke who had closure of their PFO with the Amplatzer PFO Occluder (NEJM 2013;368:1092-1100.

In the CLOSURE-I trial, closure of a PFO with a device in patients with a cryptogenic stroke or transient ischemic attack (TIA) was not superior to medical treatment (NEJM 2012;366:991-999).

The REDUCE trial, which compares the GORE Septal Occluder plus antiplatelet therapy to antiplatelet therapy alone in patients with PFO and a history of cryptogenic stroke or TIA, is still underway.

Chapter 25

NANOTECHNOLOGY-WHEN GOOD THINGS COME IN SMALL PACKAGES

July 16, 2009

Despite an increasing number of new antiepileptic drugs, approximately 30% of people with epilepsy continue to have seizures, and many suffer adverse medication effects. More effective and less toxic drugs are sorely needed. However, a recent journal article suggests that novel delivery systems may improve the efficacy and tolerability of drugs we already have (Bennewitz and Saltzman 2009).

The authors propose multiple strategies to deliver antiepileptic drugs to the brain, which include prodrugs (e.g., fosphenytoin), efflux pump inhibition, hyperosmolar blood brain barrier opening, direct drug delivery to the cerebrospinal fluid and cortex, gene and cell therapies, and nanoscale drug delivery. It was the use of nanoparticles to transport antiepileptic drugs into the brain that I found particularly intriguing.

Nanotechnology is all the rage these days-check out this press release from the Massachusetts Institute of Technology (MIT): "Professor Chad Mirken received a $500,000 prize for 'innovations that have the potential to transform the future of medical diagnostics and patient point-of-care and to ignite change across many industries from semi-conductors to healthcare'" (June 24, 2009, http://web.mit.edu/newsoffice/2009/lemelson-0624.html). And here's another one from the *New York Times*, "Collaborating for Profits in Nanotechnology," http://www.nytimes.com/2009/07/16/business/smallbusiness/16edge.html?ref=technology).

Nanotechnology may be defined as "engineering of functional systems at the molecular scale." Nanoparticles range from 10 nanometers (nm) to 1000 nm. A nanometer is really tiny, one *billionth* of a meter.

For the purpose of drug delivery, nanoparticles are typically composed of biodegradable polymers and copolymers (For more info, check out the Center for Responsible Nanotechnology: http://www.crnano.org/whatis.htm. Another resource is Michael Crichton's rather technical and fanciful novel "Prey".)

According to Bennewitz and Saltzman, the primary obstacle to achieving therapeutic antiepileptic drug concentrations in the brain from oral and intravenous (IV) routes is the blood brain barrier (BBB). Using nanotechnology, antiepileptic drugs can be encapsulated within a "nanoscale delivery system" constructed of polymer nanoparticles, liposomes, or other tiny materials, which can sneak through the brain capillary endothelial cells and astrocytes that form the BBB. Once inside, the antiepileptic drug is released as the polymer container degrades, over a period ranging from days to weeks. (The release time can be controlled by changing the polymer type or ratio of copolymers making up the nanoparticles.) Such a delivery system is likely to reduce the necessary dosage of antiepileptic drugs and decrease systemic side effects.

Many technical challenges remain, such as making the nanoparticle container large enough to carry a significant amount of drug without making it too big to pass through the BBB, preventing the carrier from getting cleared from the plasma by the reticuloendothelial system, facilitating penetration into the BBB, and making sure the nanoparticles can navigate the tortuous environment of the brain parenchyma once they pass through the BBB.

But these challenges may not be insurmountable. For example, an *in vitro* cellular model suggests that nanoparticles coated with choline are 3-4 times more likely to penetrate the BBB than uncoated nanoparticles.

Nanoparticle delivery systems are not yet available for the treatment of epilepsy, but I look forward to the time when I can write antiepileptic prescriptions and check the box, "with nanoparticles."

References

Bennewitz MF, Saltzman WM. Nanotechnology for delivery of drugs to the brain for epilepsy. Neurotherapeutics: The Journal of the American Society for Experimental NeuroTherapeutics 2009;6:323-336.

Chapter 26

IS THERE A DOCTOR ON BOARD?

May 29, 2009

I was on my way to the ACTRIMS meeting today and was squeezed into one of those tiny "regional jets" that looked like it had been designed for preschoolers. The plane was ready to take off, but an air traffic control delay held us on the tarmac for an extra thirty minutes. Unable to use my laptop, a short nap seemed the best use of my time. Soon after I drifted off into a peaceful sleep, I was rudely awakened by the loudspeaker requesting the services of a doctor on board.

I have to admit I took a second to glance around and see if any other physicians responded to the call, but no one did. I walked up the aisle to find a 61-year-old heavyset white man, diaphoretic and clammy. (In the spirit of HIPAA*, let's call him Bob.) Frankly, Bob looked like central casting for the middle aged guy having a heart attack in a B-rated airplane movie. His face was ashen, his speech was labored, and he barely moved. A soft spoken man who identified himself as a nurse was already taking Bob's pulse and quietly informed me he couldn't feel it. Graciously, he offered Bob's sweaty wrist to me.

I tried taking Bob's pulse, but couldn't feel much either. But Bob was talking, although with some effort. He said he was dizzy and denied chest pain. He had hypertension and took blood pressure medication, something that began with a "P." Recently, his doctor told him to cut the dose of his blood pressure medication by half a pill because of episodes of low blood pressure, down to 80/50-kind of like this. Bob said that usually it took about 20 minutes for these dizzy spells to go away. He denied chest pain, heart trouble, or diabetes. Bob assured me he would be all right in a few minutes. I encouraged him to drink some complimentary cranberry juice, and he gulped it down.

It was obvious that Bob did not like being the center of attention in the crowded plane, and even in his weakened state, his bulk and demeanor made him a little intimidating. After some encouragement, Bob told me that years ago he had been accepted to medical school, but decided to play professional football instead. His pulse was still hard to find. I was tempted to feel his carotid, but since Bob was still talking, I figured his heart was still beating. It seemed a little too dramatic to start palpating his neck for his carotid and too embarrassing to start groping around his groin for a femoral pulse. His breathing wasn't labored, and his respiratory rate was normal.

By this time the plane had been cleared for take off, and the flight attendant demanded my opinion: should Bob go to the hospital, or should we depart on our planned 2.5 hour flight? Clearly the most prudent course was to ask Bob to get off the plane; it was going to be a very long flight if Bob had a myocardial infarction (MI) after take off (at least for me, if not for Bob). On the other hand, Bob made a pretty good case for iatrogenic hypotension related to excessive blood pressure medication. He had survived several similar episodes, and I was pretty sure he didn't want to get off the plane.

We didn't break out the medical kit, but I was pleased to learn that it contained an automated external defibrillator, blood pressure cuff, stethoscope, 6 airways, 3 CPR masks, 3 pairs of nonlatex gloves, nitroglycerin tabs, lidocaine, epinephrine, atropine, aspirin, acetaminophen, and assorted other medical supplies. Two portable oxygen bottles designed to last 30 minutes each were available.

I reassessed Bob again. He didn't look quite so pale, seemed a bit more energetic, and said he was getting better. I gave the flight attendant the OK to take off. I imagined the headlines, "Dr. Wilner gives passenger clean bill of health minutes before fatal heart attack."

Bob slept most of the trip, and we landed safely. As the passengers in front of me disembarked, I watched Bob leave the plane, a little slowly, but under his own power. When I left, the pilots and crew thanked me.

I'm a bit embarrassed by my hesitation to get involved, but in my defense it was only momentary. In theory, in-flight medical care should be protected by the Good Samaritan laws. I had investigated this question just last year after I participated in another in-flight emergency on a 13-hour flight to Japan. That one concerned a young man who was intoxicated with sleeping pills and alcohol, and he required a lot of supervision. When we landed in Tokyo, he was still in a stupor, and I recommended that emergency services be called.

I would be very interested to learn from other doctors' experiences regarding in-flight emergencies. Have you taken care of a patient in flight? If called upon, do you volunteer? Do you feel obligated as a physician to care for a sick person on a plane? Are you concerned it might interfere with your own travel plans (e.g., having to remain with the patient after landing)? How worried are you about medical liability? As a neurologist or other specialist, how equipped are you to deal with most medical emergencies? Are there any CME programs out there on how to approach an in-flight medical emergency? What about the in-flight medical kit? Did it have what you needed? How did the patient do? Would you do it again? Please share your comments.

*HIPAA-Health Insurance Portability and Accountability Act

Chapter 27

JUST BECAUSE YOU KNOW IT'S TRUE DOESN'T MAKE IT SO

April 29, 2009

The American Academy of Neurology meeting now hosts 3 poster sessions each day for 3 days in a row, and each session has more than 100 posters. Consequently, this blog will not attempt a thorough review of the more than 300 posters presented today! Rather, I will pick just one. This poster was in the hall, and is not even listed in the abstract book. The presenter wasn't there, but the images caught my eye. There were pictures of Jean Martin Charcot, George Gilles de la Tourette, Jean Itard, and Sandor Ferenczi. Titled, "Misperceptions of Coprolalia Throughout History," the author was Erika Levy, BA, from the University of Rochester School of Medicine and Dentistry. The poster was noteworthy for several reasons:

1. The primary thesis was that coprolalia has been wrongly described as "inevitable" by none other than Charcot, "an irresistible psychic compulsion" by Tourette himself, due to "diseased will" by Itard, and an "expression of erotic emotion" by Ferenzci. One could probably accept Tourette's description, and possibly Itard's, but the others are inaccurate. The lesson: the great masters, as great as they were, were not always right.

2. The second interesting point of the poster is that coprolalia is not as common as we may have been

taught. According to the old DSM III psychiatric classification, coprolalia is present in 60% of patients with Tourette's. However, when the author examined 136 children with attention deficit hyperactivity disorder (ADHD) and tics, 16% had coprolalia according to the parents, 5% according to the teacher, and only 3% according to both the parents and the teacher. The study suggests that coprolalia is not as common as we have been led to believe. Larger studies would be welcome to confirm these findings.

3. The third point of the poster is that the dramatic nature of coprolalia has led to its exploitation by the media in TV and movies, such that the general public strongly associates coprolalia with Tourette's. The poster hints at the question of the responsibility of the media to accurately represent medical illnesses. (Along these lines, the American Academy of Neurology previously presented an award to the producer of The West Wing for the accurate representation of President Bartlett's multiple sclerosis. The popular television show was able to educate millions of people about this disease, performing an important public service.)

Let's hope Ms. Levy is a budding neurologist, for her investigation of Tourette's syndrome and coprolalia demonstrates a willingness to question what we all know is true, but may turn out not to be.

Chapter 28

THE CHEESECAKE FACTORY-A TASTE OF TOMORROW'S HEALTHCARE?

August 11, 2012

Introduction

Atul Gawande, MD, a surgeon, writer, and public health researcher, suggests in his most recent article that the practice of medicine could improve if only it learned lessons offered by the Cheesecake Factory, a successful restaurant chain (Gawande 2012).

But as brilliant a writer as Gawande is, this article left me with a severe case of indigestion. There are so many differences between the practice of medicine and a restaurant chain that I can't accept his analogy. Here are 4 big ones:

Flawed Analogy

1. Gawande, an astute observer, conveniently overlooks the fact that customers in the Cheesecake Factory actually pay their bills. Had he left the restaurant with his teenage daughters and their friends without paying the check, there would have been severe and immediate repercussions. Consequently, he ordered from the menu what he could afford. Such is not the case in the American Medical System, which for the most part provides care in an open-ended fashion, with the bill waiting somewhere down the

line. Doctors order what their patients need (and in some cases want, but don't need), without necessarily considering the cost. Further, many hospitals, unlike the Cheesecake Factory, are not-for-profit, a completely different business model.

2. A fundamental difference between the practice of medicine and the Cheesecake Factory is that the Cheesecake Factory provides a standardized product. That "salmon like butter in my mouth" Gawande extolls is prepared exactly the same way for each customer who orders it. However, every textbook of medicine and every skilled physician, including Gawande, knows that the practice of medicine must be individualized for each patient, a concept at odds with the standardized product provided by the Cheesecake Factory. For example, drugs must be chosen depending upon a patient's allergies, comorbid diseases, and concomitant medications. Doses must be adjusted depending upon body weight, kidney and liver function, and the ability to swallow a pill or capsule. A chain restaurant would never attempt to fine-tune its dishes to the unique demands of each and every customer, but that's what the American Medical System tries to do every day. And it's a lot harder than broiling a fish.

3. Another insurmountable incongruity between medical care and a restaurant chain is that people don't have to eat at restaurants. They can cook dinner and eat at home. But medical consumers can't stay home. Not only must they seek care, most patients

have little choice about when and where. For example, the patient in a motor vehicle accident rushed to the emergency room will go where the ambulance takes him. The patient newly diagnosed with cancer may do some comparison shopping, but is likely to go to the nearest hospital that can provide the necessary treatment as soon as possible.

4. There are other arguments that skewer the Cheesecake Factory analogy, not the least of which is the intangible but critical personal relationship between a patient and his or her physician, which has healing properties of its own. David Shaywitz, MD, PhD, points this out in his response to Gawande's article in *Forbes*. As attentive as the white-clad waiters in the Cheesecake Factory may be, I suspect they rarely offer such an intimate and powerful connection.

EMR-When Standardization Fails

Solutions that "standardize" procedures and aim to improve efficiency may fall short when put into practice. Perhaps the best example is the electronic medical record (EMR). What could be more simple than having each patient's record computerized, so that every piece of information would be stored and instantly retrievable? Imagine how much money that would save! In theory, it's true. And in practice, many expensive tests that would have been unnecessarily repeated have been canceled when prior test results were easily located in the EMR. But the EMR has also produced the 10 page consult note stuffed with obligatory bullet points and overflowing with so many extraneous details that the key information may never be noticed, or worse, never included in the record at all. In its blind effort to standardize medical information and include everything, the EMR often neglects the one piece of essential information that really matters. To borrow Gawande's analogy, the standardized EMR produces the perfect McDonald's hamburger, complete with mustard, ketchup, pickles, onions and a dash of salt-all on a toasted bun, perfect...except sometimes the burger goes missing.

Business 101
Could the delivery of medical care be more cost effective? Could it be a better experience for those who are sick? Could waiting times in emergency rooms be shorter? Clearly the answers to all of these questions are yes. But these are questions of management, not medicine. As Gawande states, this is 'Business 101."

Tele-Medicine
Gawande explores the concept of tele-medicine, which is a high-tech way of providing another set of eyes for a patient's care from a distant source. Tele-medicine has proven particularly effective for the management of stroke, allowing small hospitals that do not have stroke specialists to consult specialists at major centers. Tele-medicine can also assist with quality control, as Gawande states, and may have a role in assisting busy intensive care units. But this has little to do with the Cheesecake Factory and everything to do with getting the job done right by the people trained to do it, an essential component of any service industry.

Say What?

One of Gawande's assertions is incomprehensible. He states, "In medicine, we hardly ever think about how to implement what we've learned. We learn what we want to, when we want to." The evidence against this, at least in my experience, is monumental. Every patient presents management questions that must be answered, often on the spot. Implementation of learning is what the practice of medicine is all about.

One Tasty Morsel?

Gawande touches on one feature of success of the Cheesecake Factory that *could* improve the current practice of medicine. He writes, "The managers had all risen through the ranks. This earned them a certain amount of respect." Physicians are familiar with this system, as the intensive experience of 4 years of medical school, 1 year of internship, and 2 or more years of residency plus subsequent fellowship years, coupled with standardized examinations provide a common experience, bond, and context for assessment of their peers. It is during these years of hands-on learning and apprenticeship that the "best practices" of medicine that Gawande refers to are learned. The rigor and duration of this training are unmatched by any other category of "provider" or administrator in our health care system. Those who manage physicians have not risen through these same ranks, but rather earned their experience in MBA programs and the business world, credentials that carry little weight with clinicians. Consequently a huge cultural chasm separates health care managers from health care providers. Is the success of the Cheesecake

Factory telling us that those would manage hospitals and health care should have "risen through the ranks?" I could swallow that.

References

Gawande, Atul. Big Med. The New Yorker, August 13, 2012.

Shaywitz, D. Do you believe doctors are systems, my friends? Forbes, 8/6/2012.

Section 3.

Neurology and Social Media

Chapter 29

NEUROLOGISTS ON FACEBOOK?

February 18, 2010

The advent of low cost and near-instantaneous communication on the Internet has spawned a number of popular social media websites such as Facebook, Myspace and Twitter. These sites provide an informal international forum for people to share personal and professional information. Popular topics range from golf and wine to the more esoteric, such as model railroads and medieval history. Physicians can discuss medical news, challenging clinical cases, business management, and even market their practices. Other sites such as SERMO, iMedExchange, NeuroList, and Medscape's Physician Connect host medical forums. These informal discussion groups complement more traditional online medical information such as continuing medical education (CME), noncredit courses, and medical conference coverage.

Another new communication tool that has become popular is the physician blog (like this one). Examples of physician blogs include KevinMD, Dr. David's Blog, Dr. Val, and Pauline Chen's blog in the *New York Times*. Blogs differ from traditional editorial columns or Op-Ed pieces in that they allow (and encourage) reader feedback.

In a recent survey, physician usage of social media grew 50% last year, and more among younger doctors. Even a venerable institution such as the American Academy of

Neurology has its own Facebook and Twitter accounts (although the arguably more stodgy American Neurological Association has yet to embrace social networking). Medscape.com, the physician side of WebMD, also communicates with Facebook and Twitter. MedPageToday.com, another physician news and education site, can be followed on Twitter.

While one may wonder who has time for all this information, Facebook now has 350 million accounts, so if social networking is just a passing fad, it's a popular one!

The Massachusetts Medical Society offers an online CME program "Social Networking 101 for Physicians" that alerts physicians to the potential medical-legal risks of participating in online media sites such as Facebook and Twitter. Much of the advice is common sense. For example, physicians need to protect patient confidentiality when discussing cases to comply with HIPAA (Health Insurance Portability and Accountability Act) regulations. Social networking pages are not an accepted means of patient-doctor communication regarding clinical care, and physicians should have a clear policy with patients regarding all confidential communication. Physicians should also preserve professional boundaries-patients should be blocked from participating on a physician's personal Facebook page. The Massachusetts Medical Society deems the topic of social networking so important that it awards 1 hour of state-mandated Risk Management CME for physicians who pass the course.

Physicians need to be mindful that any posts to Facebook, Twitter, other Internet sites, as well as their personal and professional emails, no matter how spontaneous or casual, may be indelibly engraved in the Internet forever. These may be retrieved by anyone who knows how to use the Google search bar, which is just about anybody over 5 years old. To prevent embarrassment and potential lawsuits, you shouldn't write anything you wouldn't say in public, particularly negative comments about people or institutions (no matter how true!). Your comments will not only live forever in some giant data bank in the "Internet Cloud," but liberal use by others of the "copy and paste" edit function enables your comments to circle the globe faster than you can say "woops!" "Pause before you post" is a good maxim for self preservation.

For journalists, social networking sites can help attract a larger audience. Nicholas Kristof, one of my favorite *New York Times* correspondents, commented on his participation in social media in an interview in the latest issue of *TimeOutNewYork.com* (February 18-24, 2010). When asked why he used multiple platforms, Mr. Kristof observed, "I really think that is part of the way to continue to engage audiences. I can engage old white men in my column and then I can engage teenyboppers with my Facebook pages... We need to try to evolve, and so that's one reason why I shoot videos for the *New York Times* Website, why I blog, why I Twitter, why I Facebook, why I have a YouTube channel."

Personally, I have just scratched the surface of Facebook and Twitter and am awed by their potential. For the moment, I use them to post the title and hyperlink of my regularly appearing blogs (Wilner on Neurology), monthly epilepsy updates (Epilepsy Notes), and other articles that I write. Twitter followers can elect to receive these "tweets" on their computers, cell phones, or go to the Twitter site to see what's new. To sign up for these brief messages, click "follow" on my Twitter site (twitter.com/drwilner).

As neurologists and other physicians become more comfortable with social media, hopefully they will enjoy their online participation, avoid medical-legal entanglements, and at least some of the information they glean from communicating with their colleagues will benefit their patients.

Chapter 30

HOSPITAL PRIVILEGES TERMINATED DUE TO FACEBOOK POST

April 25, 2011

Introduction

Alexandra Thran, MD, a 48 year old emergency room physician formerly at Westerly Hospital, Westerly, RI, posted a few notable cases she had seen in the emergency room on Facebook. She avoided using patient names or ages. Apparently, "unauthorized third parties" were able to determine one patient's identity from the post. When Dr. Thran learned of this, she immediately deleted her account.

Westerly Hospital concluded that Dr. Thran used her Facebook account "inappropriately." Both the hospital and Dr. Thran agreed that she had "no intention to reveal any confidential patient information."

The hospital's solution? Terminate Dr. Thran's hospital privileges.

On April 13, 2011, the Rhode Island Board of Medical Licensure found Dr. Thran guilty of "unprofessional conduct." The Board handed out a $500 fine with instructions for her to attend a continuing medical education (CME) course dealing with physician-patient confidentiality issues.

The Unknowns

Given that Westerly Hospital is rather small (125 beds), one has to wonder how the hospital administration concluded that the patient's identity was revealed through Dr. Thran's Facebook post and not by one of the many other participants in the patient's care. Any of the following could have breached confidentiality (in alphabetical order); admission's clerk, ambulance driver, billing clerk, dietician, emergency medical technician, housekeeper, IT technician, maintenance engineer, nurse, nurse's aid, pharmacist, phlebotomist, physician, physician's assistant, respiratory therapist, security guard, social worker, xray technician, ward clerk, and the list of possible suspects goes on. One might also include the patient's friends, neighbors, relatives, or even the patient him/herself!

Confidentiality

Patient confidentiality is a basic tenet of the physician/patient relationship. If, indeed, Dr. Thran violated patient confidentiality on Facebook, it constituted an error in judgment.

According to the American Medical Association's *Principles of Medical Ethics*, "A physician shall respect the rights of patients, colleagues, and other health professionals, and shall safeguard patient confidences and privacy within the constraints of the law (AMA a)." According to the AMA, these principles "are not laws, but standards of conduct which define the essentials of honorable behavior for the physician."

The AMA has also specifically addressed the use of social media by physicians (AMA b). "Physicians should be cognizant of standards of patient privacy and confidentiality that must be maintained in all environments, including online, and must refrain from posting identifiable patient information online."

A recent article published in the *Annals of Internal Medicine* echoes this advice, "A professional approach is imperative in this digital age in order to maintain confidentiality, honesty, and trust in the medical profession...Although social media posts by physicians enable direct communication with readers, all posts should be considered public and special consideration for patient privacy is necessary" (Mostaghimi and Crotty 2011). The authors recommend that physicians may successfully use social media by creating separate online identities, one professional, one personal. Pertinent to Dr. Thran's case, the authors advise, "Refrain from posting potentially identifiable vignettes online unless you obtain patient consent."

The principle of confidentiality allows patients to communicate personal, and perhaps delicate or incriminating information to enable their physicians to properly care for them. For example, an executive might forego telling his physician that he drinks 3 scotches before lunch if he believed that information would get back to his boss (or appear on Facebook!). But withholding this information might lead to costly, time consuming and potentially invasive testing because of elevated liver function tests, which could have been easily explained had the history been complete. (An episode of the television series *House* featured the same theme; history that a patient finally provided, on her deathbed, led to her diagnosis when she admitted that she had not travelled to Hawaii (as she told her husband), but to Rio de Janeiro with a paramour, where she contracted a rare, lethal parasite...) There is no question that the principle of confidentiality is essential to the physician-patient relationship.

But as much as confidentiality is important, complete privacy in medical care is an illusion, a fantasy. For example, have you ever sat in a crowded doctor's waiting room and had your name called? (I did just this week.) Imagine the twittering behind my back-how come Dr. Wilner is at the *dermatologist's* office? What is *wrong* with his *skin?* This routine, but blatant breach of privacy happens to thousands of patients countless times a day. Within our medical system, the enforcement of patient privacy appears rather inconsistent.

However, an entry on Facebook is especially egregious for a couple of important reasons. First the post is not an essential part of the patient's medical care. Second, it differs in the matter of scale, as there are more than 500 million Facebook users.

Medical Education

The issue of confidentiality also arises when it comes to sharing patient details for the purpose of medical education. My old medical textbooks anonymized patients with a black bar across their eyes; a token effort to obscure their identities. But concerns for patient privacy have reached astounding new heights in the world of medical education. I was recently asked to write an article for a psychiatry newsletter based on several difficult cases. The newsletter targets a very specialized medical audience, and has, frankly, a rather small circulation. Nonetheless, the editor insisted on stringent guidelines regarding patient anonymity:

'If it is not possible for informed consent to be obtained, the report can be published only if all details that would enable any reader (including the individual or anyone else) to identify the person are omitted. Merely altering some details, such as age and

location, is not sufficient to ensure that a person's confidentiality is maintained.'

In the absence of patient consent, which was no longer possible to obtain, I complied as best I could by changing the age, sex, side of the lesion, and other recognizable details. I strived to keep the salient points, but each alteration chipped away at the case's veracity. If even the patient can't recognize the case, I wondered, is it still the same case? How can one possibly communicate with other physicians about patients with rules as limiting as these?

Should cases published for the purpose of medical education be viewed with a different lens? Would Dr. Thran have been sanctioned by the hospital and the medical board if she had published her patient vignettes in the *New England Journal of Medicine* rather than Facebook?

Ideally, obtaining patient consent is the way to go. But often the educational value of a particular case is not apparent until years later, when consent is no longer possible. And what if the patient says no?

Justice

In law and ethics, it is axiomatic that the "punishment should fit the crime." With respect to Dr. Thran's case, there may be details we do not know, and the Facebook post in question is no longer available for review. However, all parties agreed that Dr. Thran had no malicious intent regarding the posting, and she acted promptly to correct her error. One might conclude that Dr. Thran wrote about her patients because she couldn't stop thinking about them (on her own time, since emergency room physicians are typically shift workers), and actually cared about them.

Conclusions

For better or worse, social networking is here to stay, and physicians need to learn to manage this type of communication. Resources are available, such as the CME program, "Social Networking 101 for Physicians," which emphasizes the need to protect patient confidentiality when using social networking in order to comply with HIPAA (Health Insurance Portability and Accountability Act) as well as conventional medical ethics. Physicians should also inquire whether their hospital has a specific policy regarding online posting.

More than a year ago, I wrote a column about neurologists and social media (see Chapter 29). Since then, the use of Facebook, Twitter, Linked-In, and other social media has continued to grow, along with their potential pitfalls for healthcare providers. The actions of Westerly Hospital and the RI Medical Board demonstrate that physicians will be held strictly accountable for breaches in patient confidentiality on Facebook.

References

AMA (a). Principles of Medical Ethics. http://www.ama-assn.org /ama/pub/physician-resources/medical-ethics/code-medical-ethics/principles-medical-ethics.page?

AMA (b). Professionalism in the use of social media. http://www.ama-assn.org/ama/pub/meeting/professionalism-social-media.shtml.

Mostaghimi A, Crotty BH. Professionalism in the digital age. Annals of Internal Medicine 2011;154:560-562.

Morgan JT. Rhode Island Board disciplines six doctors, 1 for Facebook post. The Providence Journal, Tuesday, April 19, 2011, http://www.projo.com/news/content/DOCTORS_DISCIPLINED_04-19-11_8DNKMS6_v9.1a1f2d5.html.

Fine, Michael. Director of Health. State of Rhode Island Department of Health Board of Medical Licensure and Discipline. In the matter of Alexandra Thran, MD. No. C10-156, 4/13/2011.

Section 4.

Memory and Alzheimer's Disease

Chapter 31

"FRIENDS WITH BENEFITS"-AN ACCURATE PORTRAYAL OF ALZHEIMER'S DISEASE?

September 20, 2011

Introduction
In the new romantic comedy, "Friends with Benefits," two young professionals (Dylan and Jamie) experience the fun and fallout of adding sex to their platonic relationship after Dylan leaves Los Angeles to take a new job in New York City.

Alzheimer's Disease
The film features a subplot that neurologists may find particularly interesting. Back in Los Angeles, Dylan's father (Mr. Harper) has Alzheimer's disease. Annie, Dylan's sister, is the primary caretaker. Annie tells Dylan that his father is gradually getting worse, but that his condition fluctuates from normal to severely demented on a moment to moment basis. This background information sets us up for the dramatic changes in behavior exhibited by Mr. Harper.

In one scene, the father suddenly realizes that his wife is not at the restaurant with the rest of the family. When he insists on trying to find her, Dylan reluctantly tells him that his wife is not coming because she divorced him 10 years ago. Mr. Harper reacts to the news as if he is hearing it for the first time and becomes agitated and angry. He gets up and leaves the table, trips and falls, and creates a commotion in the restaurant. The family is embarrassed and saddened as this episode reinforces Annie's observation that Mr. Harper is mentally deteriorating.

In another scene, after Mr. Harper flies to New York City from Los Angeles, he and Dylan grab a bite to eat at the airport. Mr. Harper's dementia is evident as he makes himself comfortable by taking off his pants and neatly hanging them over a railing. He mistakes a passerby for "Didi," prompting Dylan to inquire about Didi's identity. Mr. Harper explains that he was still in love with Didi, a girl he dated before he married. He concedes that his enduring love for Didi may have been one of the reasons his wife left him and offers sage advice to Dylan about love. Dylan takes his father's advice, fixes his relationship with Jamie, and everyone lives happily ever after...

Your Thoughts?

Although people with Alzheimer's disease may have "good days and bad days," Mr. Harper's extreme and rapid vacillations in cognitive ability and behavior seem unrealistic. For example, in the same scene, Mr. Harper sits without his pants in a restaurant and also talks wisely to his son. How does this Hollywood depiction of Alzheimer's disease correspond with your experiences?

Chapter 32

MEMORIES TO KEEP AND THOSE TO FORGET

September 1, 2009

Introduction

Neurologists are preoccupied with memory. "Memory Disorders Clinics" have sprouted up all over the country, which cater to millions of people with mild cognitive impairment, Alzheimer's disease, depression, and other assorted memory problems. Forgetting one's keys may be a simple consequence of inattention, or the foreshadowing of a devastating, irreversible, neurodegenerative disease. Neurologists are called upon daily to tell the difference.

Memories are so important that their loss is not merely inconvenient, but emotionally upsetting. Witness the fiery arguments that may ensue when an old married couple cannot agree on the date of a shared past event, or the emotional reaction of an acquaintance when one forgets his or her name.

Without the ability to form new memories, we cannot learn, and our ability to interact meaningfully with our environment is severely limited. The paradigm for life without memory has been well studied in the accidental case of H.M., who lost much of his ability to form new memories after bilateral hippocampal resections in an effort to control his epilepsy. As a result of H.M.'s memory deficit, bilateral temporal lobe resections are now strictly avoided in the surgical treatment of epilepsy.

Trying to Remember
A recent visit to Cebu, Philippines, highlighted for me the crucial importance of memory, not just to the normal functioning of an individual, but to the fabric of our society. As it happened, I was there on August 15, the date of Japan's surrender in WWII, 64 years ago. There was a memorial service on the grounds of my hotel for the Japanese and Filipino WWII victims, sponsored by the Japanese community of Cebu, and I was able to attend.

The ceremony lasted 2 hours, was conducted entirely in Japanese, and was quite solemn. After the Philippine and Japanese national anthems, Mr. Miyagawa, the Japanese Consul at Cebu, gave a speech, followed by Mr. Kawasumi, President of the Japanese Association of Cebu. Then the attendees, approximately 200 people, offered incense and flowers at a Japanese Shrine. Mr. Ishida, President of the Japanese Association of Travel Industries, Cebu, also spoke.

Perhaps the most interesting part of the ceremony was the participation by Mr. Toyoki Akita, an 83 year old man. The same age as my father, Mr. Akita is also a WWII veteran. The memory of a war that ended 64 years ago was important enough that he had flown the 4 hours from Japan to attend this memorial service. For Mr. Akita, the war, and his role in it, demanded continued and public preservation. I couldn't help but wonder what role Mr. Akita had played in the war, and how had it compared to my father's experience in the US Army?

The ceremony concluded with a flyover by a single engine plane to commemorate the role of Japanese Kamikaze pilots. As it happened, the hotel sits on a steep hill, which allowed the plane to approach at an unnaturally low altitude. While I have no first hand memories of WWII, the distinctive drone of the plane's engine, its low approach, and its silhouette against the sun evoked vivid images from WWII movies of Japanese Zeros and their fiery crashes into US Navy Ships. Although it may seem a little silly, I was not comfortable as the plane continued its slow, deliberate approach towards me. The plane dropped confetti instead of bombs, but it was still unnerving.

The ceremony was meant to honor both Japanese and Filipinos who died in the war, but it seemed to me that the collective Japanese memory of WWII might differ from those of the Filipinos. For example, even those who are not students of WWII have heard of the Bataan "Death March," in which thousands of US and Filipino prisoners of war were brutalized or perished at the hands of the Japanese. To me, the ceremony seemed more of an "acknowledgment" than an apology. Of course, I could not understand the text of the speeches, which might have altered my perception significantly. Mr. Ogawa, a hotel employee who attended the ceremony, explained to me that, indeed, the ceremony was an apology, intended to facilitate future positive relationships between the Japanese and Filipino communities.

I wonder what will happen when Mr. Akita becomes too old to attend future memorial services, and how the memories of the war will fade as they recede in time. For how many years will the memorial services continue in Cebu, and who will attend?

Trying to Forget
Problems with memory are not all about remembering. Sometimes, there are the ones we want to forget, but can't:

Macbeth:
Canst thou not minister to a mind diseas'd,
Pluck from the memory a rooted sorrow,
Raze out the written troubles of the brain,
And with some sweet oblivious antidote
Cleanse the stuff'd bosom of the perilous stuff
Which weighs upon the heart?

William Shakespeare, Macbeth, circa 1607

Such is Lady Macbeth's affliction. She cannot forget the memory of her role in the king's murder, and it drives her to suicide. As with Lady Macbeth, for many people with post-traumatic stress disorder (PTSD), it is the memory of traumatic events that troubles them, not the failure to remember.

As "brain experts," neurologists play a crucial and unique role in the understanding and preservation of memory function. Long days in the memory clinic are not just about identifying, classifying and treating memory deficits, but about preserving our humanity. It is our memories that make us who we are, and the ability to form new memories that allows us to become who we want to be.

Section 5.

Multiple Sclerosis

Chapter 33

ZAMBONI "VENOUS INSUFFICIENCY" THEORY OF MULTIPLE SCLEROSIS- RED FLAGS WARN OF THIN ICE

April 14, 2010

Here in Canada, ice hockey is a big sport. But everyone knows you don't go skating on the pond when the ice is thin.

At the request of the National Multiple Sclerosis (MS) Society, the American Academy of Neurology hosted a prime time press conference to create a venue where the controversial theory that "chronic cerebrospinal venous insufficiency" (CCSVI) is the etiology of MS could be discussed by its leading proponents, Paolo Zamboni, MD, Director, Vascular Diseases Center, University of Ferrara, Italy, and a panel consisting of Robert Zivadinov, MD, PhD, Director of the Buffalo Neuroimaging Analysis Center, Buffalo, NY, Andrew Common, MD, Radiologist in Chief, St. Michaels Hospital, University of Toronto, Ontario, CA, and Aaron Miller, MD, Professor of Neurology and Director of the MS Center at Mount Sinai, NY, NY, and Chief Medical Officer of the National MS Society.

Spurred by Dr. Zamboni's 2009 report of 65 patients who had significant improvement in their MS after percutaneous transluminal angioplasty of their jugular or azygous veins to correct CCSVI, over 4,300 people registered to listen in to the press conference. Over 1,000 questions were submitted in advance.

Before I went to the press conference, I was skeptical. A breakthrough in MS by a vascular surgeon seemed unlikely to me (particularly since my old chief is a neuroimmunologist and pretty smart guy) but, well, who knows?

After the press conference, I was really skeptical.

Dr. Zamboni defined CCSVI as a "syndrome characterized by stenosis of the internal jugular and/or azygous veins with opening of collaterals and insufficient drainage proved by cerebral MRI perfusional study." Why venous stenosis, if it actually exists, should cause MS is unclear-the first red flag. There were at least 2 neuroimmunologists in the room, and I could see that neither one was buying Dr. Zamboni's theory that venous congestion causes leakage of red cells, deposition of iron, break down of the blood brain barrier, an immunologic response, and Voila! MS. Reversing the venous congestion would, according to Dr. Zamboni, relieve the disease's symptoms.

Apparently, there are neuroimaging criteria for diagnosing CCSVI. These were not explained during the conference, but are critical to the diagnosis. The criteria were defined by Dr. Zamboni, but it is not clear how they were validated, the second red flag.

The third red flag was the hopelessly detailed and confusing presentation by Dr. Zivadinov of the ongoing Combined Transcranial and Extracranial Venous Doppler Evaluation in Multiple Sclerosis and Related Diseases (CTEVD) Study. The press room was packed with neurologists and journalists, and the conference was specifically designed for lay listeners. I would be amazed, if anyone, including the neurologists in attendance, understood much more than the general gist of the three-phase study, which was to try and identify the prevalence of venous congestion in patients with MS, normals, and patients with other neurologic diseases by various types of imaging. Frankly, I was really frustrated, because I was eager to understand the current research in order to make some assessment about its validity, and I wanted the flags to stop waving.

The fourth red flag was Dr. Zivadinov's insistence that there had to be "scientifically rigorous research alongside respect for patients' rights and needs." I am not sure why he thought this audience needed a lecture on medical ethics, unless it was to imply that somehow this particular research needed to be rushed through. No one, least of all the attendees at the American Academy of Neurology, questions the need for better treatment of MS. Indeed, properly controlled randomized clinical trials have spawned several new powerful MS drugs that are likely to be approved in the very near future (See Chapter 36.)

The fifth red flag was the disclosure that Dr. Zamboni was working on a "proprietary" doppler machine, which would be the only machine that could really detect the problem of CCSVI.

By now, there were so many red flags waving there was turbulence in the room. I had to hang on to my seat to keep from toppling over.

Dr. Common gave a nice clear, overview for the journalists and laypeople listening-in describing interventional radiology and the treatment of venous diseases, but he admitted to no experience treating CCSVI.

To their credit, Drs. Zamboni and Zivadinov emphasized that NO PATIENT should have percutaneous transluminal angioplasty for CCSVI outside a properly controlled clinical trial.

For me, Dr. Miller said it all, "How, when, and indeed whether CCSVI has any role in the treatment of MS remains to be seen."

I look forward to revisiting this topic when there is more high quality, scientific data, and the ice is thick enough to stand on (See Chapter 34.)

Chapter 34

CCSVI-A NEW PHRENOLOGY?

June 28, 2011

Introduction
Where does the evidence stand on CCSVI as a cause of MS?

What is CCSVI?
In 2009, Paolo Zamboni, MD, a vascular surgeon, provided the first description of chronic cerebrospinal venous insufficiency (CCSVI) in a study of 65 patients with multiple sclerosis (MS) and 235 controls (Zamboni et al. 2009). Dr. Zamboni observed that CCSVI existed in 100% of those with MS, but none of the controls. Subsequent exploration of this controversial concept has provoked heated debate and consumed enormous resources of funding, research and time.

The Five Criteria of CCSVI
Dr. Zamboni described 5 critical venous flow anomalies detectable by transcranial and extracranial color doppler ultrasound that could determine the existence of CCSVI.

1. Reflux in the internal jugular veins and/or vertebral veins in sitting and supine posture

2. Reflux in the deep cerebral veins

3. High-resolution B-mode evidence of proximal internal jugular vein stenosis

4. Flow in the internal jugular veins and/or vertebral veins that is not detectable on Doppler

5. Reverted postural control of the main cerebral venous outflow pathways

In Dr. Zamboni's study, the presence of any of the 5 criteria was significantly more likely in patients with MS than in controls (p<0.0001) (Zamboni et al. 2009). None of the control patients had more than 1 of the abnormal parameters, but all of the patients with MS had at least 2 of the parameters. Venography was performed in the 65 patients with MS and revealed unilateral or bilateral stenosis of the jugular veins (91%) and abnormalities of the azygous vein (86%). Findings on venography included agenesis, annulus, atresia, closed stenosis, membranous obstruction, septum and twisting. Venography identified 4 principal patterns of CCSVI that had different types of obstruction and venous flow. The patterns correlated with the type of MS.

There was no difference in the number of extracranial venous stenoses in patients with relapsing remitting MS treated with immunosuppressant therapy (N=37) vs. those not treated with immunosuppressant drugs (N=18). None of the control patients without MS who were scheduled for venography for other reasons had stenosis in the azygous, internal jugular, or lumbar venous territories.

Limitations of Methodology
Methodologic problems with the original study include a heterogenous study group. The 65 subjects with MS included 35 with relapsing remitting MS, 20 with secondary

progressive MS, and 10 with primary progressive MS, resulting in small numbers of each type of MS. In addition, full data for each patient regarding each of the 5 venous flow parameters were not presented, the 5 parameters were not validated, and venography procedures were not blinded.

Importance of Venous Flow

Until Dr. Zamboni's provocative paper, the study of venous function in the central nervous system had been relatively neglected (Franceschi 2009). However, the possibility that intravascular stasis caused by chronic venous obstruction could lead to pericapillary iron deposition, subsequent tissue injury, and an autoimmune response resulting in MS represented an intriguing hypothesis (Franceschi 2009). MS is characterized by perivenous white matter lesions, supporting the possibility of a venous etiology (Mayer et al. 2011). Dr. Zamboni's work sparked interest in the concept of "vascular immunology" and revived interest in long-forgotten papers that suggested a link between MS and vascular pathology (Putnam 1935).

Dr. Zamboni immediately followed this study with an open-label therapeutic study of transluminal angioplasty of the stenoses identified in the same 65 patients (Zamboni et al. 2009). All of the patients survived with minimal complications. Venous pressures were similar in stenotic or normal vessels, but after treatment, venous pressures were significantly lower (p<0.0001). However, restenosis in the internal jugular vein was 47% at 18 months, 16 times higher than restenosis in the azygous vein. Significantly more patients were relapse free (50%) compared with the year prior to the procedure (27%, p<0.0014), but the annualized relapse rate did not change. On MRI, the number of active gadolinium-enhanced lesions decreased from 50% to 12% (p<0.001). Mental and physical quality of life improved significantly in patients with relapsing remitting MS. All of the clinical and radiologic assessments were unblinded, and there was no placebo or sham-treated MS control group.

Desperate Patients Seek Treatment
Despite the lack of agreement among experts regarding whether CCSVI exists, or if it does, whether it plays a role in the pathogenesis of MS, and if it does play a role, whether reversing it with angioplasty or stents might improve symptomatology, enthusiasm for CCSVI engulfed the MS community. Interest spread quickly, in large part because of vocal patient advocacy and Internet forums such as www.thisisms.com. There is even the website, LiberationProcedureCCSV.com.

Michael Dake, MD, Professor of Cardiothoracic Surgery and Chief of the Catheterization and Angiography Center at Stanford Medical Center in Stanford, California, performed more than 35 endovascular procedures for CCSVI (Samson 2010). However, after one patient on warfarin anticoagulation following placement of an internal jugular venous stent had a fatal brain stem hemorrhage and another patient required emergency heart surgery for a dislodged stent, all CCSVI procedures were suspended at his institution.

Because endovascular procedures for CCSVI are not approved in the United States or Canada, many patients seek treatment outside North America at their own expense. Patients may receive endovascular balloon angioplasty alone or in combination with venous stenting (Ludyga et al.

2010). There is no central registry to track these patients, their results, or their adverse events. One patient treated in Costa Rica died from complications.

To accommodate these patients, TraveloMed, a medical tourism company, offers a "Liberation Treatment Package," including flight, hotel, local taxi and treatment beginning at 4500 Euros. Their website encourages patients to "Sign up now to get the procedure done this month!"

A "nonprofit" venture, the CCSVI Clinic, also arranges a medical travel package. Balloon venoplasty and stenting are available for $15,000 at Noble Hospital in Pune, India. Their website includes a disclaimer, "CCSVI Clinic can accept no responsibility or liability whatsoever for medical procedures, advice, opinions and services provided by others."

Numerous testimonials to the success of these procedures have appeared on YouTube, including one from Ginger, who sought treatment in Poland. Other patients have been treated in Bulgaria, Costa Rica, India and Mexico. Ginger enthusiastically describes improvement in her symptoms, but nothing to suggest a cure. Given the relapsing remitting nature of MS, it is impossible to determine from this and other anecdotal reports whether any improvement after CCSVI treatment is related to the procedure, a placebo effect, or simply the natural history of a relapsing remitting disease. Nonetheless, many patients have embraced this treatment as an MS cure. Patients are so invested in this therapy that one woman who experienced transient improvement of her balance, fatigue, and mobility after treatment in India attributed the return of her symptoms 6 weeks later to a return of the "blockages" rather than a failure of the therapy.

To date, no testimonial to the success of CCSVI procedures for MS in the form of a randomized, controlled, clinical trial has appeared in any peer-reviewed publication. Until a prospective, randomized, sham treatment trial demonstrates the value of endovascular treatment for CCSVI, the Cardiovascular and Interventional Radiological Society of Europe has recommended that this treatment "should not be offered to MS patients" (Reekers et al. 2011).

Conspiracy Theory
Some patients endorse a conspiracy theory, believing that neurologists, the national MS societies of the United States and Canada, and pharmaceutical companies are suppressing CCSVI because a cure for MS would mean a loss of business and profits. According to one blogger whose wife has MS, "They (the MS societies) have become a new enemy that we have to fight against, in addition to MS, and we must be determined." As Ginger declared in her video, "We're going to win this."

Diagnostic Trials: Can the Results Be Duplicated?
In response to patient demand for treatment of CCSVI, the National Multiple Sclerosis Society allocated $2.4 million for 7 pilot research studies. The MS Society of Italy also appropriated approximately $1 million for CCSVI epidemiologic research. So far, no one has been able to duplicate Dr. Zamboni's astonishing results (Khan and Tselis 2011).

A study of 25 patients with MS and 25 controls demonstrated CCSVI in 84% of those with MS and none of the controls (Al-Omari and Rousan 2010). Another study identified

CCSVI in 63 of 70 (90%) patients, but there was no control group (Simka et al. 2010).

A blinded diagnostic research trial by Zivadinov and colleagues, the Combined Transcranial and Extracranial Venous Doppler evaluation in MS and related diseases (CTEVD) trial, compared the frequency of CCSVI in a total of 499 patients, including those with MS (N=289), a control group who had no neurologic disorders (N=163), patients with other neurologic disorders (N=26), and patients with clinically isolated syndrome (CIS, N=21) (Zivadinov et al. 2011). CCSVI was present in 56.1% of patients with MS, in 42.3% of those with other neurologic diseases, in 38.1% of those with CIS, and in 22.7% of healthy controls. Sensitivity was 56.1%, specificity was 77.3%, the positive predictive value was 81.4%, the negative predictive value was 49.8%, and the odds ratio was 4.33 for CCSVI relative to controls. CCSVI prevalence was higher in patients with progressive MS and in those with neuromyelitis optica than in patients with relapsing remitting MS or CIS.

A triple-blinded sonographic study of 20 patients with MS and 20 healthy controls failed to replicate any of the findings in Zamboni's original study (Mayer et al. 2011). None of the patients or controls fulfilled anomalous venous outflow criteria 1, 2, or 4. More controls (N=16) than patients (N=13) fulfilled criterion 3, and 1 control subject fulfilled criterion 5. None of the MS patients fulfilled 2 criteria for CCSVI.

In a study of 56 patients with MS and 20 controls, none of those with MS fulfilled more than 1 of the 5 criteria (Doepp et al. 2010). A case control study of 21 patients with relapsing remitting MS and 20 healthy controls evaluated with phase-contrast MRI found no differences between the 2 groups regarding internal jugular venous outflow, aqueductal cerebrospinal fluid flow, or internal jugular reflux. However, 3 patients with MS had internal jugular stenoses on MR angiography (Sundstrom et al. 2010).

It could be postulated if CCSVI is responsible for the development of MS, then it should be present in patients with CIS because clinically definite MS will develop in most of these patients. However, a study of 50 patients with CIS identified only 8 (16%) who fulfilled CCSVI criteria. Selective venography in all 7 who agreed to the procedure failed to confirm any venous anomalies (Baracchini et al. 2011).

A Treatment Trial is Underway

The first (and only) prospective, randomized, double-blind study of endovascular treatment of CCSVI for patients with MS, the Prospective Randomized Endovascular therapy in Multiple Sclerosis (PREMISe) trial is ongoing at the State University of New York in Buffalo. Researchers will randomly assign 20 patients to balloon endovascular treatment of CCSVI or a sham angioplasty, where patients will undergo catheter insertion but without balloon inflation. During the sham procedure, a video fluoroscopy of a different balloon angioplasty procedure will be shown in the operating room to provide realism. The patient will be blinded as will the clinician performing the clinical assessment following the procedure. The principal investigator will be Adnan Siddiqui, MD, Assistant Professor of Neurosurgery at the University of Buffalo School of Medicine and Biomedical Sciences in Buffalo, New York.

Experts Weigh In

At the 2010 American Academy of Neurology (AAN) meeting in Toronto, Canada, the AAN hosted a press conference to provide information about CCSVI (see Chapter 33). Facilitated by stories on the Internet, interest was high, with more than 4000 people registered online and a packed conference room on site. Speakers included Paolo Zamboni, MD, Director, Vascular Diseases Center, University of Ferrara, Italy; Robert Zivadinov, MD, PhD, Director of the Buffalo Neuroimaging Analysis Center, Buffalo, New York; Andrew Common, MD, Radiologist in Chief, St. Michaels Hospital, University of Toronto, Ontario, Canada; and Aaron Miller, MD, Professor of Neurology, Director of the MS Center at Mount Sinai, NY, NY. Dr. Miller is also the Chief Medical Officer of the National MS Society. At the end of the conference, Dr. Miller concluded, "How, when, and indeed whether CCSVI has any role in the treatment of MS remains to be seen."

Expert clinicians have been skeptical. For example, Randall Shapiro, MD, Clinical Professor of Neurology at the University of Minnesota, likened CCSVI therapy to other MS "cures" that have come and gone, such as bee stings, colustrum, cobra venom, goat serum, hyperbaric oxygen, mercury amalgams, vertebral stenosis surgery, and vitamin therapy. According to Dr. Shapiro, the proposed rationale of CCSVI as an MS etiology "would appear to defy logic and reason..."

Jeffrey Dunn, MD, Associate Director of Stanford's MS Center, commented on CCSVI procedures, "...Patients remain insufficiently aware of the active and serious risks, and our colleagues have felt insufficiently equipped to defend their cautionary advisories...If I can do anything to protect MS patients from the potentially devastating effects of false hopes or the risks of invasive and unproven treatment, I am happy to do so" (Samson 2010).

Victor Rivera, MD, Director of the Maxine Mesinger MS Clinic at Baylor College of Medicine in Houston, Texas, moderated a debate between Dr. Zivadinov and Mark Freedman, MD, Director of the Multiple Sclerosis Research Unit at Ottawa Hospital in Ottawa, Ontario, Canada, at the recent Consortium of Multiple Sclerosis Centers Annual Meeting in Montreal, Canada, June 1-4, 2011. Dr. Zivadinov suggested that CCSVI might contribute to MS in a manner similar to environmental factors such as latitude, viral exposure, Vitamin D levels, or genetic predisposition, but that CCSVI was not the sole cause of MS. Dr. Zivadinov conceded, "CCSVI is neither necessary nor sufficient to cause MS."

Animal models, which would be a logical part of the research process, have not been developed to aid in the diagnosis of CCSVI or to test the effects of endovascular treatment. According to Dr. Zivadinov, the development of a CCSVI animal model is "too difficult."

If intracerebral venous congestion leads to MS, disorders that cause cerebral venous congestion such as cerebral venous thrombosis, chronic obstructive pulmonary disease, idiopathic intracranial hypertension, or radical neck dissection that results in internal jugular vein removal might be expected to be associated with an increase in MS. However, they are not (Doepp et al. 2010).

CCSVI Interventions

Although endovascular interventions rarely result in life-threatening complications (Samson 2010), invasive procedures are not without risks. The relative safety of endovascular treatment of 331 patients with CCSVI, including balloon angioplasty and stenting, has been reported (Ludyga et al. 2010). There were no deaths, cerebral strokes, or instances of stent migration. Stent thrombosis occurred in 2 (1.2%) patients, and 1 (0.3%) patient required surgical removal of an angioplastic balloon. Local bleeding occurred in 4 patients (1.2%), difficulty removing balloon or delivery system occurred in 4 patients (1.2%), unsuccessful catheterization occurred in 4 patients (1.2%), problems with stent placement occurred in 4 patients (2.3% of stents), transient cardiac arrhythmia occurred in 2 patients (0.6%), and minor gastrointestinal bleeding occurred in 1 patient (0.3%).

Conclusions and Recommendations

The theory that CCSVI leads to venous congestion, increased pericapillary iron deposition, an autoimmune response, and MS is a tantalizing one, but it is scantily supported by objective data. More than a year, millions of dollars, and a myriad of publications later, Dr. Miller's assessment that the role of CCSVI in MS remains to be seen still holds true.

Dr. Zamboni may have invented a new phrenology, a seemingly rational series of observations and measurements that has no significant relationship to the physiology under study. The CTEVD study did reveal an increased prevalence of CCSVI in people with MS, but also found CCSVI in healthy controls, patients with CIS, and those with other neurologic diseases (Zivadinov et al. 2011).

CCSVI may be nothing more than normal anatomic venous variation coupled with nonspecific venous changes associated with the neurodegeneration of MS and other diseases. A sham treatment study, PREMiSE (Prospective Randomized Endovascular Therapy in Multiple Sclerosis) is underway to clarify the value of reversing the features that define CCSVI.

Although further studies regarding the role of venous circulation in the etiopathogenesis of MS may be informative, endovascular "treatment" at this time is inappropriate. Patients requesting CCSVI procedures should be referred to centers doing clinical trials. Both Dr. Zamboni and Dr. Zivadinov endorsed this recommendation at the 2010 AAN press conference. Those who subject patients to endovascular procedures for CCSVI outside of clinical trials exploit the fears, hopes, and wallets of desperate patients and their families and put these patients at risk for procedure-related complications that may, albeit rarely, be fatal.

Time will tell whether CCSVI represents a phenomenal medical breakthrough for patients with MS or a failed hypothesis. Accumulating evidence suggests the latter.

References

Zamboni P, Galeotti R, Menegatti E et al. Chronic cerebrospinal venous insufficiency in patients with multiple sclerosis. J Neurol Neurosurg Psychiatry 2009;80:392-399.

Franceschi C. The unsolved puzzle of multiple sclerosis and venous function. J Neurol Neurosurg Psychiatry 2009;80:358.

Mayer CA, Pfeilschifter W, Lorenz MW et al. The perfect crime? CCSVI not leaving a trace in MS. J Neurol Neurosurg Psychiatry 2011;82:436-440.

Putnam T. Studies in multiple sclerosis: encephalitis and sclerotic plaques produced by venular obstruction. Arch Neurol Psychiatry 1935;33:929-940.

Zamboni P, Galeotti R, Menegatti E et al. A prospective open-label study of endovascular treatment of chronic cerebrospinal venous insufficiency. J Vasc Surg 2009;50:1348-1358.

Samson K. Experimental multiple sclerosis vascular shunting procedure halted at Stanford. Ann Neurol 2010:67:A13-A15.

Ludyga T, Kazibudzki M, Simka M et al. Endovascular treatment for chronic cerebrospinal venous insufficiency: is the procedure safe? Phlebology 2010;25:286-295.

Reekers JA, Lee JM, Bellie AM, Barkhof F. Cardiovascular and Interventional Radiological Society of Europe commentary on the treatment of chronic cerebrospinal venous insufficiency. Cardiovasc Intervent Radiol 2011;34:1-2.

Khan O, Tselis A. Chronic cerebrospinal venous insufficiency and multiple sclerosis: science or science fiction? J Neurol Neurosurg Psychiatry 2011;82:355.

Al-Omari MH, Rousan LA. Internal jugular vein morphology and hemodynamics in patients with multiple sclerosis. Int Angiol 2010;29:115-120.

Zivadinov R, Marr K, Cutter G et al. Prevalence, sensitivity, and specificity of chronic cerebrospinal venous insufficiency in MS. Neurology 2011, Apr 13 (Epub ahead of print).

Doepp F, Friedemann P, Valdueza JM et al. No cerebrocervical venous congestion in patients with multiple sclerosis. Ann Neurol 2010;68:173-183.

Sundstrom P, Wahlin A, Ambarki K et al. Venous and cerebrospinal fluid flow in multiple sclerosis: a case-control study. Ann Neurol 2010;68:255-299.

Baracchini C, Perini P, Calabrese M et al. No evidence of chronic cerebrospinal venous insufficiency at multiple sclerosis onset. Ann Neurol 2011;69:90-99.

Update May 19, 2013

Discussion of CCSVI on the website www.thisisms.com totaled 103,841 posts to date, more than 10 times any other topic.

TraveloMed now advertises "IVUS: Latest Technology in MS." (IVUS=intravenous ultrasound, used to diagnose CCSVI.) A travel package, complete with CCSVI procedure, hotel accommodations, meals, and transportation from the airport is available for 6,800 Euros.

The website, LiberationProcedureCCSV.com no longer exists.

Initial results of the PREMiSE study presented at this year's American Academy of Neurology meeting (2013) by Adnan Siddiqui, MD, PhD, Principal Investigator of PREMiSE, revealed that the patients with MS who received angioplasty for CCSVI had "increased disease activity" compared to controls who received the sham procedure (http://www.youtube.com/watch?v=94gLM4QlU_A&feature=youtu.be).

Comment: So, not only did the "Liberation Procedure" not make patients with MS better, it made them worse! Could there ever be a better example of why potentially dangerous and costly procedures such as this should not be available to patients before proper scientific investigation?

An article at CCSVIclinic.ca concedes, "...many of these patients have not experienced long-term benefits after surgery...About 60-70,000 patients have paid hundreds of millions of dollars to get this done-not counting the cost of airfare and accommodations, as the therapy has only been available in far flung locations..." The article concludes, "While we believe we are on the right track with free flowing drainage of the central nervous system, perhaps the solution to permanent cure for MS is more complex than popping a balloon in a weakened vein and hoping for the best."

You think?

Chapter 35

EYE PROBLEMS IN MULTIPLE SCLEROSIS-AN OPHTHALMOLOGIST'S VIEW

September 24, 2012

Introduction

In these days of multitudinous, multi-author, multi-center, multi-national, randomized, double blind, placebo controlled trials*, I stumbled upon a gem of an article from the Department of Ophthalmology, Nationaal Multiple Sclerosis Centrum, Melsbroek, Belgium (Roodhooft 2012). Dr. Roodhooft, an experienced clinician, personally examined 284 adults (173 females, 111 males) referred to the multiple sclerosis (MS) clinic between 2007-2010. Dr. Roodhooft summarized his observations in an easy to read, single author article.

Indications

Most of the MS patients had an ophthalmologic examination to assess for refractive errors. Other indications included acute optic neuritis, anisocoria, arterial hypertension, blepharoconjunctivitis, cataracts, diabetes, diplopia, dry eye, headache, intraocular pressure, nystagmus, photophobia, uveitis and visual failure.

Findings

Of the 284 patients, 51 (27 females, 24 males) had functional visual loss (<6/20). There were 129 eyes with temporal pallor of the optic nerve head, 110 with global pallor, 70 with pathological excavation, and 29 with a chalky white color. None of the patients had papilledema. Nystagmus of various types (e.g., gaze-evoked, rotatory, pendular, jerk) was observed in 104 patients, with primary gaze nystagmus in 28 patients. Diplopia occurred in 51 and oscillopsia in 17 patients. Two patients had bilateral active uveitis. In addition, 65 patients had facial palsy and 19 had trigeminal neuralgia.

Dr. Roodhooft noted that 4-aminopyridine may cause diplopia "either by itself or through an overdose or a change in dose." Given the widespread use of 4-aminopyridine marketed as dalfampridine (Ampyra) to improve walking in MS, physicians should be alert to this possibility. This observation deserves more attention as diplopia is not listed as one of the "common adverse events" on the Ampyra website or in the package insert.

Treatment

The paper discusses, "How to help MS patients with ocular problems." Practical recommendations include:

1. Treat acute optic neuritis with steroids.

2. Correct refractive errors.

3. Treat dry eyes and evaluate for causes, such as anticholinergic medications or poor blinking.

4. Heat, exercise, fever and stress may temporarily worsen vision, diplopia and oscillopsia, and patients should be counseled accordingly.

5. Fresnel lenses may correct diplopia.

6. Gabapentin or memantine may help nystagmus.

7. Sunglasses may be a simple solution for photophobia.

8. Cataracts secondary to steroid use or other causes may be a correctable form of decreased vision.

9. Uveitis may cause blindness and needs to be diagnosed and treated.

10. Fatigue in MS patients is multifactorial (e.g., depression, medications, sleep disturbances) and may affect vision.

Limitations

This article does not include data from optical coherence tomography (OCT), which may soon become part of the routine evaluation of patients with MS. Follow-up regarding the clinical course of individual patients is not provided.

New Journals for Case Reports

Detailed clinical observations such as these, as well as case reports (long denigrated as "anecdotal"), may be experiencing a renaissance. As new treatments enter clinical practice, it is important to publish case reports of successes, failures, and idiosyncratic reactions. The management of complex patients and complications related to new therapies may also lend itself to publication. A new journal, *Neurology: Clinical Practice*, was recently launched as a "spoke" journal of *Neurology*. According to editor John R. Corboy, MD, FAAN, *Neurology: Clinical Practice* includes peer-reviewed articles targeted at clinical practitioners, including images and full case reports. The first edition of *Neurology: Clinical*

Practice, was published in December 2011. The most recent issue included 5 cases (September 2012).

In the field of epilepsy, a new clinical journal has also recently been created. According to the publisher, Elsevier, "*Epilepsy & Behavior Case Reports* is a new, online-only, Open Access journal devoted to the rapid publication of case reports on the behavioral aspects of seizures and epilepsy."

Epilepsy & Behavior Case Reports is a companion journal to *Epilepsy & Behavior*, which has achieved high standing in the epilepsy community since it's first publication a dozen years ago. Similar journals focusing on clinical cases may evolve in other specialties as well.

Conclusions

Whether the eye represents a "window to the soul" may be debated, but it certainly serves as a convenient portal to inspection of the optic nerve and many critical central nervous system pathways. While large, controlled trials are essential to test new therapies and establish an evidence base for clinical practice, it is a breath of fresh air to see that one needn't participate in a research juggernaut in order to make useful academic contributions. At least two new journals, *Neurology: Clinical Practice* and *Epilepsy & Behavior Case Reports* offer platforms for publication of case reports and may lead to a resurgence of academic interest in clinical phenomena. Dr. Roodhooft's well-organized observations are testimony that skilled examination of individual patients in the hospital or clinic, coupled with intellectual curiosity, can still yield useful scientific information. Bravo Dr. Roodhooft!

*There has been an explosion of articles on MS, including 2 important randomized, clinical trials just published in the *New England Journal of Medicine* on dimethyl fumarate (BG-12) (Fox et al. 2012, Gold et al. 2012). These positive trials suggest imminent Food and Drug Administration (FDA) approval of BG-12 for relapsing MS, and are worth a look, as is the accompanying editorial by Ropper (Ropper 2012).

References

Fox RJ, Miller DH, Phillips JT et al. NEJM 2012;367:1087-1097.

Gold R, Kappos L, Arnold DL et al. NEJM 2012;367:1098-1107.

Roodhooft JM. Summary of eye examinations of 284 patients with multiple sclerosis. Int J MS Care 2012;14:31-38.

Ropper AH. The "Poison Chair" treatment for multiple sclerosis. NEJM 2012;367:1149-1150.

Update May 20, 2013

On March 27, 2013, dimethyl fumarate (BG-12) received FDA approval for the treatment of relapsing MS.

Chapter 36

"ALL ABOUT MULTIPLE SCLEROSIS, ALL THE TIME"

April 30, 2009

A colleague wrote to ask me what were the "hot topics" of this year's American Academy of Neurology meeting. The answer was easy: multiple sclerosis, multiple sclerosis, and multiple sclerosis! Of course, there are advances in headache, epilepsy, stroke and all the rest, but the buzz and tension has been all about multiple sclerosis. There were many important presentations on multiple sclerosis, but I've chosen to report on two of the big ones that I attended yesterday.

The first was the TRANSFORMS study, which compared the new oral agent, fingolimod, a sphingosine 1 phosphate receptor modulator (0.5 or 1.25 mg/day), to an injectable interferon (Avonex, 30 ug IM/week) in relapsing remitting multiple sclerosis (RRMS) in 1,284 patients over 12 months in a randomized, double blind, double dummy, active control, parallel group protocol. Fingolimod depletes lymphocytes by sending them back into the lymph nodes, hopefully decreasing their harmful effects of inflammation. The ballroom was so packed they sent the overflow (including me) to the other wing of the convention center to watch the presentation on a monitor.

It was kind of creepy to hear the thunderous applause at the end of the presentation through the speakers, but observing no one clapping in our little satellite viewing room. I guess it's hard to clap when you can't see the presenter.

Bottom line: Superiority in relapse rate for both oral doses of fingolimod compared to Avonex, as well as better MRI results. Very impressive!

One caveat, about 1/3 of the patients had already failed Avonex, so is it fair to put them in the study, kind of an "enriched failure" group?

And of course, there were various safety concerns, including an increase in Herpes virus infections, more skin cancers, and macular edema in <1% of the patients. As we've learned from painful experience, long term safety data are crucial, and we don't have that yet.

The other big news is the CLARITY study, which pitted cladribine (2-chlorodeoxyadenosine), a chemotherapy agent used for hairy cell leukemia, against placebo in patients with RRMS. The protocol was double blind, placebo controlled, with 1,326 patients randomized 1:1:1 to cladribine 3.5 mg/day, 5.25 mg/day, or placebo. But here's the cool thing about cladribine, you only take it for about 10 days a year! Cladribine gets into the lymphocyte and B cell DNA and knocks them out of commission for a good, long time.

Bottom line: Relapse rate and all MRI measures were statistically better than placebo. The drug was pretty well tolerated. There were 4 cases of malignancy in the cladribine group and none in the placebo group, but this did not reach statistical significance. I spoke with company representatives later that evening and they were very pleased with the results. I could almost hear the champagne corks popping.

Neither fingolimod or cladribine are FDA approved, but they are clearly headed in that direction. Are you ready?

Update May 20, 2013

Fingolimod received FDA approval for the treatment of relapsing multiple sclerosis on September 22, 2010, and is marketed as Gilenya.

Cladribine was not approved by the FDA or European Medicines Agency. The manufacturer abandoned plans for global approval. Safety concerns appeared to be the reason.

Section 6.

Psychiatry

Chapter 37

PSYCHIATRY 101-I NEED HELP!

June 21, 2010

This week I consulted on 3 great neurology cases; a 50 year old woman who had a "wave" sensation come over her head and down into her arms with presumed epilepsy, a 34 year old man with ascending paralysis and diplopia with presumed Guillain Barre, and an 18 year old girl with recurrent syncope, hemiparesis, and unilateral blindness, with a presumed young stroke of cardiac origin.

They were all great neurology cases, except they weren't.

After multiple careful neurologic examinations, a lot of listening, and way too many expensive neuroimaging and other tests, all 3 of these patients were diagnosed with some kind of psychiatric disorder. Maybe the first one had "panic disorder" and the last two had "conversion disorder?"

When I offered the suggestion that "stress" might play a role in their symptoms, the first two readily embraced the idea, which supported my diagnosis. The last patient insisted she had no problems at all and exhibited "la belle indifference," which also supported my diagnosis. (After all, who has no problems?)

After making the psychiatric diagnoses, I really didn't know what to do next beyond call a psychiatry consult. I reassured the first woman, and she seemed OK with that. The next two were far more difficult because they were convinced they had severe neurologic disease.

I am a neurohospitalist, and weeks like this are not unusual. Probably most of you have a framed diploma in your office from the American Board of *Psychiatry* and Neurology. I don't actually remember any training by psychiatrists during my residency. Do you? Maybe that's a typo on the diploma?

I wish I had more tools to deal with patients with psychiatric illness masquerading as neurologic disease. When all the tests come up negative, I gently suggest that "stress" might play a role. Today I came up with the line, "I think it is a problem with your "mind," not your "brain." And as a chaser I added, "and that's good news, because brain problems can be very serious."

But psychiatry problems are very serious, too, as evidenced by just these 3 patients seen in the last week. These people missed work or school, worried family members, and spent bundles of health care dollars. Luckily, none of them suffered any iatrogenic complications.

One of my neurology colleagues who has an office practice says that identifying and treating psychiatric problems is a big problem for him, too. He lamented the paucity of training that we neurologists received with respect to psychiatric therapeutics. He thinks he has seen more patients with somatization disorder recently as a result of the bad economy and more "psychosocial stressors." Has anyone else witnessed an increase? Do tough economic times influence the incidence of psychiatric problems like these?

I wish some psychiatrists would weigh in on this problem. What is the best treatment approach for these patients? How can you best diagnose and treat somatization disorder? Is that the right term? Is the Diagnostic and Statistical

Manual of Mental Disorders (DSM-IV) going to help me? What do you do when a patient keeps coming up with new symptoms, hemiparesis one day, blindness the next? What's the best way to get a psychiatrist involved?

While some neurologists may not be enraptured about spending more time learning about psychiatry, it seems to be a requirement to properly do our jobs. Where is the best place for continuing education for neurologists to learn more psychiatry? Do other neurologists feel the need for more training in this area?

Chapter 38

AN EXPLANATION FOR MASS HYSTERIA?

July 11, 2012

Introduction: Mirror Neurons

In January of this year, a group of teenagers, nearly all girls, in the small town of Le Roy in western New York suddenly came down with severe Tourette-like symptoms. The case attracted extensive media attention and has been the subject of articles in the *Huffington Post* and *New York Times*, stories on local news stations, as well as YouTube and Facebook posts. Two of the girls also appeared on the *Today Show*, accompanied by their distraught mothers. Environmental toxins from the town's old Jell-O factories, a 1970 toxic train accident, PANDAS (pediatric autoimmune neuropsychiatric disorders associated with Streptococcus infection), and other unlikely etiologies have been put forward as possible explanations for this unusual phenomenon, but neurologists have confidently diagnosed conversion disorder. It is a classic case of mass hysteria.

Conversion Disorder and Mass Hysteria

Conversion disorder, or hysteria, dates back at least to the days when Egyptians were writing on papyrus rather than tweeting on Twitter. The term indicates, "a disturbance of body function that is characterized by neurological, sensory, or motor symptoms for which the available medical explanations either do not explain, or fail to account for the severity of, the patient's impairment" (Kozlowska and Williams 2005). Conversion disorder affecting groups of people (mass hysteria) often occurs in schools or other closed communities (Illis 2002). Odors or gas leaks (perceived or real) are common contemporary triggers (Boss 1997).

Neurobiology of Conversion Disorder

To understand conversion disorder from a neurobiological standpoint, one must accept that the mind is the product of the brain. Multiple models have been proposed to explain conversion reactions. Freud proposed the concept of "conversion" of intolerable memories into somatic symptoms (Illis 2002). The concept of "neodissociation" has been suggested, in which a patient with loss of function, such as hysterical visual loss, still processes visual stimuli that influences his or her behavior, yet he or she is not consciously aware of the visual input. Conversion symptoms have also been attributed to "rogue representations" of sensory data that are mistakenly integrated into consciousness.

Another theory suggests that conversion states are a protective strategy that invoke a prelearned behavioral state. One complex hypothesis implicates "false body mapping," requiring dysfunction in a circuit that contains the cingulate cortex, insula, thalamus, brainstem nuclei, amygdala, ventromedial prefrontal centers, supplemental motor area, and other key areas. Another postulate is dysfunction of the striatothalamo-cortical pathways, which control sensorimotor function and voluntary motor behavior. Advances in neuroimaging, such as functional MRI (fMRI), magnetoencephalography (MEG), single photon emission computed tomography (SPECT), and transcranial magnetic stimulation (TMS), are supplying the tools to scientifically investigate the neurologic circuitry involved.

Are Mirror Neurons the Answer?

Recently, Lee and Tsai suggested that mirror neurons may play a role in the pathogenesis of mass hysteria (Lee and Tsai 2010). The mirror neuron circuit refers to "neurons in the frontal, parietal and temporal cortex of the monkey, that discharge both when a movement is executed and when the same movement is observed" (Alegre et al. 2011). Although less well characterized, it is believed the mirror neuron system exists in humans as well. This mirror neuron system may help us understand the actions of others (Alegre et al. 2011). An inhibitive feature of the mirror neuron system keeps us from imitating everything we see. The existence of mirror neurons has been used to design more effective rehabilitation for stroke (Small et al. 2012) and may explain some of the cognitive deficits of Parkinson disease (Alegre et al. 2011).

According to Lee and Tsai, 4 characteristics of the mirror neuron system could contribute to their role in the pathogenesis of mass hysteria. First, failure of the inhibitory component in certain individuals might predispose them to imitate others. Second, transmission of mass hysteria symptoms typically occur by visual and auditory means, both of which are processed by mirror neurons. Third, mirror neurons may play a role in emotional contagion, which allows us to "catch" and feel the emotions of others. Finally, mirror neuron activity is more active in females, a group consistently overrepresented in episodes of mass hysteria.

Conclusions

Incidents of mass hysteria have been a feature of human society for thousands of years, and its cause remains unexplained. Continued research with improved neuroimaging (fMRI, MEG, SPECT) and neurostimulation (TMS) may soon bridge the ever-narrowing chasm between the mind and the brain and provide a neurobiological explanation for mass hysteria. In the meantime, we are left to struggle with unproven hypotheses and propose empiric treatment for patients with symptoms that place them in the uncomfortable borderland between neurology and psychiatry.

References

Kozlowska K, Williams LM. Self-protective organization in children with conversion symptoms: a cross-sectional study looking at psychological and biological correlates. Mind & Brain, The Journal of Psychiatry 2005;1:43-57.

Illis LS. Hysteria. Spinal Cord 2002;40:311-312.

Boss LP. Epidemic hysteria: a review of the published literature. Epidemiol Rev 1997;19:233-243.

Lee YT, Tsai SJ. The mirror neuron system may play a role in the pathogenesis of mass hysteria. Med Hypotheses 2010;74:244-245.

Alegre M, Guridi J, Artieda J. The mirror system, theory of mind and Parkinson's disease. J. Neurol Sci 2011;310:194-196.

Small SL, Buccino G, Solodkin A. The mirror neuron system and treatment of stroke. Dev Psychobiol 2012;54:293-310.

Section 7.

Sleep Apnea

Chapter 39

SHAQ SNORES!

May 23, 2011

Snoring is more than a nuisance when it signals the presence of sleep apnea. A recent short video produced by Harvard Medical School and the WGBH Educational Foundation features Shaquille O'Neal and his girlfriend Nikki "Hoopz" Alexander on a visit to the local Harvard sleep center. When they meet with the sleep specialist, Nikki recounts that Shaq tends to snore when he sleeps on his back. She imitated his reverberating "deep snore" that she said often woke him up, although Shaq couldn't recall any such events. Not only did Shaq snore, he would stop breathing as well, prompting Nikki to tell him, "Dude, you just stopped breathing in your sleep!"

Based on her history, it appeared that Shaq had frequent nighttime awakenings and apneic episodes, sufficient symptoms to warrant a sleep study.

Shaq eagerly does his homework, learns the difference between REM and NREM, and submits to the multiple electrode hookup necessary for an all night polysomnogram in the sleep center. The results indicate that he has "moderate sleep apnea." In the next scene, the doctor explains that treatment options include a mask, mouthpiece, or surgery. Shaq tries on the CPAP (continuous positive airway pressure) mask, doesn't seem to mind it too much, and says he'll try it.

After using CPAP, Shaq tells us he's sleeping 7-9 hours/night, "feels good," has "lots of energy," "relationship is good," and "everything is working." Sounds like a real success story. Who knows, CPAP might even add a few years to his game!

Sleep apnea is characterized by arousals from sleep, sleep fragmentation, and arterial oxygen desaturation, which can be significant (Hukins 2006). Daytime sleepiness is the predominant complaint, which may be evidenced by deficits in alertness and attention. Risk factors include male sex, increasing age, and obesity. Sleep apnea and hypersomnolence affect 4% of middle-aged men (Hukins 2006). Sleep apnea is associated with an increase in coronary artery disease, hypertension, metabolic syndrome, motor vehicle accidents, and decreased quality of life. Evaluation and treatment cross many medical disciplines-sleep specialists include neurologists, psychiatrists, pulmonologists, and others. Although tolerability may limit its use, CPAP is considered the "gold standard" for sleep apnea treatment (Hukins 2006).

At lest 80% of people with moderate to severe sleep apnea remain undiagnosed (Hukins 2006). Perhaps Shaq's participation in this educational video might encourage other sleep apnea sufferers to get treatment, sleep better, and improve their daytime function. It should also inspire sleep partners, like Shaq's girlfriend, to nudge their snoring partners in the direction of a sleep center for evaluation. Both of them may end up getting better sleep.

Shaq, thanks for sharing!

References

Hukins CA. Obstructive sleep apnea-management update. Neuropsychiatric disease and treatment 2006;2(3):309-326.

Video: http://sports.yahoo.com/nba/blog/ball_dont_lie/ post/Shaquille-O-8217-Neal-8217-s-girlfriend-school?urn=nba-wp3654#video.

Section 8.

Parkinson's Disease

Chapter 40

DANCE THERAPY FOR PARKINSON'S DISEASE

January 24, 2012

Introduction

Can people with Parkinson's disease really waltz their symptoms away?

Dance is one of many complementary therapies that have been tried to alleviate the symptoms of Parkinson's disease (Zesiewicz and Evatt 2009). Two recent studies suggest that dance therapy improves balance, bradykinesia, gait, motor functioning, postural instability, quality of life and other functional measures (Duncan et al. 2011, Heiberger et al. 2011).

Two Studies

In the first study, 62 subjects (35 males, 27 females, aged 48-49 years) were randomized to twice weekly, 1 hour, community-based Argentine Tango classes for 12 months or to a control group with no prescribed exercise (Duncan and Earhart 2011). The study was not for everyone, as 16/32 (50%) tango subjects dropped out as well as 11/30 (37%) controls. At 12 months, symptoms significantly better in the tango than the control group included the primary variable, the Movement Disorder Society-Unified Parkinson Disease Rating Scale 3 (MD-UPDRS-3), MiniBESTest (balance), bradykinesia, rigidity, postural instability/gait disorder

(PIGD), 6 minute walk, and nine-hold-peg test. All measurements were made off medication.

In a second study, 11 (6 women, 5 men, 58-85 years) people with moderate to severe Parkinson's disease participated in weekly 1.15 hour dance classes for 8 months (Heiberger et al. 2011). The classes were led by a professional dance teacher and included movements from ballet, choreographic elements, dance theater, contemporary dance and jazz. Dance exercises were designed so that some could be performed while sitting, enabling people with balance problems to participate. As evidenced by their engagement and smiles on a sample video, the subjects enjoyed the classes (perhaps reason enough to attend).

Motor testing performed 1 hour after class revealed short-term improvement of the UPDRS motor score from 23.7 to 15.5 (p=0.001). The best improvements were in rigidity (p=0.002), hand movements (p=0.002), finger taps (p=0.02) and facial expression (p=0.01). In addition, 10/11 (91%) subjects felt that their mobility was improved.

Why Does Dance Therapy Work?

Another study of healthy individuals without Parkinson's disease compared 24 amateur dancers (19 females, 5 males, 71 years) with an average dancing experience of 16.5 years to 38 nondancer controls (30 females, 8 males, 71 years) on a variety of cognitive and physical tasks (Kattenstroth et al. 2010). As one might expect, the dancers performed better on posture and balance testing, but also had better cognition, reaction time, motor and tactile performance. One facile explanation for these results is that the dancers were a superior self-selected group from the start. On the other hand, the authors postulate that the combination of sensory stimulation, physical activity, and cognitive challenges, not to mention the pleasure of dancing, may have stimulated neurotrophins, such as brain-derived neurotrophic factor, resulting in enhanced neuroplasticity and improved brain functioning that countered the degenerative effects of aging. In favor of this appealing hypothesis are the findings of improvements in upper extremity function, such as the 9-hole-peg test (Duncan and Earhart 2011) and hand movements, finger tapping, and facial expression (Heiberger et al. 2011) that are not obvious effects of the physical demands of dancing.

Conclusions

Dance lessons offer cognitive challenges, music therapy, physical exercise and a reason to get up in the morning. In the two studies described, subjects received dance instruction once or twice a week that included personal attention and social interaction. These factors may have possibly contributed to motor benefits otherwise attributed to increased movement and exercise.

While symptomatic medication therapy remains the mainstay of Parkinson's treatment, its effects are limited in improving balance and preventing falls. Adjunctive dance therapy appears to offer significant benefits and should be considered as part of the evolving therapeutic regimen of this relentless neurodegenerative disorder. Why it works deserves further exploration.

In terms of dissecting out the key salutary elements of the dance program, a future study where the control group attended a book club instead of a dance class, for example, could help distinguish gains related to exercise, music and movement from the more intangible gains related to goal achievement and increased socialization. The value of "cues" to movement provided by music also needs further analysis (Hackney and Earhart 2009).

To optimize results, dance therapy probably needs to be tailored to the individual patient regarding their stage of disease and resultant disabilities. Individualizing the program may help counter the 50% dropout rate seen in the 12 month tango study. The duration, frequency, intensity and type of dance therapy that have the greatest potency for the patient's specific neurological deficits need to be determined in future studies, including the advantages of partnered vs. unpartnered dance (Hackney and Earhart 2009). The extent to which measured gains transfer to the mobility challenges of everyday life and the duration of these gains after dance therapy are also important questions. Whether too much exercise or exertion might have a detrimental effect on the progression of Parkinson's disease must also be considered. The patient's interest level, appreciation for different types of music and dance, and the availability of a suitable partner are all factors likely to contribute to the activity's success or failure. Benefits may potentially extend beyond motor symptoms to nonmotor symptoms of Parkinson's disease, such as anxiety, depression, fatigue, pain and sleep disorders. Whether dance therapy has any "neuroprotective" as well as symptomatic effect remains to be demonstrated.

The time commitment in the above studies was modest, a 1 hour class twice a week (Duncan and Earhart) or a weekly 1.15 hour class (Heiberger et al. 2011); costs should be commensurate.

People with Parkinson's disease should consider dance therapy as a reasonable complementary therapy to their medical regimen. It just might be two steps in the right direction.

References

Duncan RP, Earhart GM. Randomized controlled trial of community-based dancing to modify disease progression in Parkinson disease. Neurorehabilitation and Neural Repair;2011;DOI:10.1177/1545968311421614.

Hackney ME, Earhart GM. Effects of dance on gait and balance in Parkinson's disease: A comparison of partnered and nonpartnered dance movement. Neurorehabilitation and Neural Repair 2009;24(4):384-392.

Heiberger L, Maurer C, Amtage F et al. Impact of a weekly dance class on the functional mobility and on the quality of life of individuals with Parkinson's disease. Frontiers in Aging Neuroscience 2011;3(14):1-15.

Kattenstroth JC, Kolankowska I, Kalisch T, Dinse HR. Superior sensory, motor, and cognitive performance in elderly individuals with multi-year dancing activities. Frontiers in Aging Neuroscience 2010;2(31):1-9.

Zesiewicz TA, Evatt ML. Potential influences of complementary therapy on motor and non-motor complications in Parkinson's disease. CNS Drugs 2009;23(10):817-835.

Section 9.

Stroke

Chapter 41

A LINK BETWEEN SEIZURE AND STROKE

August 2, 2012

Introduction

In a recent study, acute symptomatic seizures occurred in 6.3% of patients admitted to the hospital with a first stroke (Beghi et al. 2011). This large, prospective study included 714 patients (315 women, 399 men, age range, 27-97 years) with a first stroke hospitalized in one of 31 Italian centers. Acute symptomatic seizures were defined as those that occurred within 7 days of the stroke. Patients with a history of seizures or prior strokes were excluded.

The authors identified 2 independent predictors for acute symptomatic seizures in this stroke population: hemorrhagic stroke and cortical involvement. Those with primary intracerebral hemorrhage had the highest incidence (16.2%), while those with pure ischemic stroke had the lowest (4.2%). Patients with ischemic stroke with hemorrhagic transformation had an intermediate risk (12.5%). In addition, patients with cortical infarction had an odds ratio of 3.4 for a seizure compared to those with subcortical lesions.

The most common seizure types were simple partial (37.2%), complex partial (18.6%), and secondarily generalized (14%). Electroencephalograms (EEGs) were performed in 34 (75.6%) patients with seizures. Just over a third of the EEGs showed epileptiform activity (35.3%). The other findings were slow waves (41.2%) and aspecific findings (20.6%). Only 1 (2.9%) EEG was normal.

Nearly three quarters of the patients who had seizures did so within the first 24 hours of their stroke. Patients with seizures had a 30-day mortality rate that was nearly double the rate in patients without seizures; 12.5% vs. 6.3%, respectively.

Discussion

Stroke is one of the most frequent reasons for neurologic consultation in the hospital, and stroke is the most common cause of seizures in the elderly. However, the vast majority of strokes are not accompanied by acute symptomatic seizures, which occurred in only 6.3% of stroke patients in this study. This incidence is slightly higher than prior prospective studies, which ranged from 1.8% to 5.5%. The relatively low incidence of seizures in this large stroke population highlights the importance of pinpointing risk factors for seizures in specific patients. In this study, independent risk factors for acute symptomatic seizures were hemorrhagic stroke and cortical location. These findings are consistent with prior textbook teaching that blood is epileptogenic, and cortical lesions are more epileptogenic than subcortical lesions (Pohlmann-Eden and Newton 2008, Sisodiya 2010, Verhaert and Scott 2010).

As one would expect from the focal nature of stroke, partial seizures accounted for the majority (68.1%) of the identified seizure types. Tonic clonic, myoclonic, and non-specified seizure types also occurred but less frequently. Two patients had partial complex status epilepticus.

Twelve patients (1.7%) had a family history of seizures. Of these, 4 (33%) had seizures, 2 secondary to an infarct with hemorrhagic transformation and 2 secondary to a primary cerebral hemorrhage. However, the authors did not confirm family history as an independent risk factor for acute symptomatic seizures.

Historical risk factors not confirmed in this study were stroke size and persistent motor deficits. The risk for seizure did correlate with stroke size-small (< 1 cm, 4.6%), medium (> 1 to < 3 cm, 6.8%), and large (> 3 cm, 9.9%) - but stroke size was not confirmed as an independent predictor. Persistent motor deficits were not assessed, as this study was limited to seizures occurring within 1 week. The authors plan to report late seizure outcomes in a future publication.

Conclusions

Although only a minority of patients with acute stroke will have a seizure in hospital, identifying at-risk patients may improve their management. Physicians may wish to place patients with hemorrhagic and/or cortical strokes under closer observation with more frequent neuro checks, continuous vital sign and cardiac monitoring, and seizure precautions. One could consider an EEG in this high-risk group because electroencephalographic epileptic activity in patients with stroke might indicate a greater risk for a clinical seizure. If seizures occur, knowledge that they are likely focal in origin will assist in the selection of an antiepileptic drug effective for that seizure type. One might also consider prophylactic antiepileptic drugs in this high-risk group, although the value of this intervention has not been proven. Because stroke patients with acute symptomatic seizures suffered twice the mortality of those without seizures, more intensive management may be necessary in this population.

References

Beghi E, D'Alessandro R, Beretta S et al. Incidence and predictors of acute symptomatic seizures after stroke. Neurology 2011;77:1785-1793.

Pohlmann-Eden P, Newton M. First seizure: EEG and neuroimaging following an epileptic seizure. Epilepsia 2008;49(Suppl 1):19-25.

Sisodiya SM. Etiology and pathology of epilepsies: overview. In: Panayiotopoulos CP, Ed. Atlas of Epilepsies. London UK: Springer-Verlag, London Limited, 2010.

Verhaert K, Scott RC. Acute symptomatic epileptic seizures. In: Panayiotopoulos CP, Ed. Atlas of Epilepsies. London UK: Springer-Verlag, London Limited, 2010.

Chapter 42

STROKE IN ANTARCTICA-A MEDICAL EMERGENCY?

October 10, 2011

Introduction

On August 27, 2011, Ms. Renee-Nicole Douceur was sitting at her computer when she suddenly noticed "half the screen is missing." Under normal circumstances, the 58 year old woman would have called 911 and gone to the emergency room. But Ms. Douceur is the Winter Site Manager of the Amundsen-Scott South Pole Station for the Raytheon Polar Services Company...

An evaluation by a physician, Dr. Patricia McGuire, also working at the South Pole, concluded that the likely diagnosis was an occipital lobe stroke that resulted in partial visual loss in both fields, memory changes, and "brain fatigue." Ms. Douceur also had become irritable, attributed to "brain swelling."

Six weeks later, she's still at the South Pole. Ms. Douceur wrote on her website:

The stroke has affected my stereo vision. Though I see OK far but when I try to read I only see the first few words of a sentence before I need to shift and refocus on the next several words. When I read paragraphs I get easily mixed up trying to distinguish sentences. Obviously this has affected my speed reading ability (basically nil) so it takes a long time to read an article or anything.

This is also worse when I don't get enough sleep which down here is nearly impossible to get good rest because nearly everybody has difficulty sleeping (don't know of anybody that sleeps like a baby). I have been slowly improving, especially when the stroke first occurred I could only see half a face. Now I can see the whole face but when up close it tends to momentarily fade in and out. When I watch a movie I have to concentrate on it which makes enjoyment a lot less. It seems I have been progressively getting worse in my left eye use to be 20/20 vision now as bad as 20/50 on some days. My right eye (dominate) seems to be OK between 20/20 to 20/30, again dependent on sleep. Also, it seems I've been seeing more missing pixels (as I call it the satellite TV scramble signal syndrome) as time progresses.

Her physician discussed the case with neurological and ophthalmological consultants at the University of Texas via telemedicine, and it appears that her condition has been stable for the last 6 weeks. A "computer-based rehabilitation program" was ordered, but due to technical problems, Ms. Douceur has not been able to use it.

Patient Wants to Leave!

That's not good enough for Ms. Douceur. She hired an attorney and contacted United States Senator Jeanne Shaheen of New Hampshire to try and speed up her rescue. (The Senator is involved because the National Science Foundation manages the U.S. Antarctic Program.) According to Ms. Douceur, her doctor told her that she needs more sophisticated medical treatment "as soon as possible." She is also concerned that the relatively low oxygen concentration at the Antarctic station due to its high altitude, resulting in

89% blood oxygen levels, might impair her recuperation. She is currently receiving supplemental oxygen. She also worries that the harsh Antarctic climate has impaired her neutrophil function, which might also slow her recovery. Her attorney suggested that the delay in her evacuation was "made in haste and solely on economic grounds."

Raytheon's attorney responded, "Following a medical examination and assessment, the medical staff at the Station concluded that her condition was not life-threatening and was clinically stable. Accordingly, the medical staff recommended a non-emergency medical administrative movement when it becomes available...Looking forward, the current plan is to transport Ms. Douceur from the South Pole Station to McMurdo Station for further transport to Christchurch, New Zealand, as soon as practicable once the South Pole Station is able to reopen for normal air operations, which is expected to occur on or about October 15th. Once Ms. Douceur arrives in Christchurch, she will be referred for a CT scan and repeat neurologic and ophthalmologic evaluations."

The National Science Foundation responded to The Honorable Jeanne Shaheen, "It is currently winter at the South Pole, with the sun only just coming up and temperatures too cold* for routine aircraft operations...For all medical evacuations, the overall risk to all concerned must be carefully weighed against the potential benefit to the patient. Raytheon recommended, and NSF has already determined, that Ms. Douceur should be transported from the South Pole on the first available flight..."

Ms. Douceur's attorney objected, "Every day there is a delay in positioning aircraft increases Ms. Douceur's suffering, adds needless additional stress (in an already highly stressful environment), inhibits proper healing, and most importantly, lessens her chance for a full recovery. If anything, NSF and RPSC are ensuring permanent and irreversible damage will set in."

Ms. Douceur is also concerned that should she ever get a flight home, her brain might suffer further damage if the plane is not pressurized. She wonders whether she needs supplemental oxygen for the flight as well.

Psychosocial Aspects

Ms. Douceur's attorney attributed an exacerbation of her irritable bowel syndrome and insomnia to "extraordinary stress" resulting from a "buildup of tension on station amongst the staff." The attorney explained that this tension resulted from Ms. Douceur's job "performing due diligence reviews of possible fraud and falsification of documents." This stress "undoubtedly contributed significantly to her stroke" and "...harassment continues even to this day..."

Questions

1. Given that we don't know whether the patient had an ischemic stroke or hemorrhagic stroke, or has an underlying lesion like a brain tumor, arterio-venous malformation or other mass, should she be immediately transported out of Antarctica?

2. Could she have atrial fibrillation (no mention of an EKG in her work up) and require anticoagulation to prevent a second stroke?

3. Should she be on aspirin given the high likelihood of an ischemic stroke (statistically speaking)?

4. Does she need oxygen for the ride home?

5. Given that she's getting better, would you agree with Raytheon and the NSF that it is not prudent to risk additional lives and resources with a potentially unsafe rescue until the weather improves?

6. For those with medical evacuation experience, is it common for there to be a disagreement between the patient and the sponsoring agency as to the urgency of an evacuation?

7. There appear to be significant psychosocial factors in this case. Could they have contributed to the stroke?

8. If you were her doctor at the South Pole, what would you recommend?

N.B.

This blog is based on a *New York Times* article and documents posted for public review on a website created by Ms. Douceur's niece: www.SaveRenee.org.

*The temperature today at the South Pole is -72 F (-58 C), but it feels colder. With the wind chill factor, it's -110F (-79 C).

Update May 21, 2013

Ms. Douceur was evacuated by a Basler aircraft from the South Pole on Monday, October 17, 2011, along with a medical escort to McMurdo Station, Antarctica. The temperature was -73.8 F. Later that day she flew from McMurdo Station to Christchurch, New Zealand. According to the patient, an MRI the next day revealed a subcortical lacunar stroke. She returned to the United States on October 24, 2011, where she had another evaluation at Johns Hopkins Hospital. On October 28, 2011, she gave a press conference and said that her vision and speech were improving. She planned to get rehabilitation services in Vermont.

The website, www.SaveRenee.org, is no longer functioning.

Additional References

CNN News: http://edition.cnn.com/2011/10/29/us/maryland-south-pole-rescue/index.html.

http://www.southpolestation.com/trivia/10s/renee.html.

http://tvnz.co.nz/world-news/us-scientist-rescued-antarctica-4469441/video.

Chapter 43

SERENE BRANSON-TIA ON TV?

February 18, 2011

Introduction

Serene Branson, A CBS2 news reporter, spoke "gibberish" on live TV while broadcasting from the Grammy Awards last Sunday night (February 12th, 2011). http://www.hollywoodreporter.com/news/cbs-2-reporter-serene-branson-99449

TIA on TV?

The video reveals an abrupt onset of fluent expressive aphasia without dysarthria. During the brief episode, which we can observe for about 10 seconds, there is no facial asymmetry and no weakness of the right hand in which Ms. Branson holds her microphone. Multiple literal paraphasias, such as "virtation" and "darison," make her speech incomprehensible. It is unclear whether she is aware of the errors, but it appears she is trying to repeat herself, perhaps in an effort to self-correct.

According to a news report, Ms. Branson was assessed by paramedics, had normal vital signs (and presumably resolution of her symptoms), and went home. Sometime later, she followed up with a doctor for testing. (The results have not been published.)

Diagnosis?

While "diagnosis at a distance" is fraught with peril, Ms. Branson appears to have had an episode of Wernicke's aphasia, a transient malfunction of her superior temporal gyrus, possible due to vascular insufficiency of the left middle cerebral artery (Kirshner and Jacobs 2009). The sudden onset and prompt resolution are consistent with a transient ischemic attack (TIA). Other etiologies, such as a partial seizure or complicated migraine are also in the differential.

With respect to vascular risk factors, Ms. Branson appears relatively young for a TIA, but we do not have any information regarding her past medical history and possible risk factors such as recent trauma that may have predisposed to carotid artery dissection, clotting disorders, cardiac disease (patient foramen ovale?), diabetes, family history, fibromuscular dysplasia, hypertension, intracerebral lesions such as an arterio-venous malformation or brain tumor, or even illicit drug use with cocaine.

Proper Treatment?

Even though her speech returned to normal, I would have rushed her to the hospital. Sometimes TIA symptoms wax and wane, and they may have recurred while she was at home. Inpatient observation with cardiac monitoring for arrhythmias, frequent blood pressure monitoring, a complete neurological history and examination, accompanied by MRI, would have been the protocol at my hospital. According to the American Stroke Association, TIA is a "medical emergency" and patients should call 911.

Comprehensive Practice Guideline

A recent practice guideline on the management of extracranial carotid and vertebral disease published in the Journal of the American College of Cardiology and endorsed by the American Heart Association Task Force on Practice Guidelines, American Academy of Neurology, American Stroke Association, and numerous other staid organizations, addressed the issue of TIA. The guidelines point out that typical TIA symptoms last less than 15 minutes, but the definition includes symptom duration up to 24 hours. TIA is a common health problem, with at least 240,000 TIAs occurring annually in the US. TIA is an important risk factor for stroke, which is the most frequent neurologic problem requiring hospitalization.

Stroke remains the #1 cause of disability and the 3rd leading cause of death in the United States. In dollars, the direct and indirect cost of stroke in 2009 was estimated at $68.9 billion. Early recognition of TIA and risk factor modification can decrease the risk of stroke.

Stroke Education

For effective treatment with tPA for stroke, there is a great urgency for symptom recognition and prompt presentation to the hospital. Educational materials are available from the American Heart Association and the American Stroke Association regarding TIA that stress the need for immediate care. The Stroke Collaborative Campaign of the American Academy of Neurology, American College of Emergency Physicians, American Heart Association and American Stroke Association provides resources on stroke education for patients and physicians.

Celebrities

Three time superbowl veteran Tedy Bruschi of the New England Patriots had a stroke in 2005 and subsequent patent foramen ovale repair. In 2008, Mr. Bruschi received a public leadership award from the American Academy of Neurology for his role as an educational spokesman for stroke. Bruschi wrote about his stroke in his autobiography, *Never Give Up: My Stroke, My Recovery, and My Return to the NFL.* His celebrity status has no doubt assisted the public health goal of stroke reduction.

If Serene Branson did have a TIA, hopefully she has received an appropriate medical work up and will soon resume her reporting. The wide exposure on the Internet of her videotaped neurologic event provides a golden opportunity for neurologic teaching. Perhaps Ms. Branson would be willing to lend her considerable communication skills as an educational spokesperson regarding the risk of TIA and stroke?

In the meantime, best wishes to Serene for a speedy and complete recovery.

References

Brott TG, Halperin JL, Abbara S et al. 2011. ASA/ACCF/AHA/AANN/AANS/ACR/ASNR/CNS/SAIP/SCAI/SIR/SNIS/SVM/SVS Guideline on the management of patients with extracranial carotid and vertebral artery disease. Journal of the American College of Cardiology 2011;57:1002-1044.

Kirshner HS, Jacobs DH. Aphasia. eMedicine Neurology 2009;http://emedicine.medscape.com/article/1135944-overview.

Update May 21, 2013

In an interview with CBS2 anchor Pat Harvey six days later, Serene Branson explained that prior to the newscast she felt nauseous and dizzy, her head was pounding, and was very uncomfortable. When she started speaking, she felt "frustrated and terrified because the words were not coming out." Her right cheek and hand went numb. Paramedics arrived and evaluated her. As her symptoms improved, they let her go home, where she fell asleep. The next day, her mother persuaded her to go to the hospital. An evaluation at UCLA Medical Center concluded that she had a "migraine with aura" rather than a TIA. Migraine can run in families, and Ms. Branson observed that her mother had similar episodes. Branson is back at work at CBS2 and speaks on behalf of the National Headache Foundation to raise awareness about migraine.

Additional References

Braxton G. Stricken reporter Serene Branson recalls her on-air terror. http://articles.latimes.com/print/2011/feb/18/entertainment/la-et-serene-branson-20110218, *Los Angeles Times,* February 18, 2011.

A year later, CBS2 reporter Serene Branson looks back on her on-air medical emergency. http://losangeles.cbslocal.com/2012/02/13/a-year-later-cbs2-reporter-serene-branson-looks-back-at-her-on-air-medical-emergency/, February 13, 2012.

Chapter 44

DWI-BEST EARLY PREDICTOR OF ACUTE ISCHEMIC STROKE SIZE

November 12, 2010

According to the American Academy of Neurology's recent evidence-based guideline (Schellinger et al. 2010), diffusion-weighted imaging (DWI) magnetic resonance imaging (MRI) is more accurate than noncontrast computerized axial tomography (CT) for the diagnosis of acute ischemic stroke (Level A). This conclusion was based largely on a Class I study that unequivocally demonstrated superiority of MRI (DWI and gradient echo) compared to CT (p<0.0001). The lack of sensitivity for early stroke on CT will come as no surprise to the many physicians who have cared for patients presenting with a dense hemiparesis, aphasia and a "negative" CT scan.

In the emergency room at my hospital, patients with suspected acute stroke are immediately evaluated with a noncontrast CT as part of a "Code BAT" protocol to help determine eligibility for intravenous tissue plasminogen activator (tPA). CT scanning can be done within minutes and requires minimal patient cooperation. If the CT scan reveals an absence of hemorrhage, tumor, or other contra-indication, the patient can proceed through the remaining gauntlet of criteria before receiving tPA.

MRI on the other hand, requires the patient to remain motionless for optimal images. Patients must be screened ahead of time for metal implants; an ever-increasing number of patients are ineligible for MRI because of implanted cardiac pacemakers and/or defibrillators. Many patients also have relative contraindications such as cochlear implants, hemostatic clips, insulin pumps and nerve stimulators.

In addition to the findings on the physical and neurological examination, neuroimaging can help with prognosis. DWI, which measures the net movement of water in tissue due to random molecular motion, reveals hyperintense ischemic tissue damage within minutes to hours after acute stroke. For anterior circulation ischemic strokes, baseline DWI volumes probably predict final infarct volumes (Level B). For vertebrobasilar artery territory strokes, they are less precise. In conjunction with T1 weighted images and apparent diffusion coefficient (ADC) maps, DWI can differentiate acute from less acute lesions. To the extent that infarct size correlates with clinical outcome, DWI may also assist with long-term prognosis in anterior circulation stroke syndromes (Level C). The value of perfusion-weighted imaging (PWI) in diagnosing acute ischemic stroke is less clear (Level U).

Improved diagnostic imaging will help eliminate false negative CT scans and provide an earlier, more certain diagnosis of acute ischemic stroke. False-negatives are less common with DWI, but may also occur. In addition, more sensitive imaging will decrease the misdiagnosis of acute ischemic stroke in patients with conversion disorder, postictal paresis, Bell's palsy, or other conditions that may be mistaken for stroke in the emergency room. Misdiagnosis is particularly worrisome because some of these patients may receive tPA, a drug with considerable potential morbidity.

MRI with DWI may be preferable to noncontrast CT for cooperative patients when the diagnosis of acute ischemic stroke is in question.

References
Schellinger PD, Bryan RN, Caplan LR et al. Evidence-based guideline: The role of diffusion and perfusion MRI for the diagnosis of acute ischemic stroke. Report of the Therapeutics and Technology Assessment Subcommittee of the American Academy of Neurology. Neurology 2010;75:177-185.

Chapter 45

STENT OR CAROTID ENDARTERECTOMY? CARDIOLOGISTS SMILE AFTER CREST

February 28, 2010

Results of the CREST (Carotid Revascularization Endarterectomy versus Stenting Trial) just reported at the International Stroke Conference in San Antonio, TX, revealed that carotid stenting had similar long-term results to carotid endarterectomy in symptomatic and asymptomatic patients with carotid artery disease. The composite endpoint of stroke, myocardial infarction or death was 7.2% with stenting vs. 6.8% with carotid endarterectomy, a nonsignificant difference.

These results were discussed by Ralph Sacco, MD, Chief of Neurology at the University of Miami, Miami, Florida, a stroke expert and President-Elect of the American Heart Association. Dr. Sacco explained that carotid endarterectomy had slightly higher 30-day incidence of myocardial infarction, but slightly lower 30-day risk of stroke. Long-term results were similar with both strategies. CREST included 2,502 patients from 117 US and Canadian centers followed for up to 4 years.

Dr. Sacco observed that it is difficult to compare the results of the CREST trial to the European ICSS (International Carotid Stenting Study) just published in *The Lancet* because the latter trial had an endpoint of 120 days, was not performed at US centers, was restricted to symptomatic patients, and used multiple types of stents. The ICSS study concluded that endarterectomy was significantly safer than stenting at 120 days with respect to stroke, death or procedural myocardial infarction (5.2% vs. 8.5%, respectively). Three-year follow up results will be reported. *The Lancet* article also reviews previous endarterectomy and stent trials.

Results from CREST suggest that carotid stenting is a legitimate option for carotid stenosis and had at least one of my cardiology colleagues very excited. Which procedure will you recommend to your patients?

Section 10.

Epilepsy

Chapter 46

EZOGABINE: A NEW DRUG FOR SEIZURE CONTROL

June 30, 2011

Introduction

One June 10, 2011, the US Food and Drug Administration (FDA) approved ezogabine (Potiga) as an adjunct medication for partial seizure control (FDA 2011). Previously known as retigabine, it received approval from the European Medicines Agency March 28, 2011, under the trade name Trobalt. GlaxoSmithKline and Valeant Pharmaceuticals co-developed this new antiepileptic drug (AED).

Ezogabine is the first new AED since 2008, when the FDA approved lacosamide (Vimpat) for partial seizures and rufinamide (Banzel) for Lennox-Gastaut syndrome. New therapeutic options are always welcome for the 30% of people with epilepsy and unsatisfactory seizure control.

Phase 3 Results

Jacqueline French, MD, Professor of Neurology, NYU School of Medicine, and Director of the Epilepsy Study Consortium, NY, NY, was the lead author of the recently published phase 3 multicenter, double blind study of 305 adult patients randomized to ezogabine (N=153) 1200 mg/day (administered 3 times daily) or placebo (N=152) (French et al. 2011). A previous similar phase 3 study demonstrated effectiveness at lower doses of 600 mg/day and 900 mg/day (Brodie et al. 2010).

Martin Brodie, MD, Professor of Medicine and Clinical Pharmacology at the University of Glasgow, Scotland, observed, "Retigabine (ezogabine) is an interesting first-in-class antiepileptic drug, but not a breakthrough treatment."

Dr. French added, "It is early in terms of finding the 'niche' population where ezogabine will be most effective. There are many populations in which we have no experience yet. But clearly some patients with partial-onset seizures responded to this drug when they have failed a number of other drugs."

In Dr. French's study, the patients who tolerated ezogabine titration and entered the maintenance phase had a median percent reduction in seizure frequency of 54.5% vs. placebo of 18.9% ($p < 0.001$). In addition, responder rates ($\geq 50\%$ reduction in total partial seizure frequency) were 55.5% for ezogabine vs. 22.6% for placebo ($p < 0.001$). More than 30% of patients in the maintenance phase had >75% seizure reduction compared with their baseline measurements. However, only 3.3% became seizure-free.

Unique Mechanism of Action

Ezogabine was first identified in 1991 by the National Institutes of Health anticonvulsant screening program where it demonstrated a broad spectrum of activity in animal models of epilepsy (Landmark et al. 2010). Ezogabine opens KCNQ2/3 (Kv7.2/7.3) voltage-gated potassium channels on neurons and activates M-current, which regulates neuronal excitability and suppresses epileptic activity (French et al. 2011, Porter et al. 2007).

Tolerability

As with all AEDs, tolerability may be an issue. In Dr. French's phase 3 study, 26.8% of patients discontinued the trial due to adverse events. The most common side effects were dizziness (40.5%), somnolence (31.4%), fatigue (15.7%) and confusional state (14.4%). Hallucinations occurred in 2%-3% of patients. Mean body weight increased by 2.6 kg (3.5%). In both phase 3 studies, adverse events were more common during titration and tended to disappear in the maintenance phase. Depression, often seen with AEDs, occurred less often in the ezogabine than placebo-treated patients.

Urinary Tract

One of ezogabine's side effects, urinary retention, may be due to its effects on KCNQ channels in the detrusor muscle of the bladder (Landmark et al. 2010). Fifteen patients had a post-void residual volume > 100 ml from baseline compared with 6 placebo-treated controls. Urinary tract infection, urinary hesitation, dysuria and chromaturia were more common in ezogabine-treated patients, but were not serious. With respect to the possibility of teratogenicity, no human pregnancy data are available (Landmark et al. 2010).

Pharmacokinetics

Ezogabine is metabolized in the liver and excreted by the kidney. Carbamazepine and phenytoin may increase ezogabine clearance by about 30%, but ezogabine does not alter carbamazepine, phenytoin, topiramate, or valproic acid pharmacokinetics (Landmark et al. 2010). Lamotrigine may mildly increase the half-life of ezogabine, and ezogabine increases lamotrigine clearance by about 20%. Ezogabine does not alter the metabolism of hormonal birth control.

New Drugs in the Pipeline and Conclusions

Multiple antiepileptic drugs are in development, including others with unique mechanisms of action such as perampanel, a noncompetitive antagonist of AMPA (alpha-amino-3-hydroxy-5-methyl-4-isoxazole propionic acid) receptors. In addition, a second-generation selective opener of neuronal KCNQ (Kv7) potassium channels, ICA-105665, has begun early trials (Prunetti and Perucca 2011). As different strategies toward the development of new AEDs are used, even more effective drugs may result (Schmidt 2011).

References

FDA News Release. FDA approves Potiga to treat seizures in adults, http://www.fda.gov/NewsEvents/Newsroom/PressAnnouncements/ucm258834.htm, June 13, 2011.

French JA, Abou-Khalil BW, Leroy RF et al. Randomized, double-blind, placebo-controlled trial of ezogabine (retigabine) in partial epilepsy. Neurology 2011;76:1555-1563.

Brodie MJ, Lerche H, Gil-Nagel A et al. Efficacy and safety of adjunctive ezogabine (retigabine) in refractory partial epilepsy. Neurology 2010;75:1817-1824.

Landmark CJ, Johannessen SI, Chung SS. Chapter 288. Newest AEDs: brivaracetam, carisbamate and retigabine.

In: Panayiotopoulos CP, ed. Atlas of Epilepsies. New York, Springer, 2010.

Porter RJ, Nohria V, Rundfeldt C. Retigabine. Neurotherapeutics 2007;4:149-154.

Prunetti P, Perucca E. New and forthcoming anti-epileptic drugs. Curr Opin Neurol 2011;24:159-164.

Schmidt D. Antiepileptic drug discovery: does mechanism of action matter? Epilepsy & Behavior 2011, in press.

Wilner N. Pharmacopoeia of antiepileptic drugs: overview. In: Panayiotopoulos CP, ed. Atlas of Epilepsies. New York, Springer, 2010.

Update May 21, 2013

Perampanel received FDA approval for the adjunct treatment of partial seizures in patients at least 12 years old on October 23, 2012. It is marketed under the trade name, "Fycompa."

An unusual new side effect has been reported with ezogabine (see Chapter 47.)

Chapter 47

BLUE PERSON SYNDROME

May 10, 2013

Introduction: A Startling New Side Effect
The US Food and Drug Administration (FDA) issued a drug safety communication (FDA 2013) on April 26, 2013, alerting the medical community that ezogabine (Potiga, GlaxoSmithKline, Research Triangle Park, North Carolina), one of the newest antiepileptic drugs, may cause blue-gray skin discoloration and retinal pigment changes.

Ezogabine
Ezogabine, formerly known as retigabine, received FDA approval as Potiga for adjunctive treatment of partial on-set seizures in adults on June 10, 2011. Ezogabine is a positive allosteric modulator of KCNQ2-5 potassium channels that inhibits high-frequency action potential firing, a unique mechanism of action for an antiepileptic drug (Gunthorpe et al. 2012). Ezogabine was co-developed by GlaxoSmithKline and Valeant Pharmaceuticals and marketed as Trobalt in the European Union. An article about ezogabine that included a summary of 2 phase 3 clinical trials appeared in this column shortly after the drug received FDA approval (Wilner 2013).

New FDA Advisory
To date, approximately 2,900 patients have received a prescription for ezogabine in the United States and 6,000

globally. Blue-gray pigmentation, observed on the sclera and conjunctiva, lips, nail beds of fingers and toes, and more widespread on the body has occurred in 38 (6.3%) of 605 patients followed in clinical trials. Nearly all of the patients who had skin discoloration, 36 of 38 (95%), had taken the drug for at least 2 years.

Of 36 patients still in ongoing studies who had eye examinations, 11 (31%) had retinal pigment abnormalities. Four of the 11 (36%) did not have skin discoloration. Although 5 patients had worse than 20/20 visual acuity, baseline values for visual acuity were not available for comparison. Consequently, it is not known whether the retinal pigment changes resulted in visual loss. One patient, who received a full panel of retinal tests, had findings consistent with "retinal dystrophy." All cases of retinal abnormalities were exposed to ezogabine for at least 3 years.

The Price of Early Adoption
Pigment changes with ezogabine had not been observed during the 2 pivotal phase 3 clinical trials and are only becoming apparent 2 years after FDA approval of the drug. This scenario is reminiscent of retinal toxicity resulting in permanent peripheral visual field defects in patients taking vigabatrin (Sabril, Lundbeck, Deerfield, Illinois). These field defects were not reported until 1997, even though the drug had been approved in the United Kingdom since 1989 (Ben-Menachem 2009). Vigabatrin's toxicity appears to be dose- and duration-dependent. The product label now carries a "boxed warning," and vigabatrin's clinical use has been severely limited. Another example of significant side effects detected after approval in an epilepsy drug is the

rare occurrence of aplastic anemia and hepatic failure with felbamate, which surfaced after approximately 1 year of clinical use. Felbamate is now rarely used in clinical practice except in the most refractory cases.

Eye Sensitivity

The eye appears to be a sensitive substrate for adverse events induced by antiepileptic and other drugs. The occurrence of retinal abnormalities with vigabatrin and ezogabine (as well as acute myopia and secondary angle-closure glaucoma with topiramate and macular edema with fingolimod, a new drug for multiple sclerosis) suggests that future clinical trials may need to include baseline and periodic ophthalmologic examinations.

A Numbers Game

Despite the clinical rigor of phase 3 clinical trials, if an adverse effect is related to treatment duration, it may easily be missed in trials that last only a few months. Alternatively, phase 3 trials may also miss rare adverse effects. For example, an idiosyncratic side effect that occurs in only 1/10,000 or 1/100,000 patients may not occur in a study that includes less than 1,000 patients. Of note, the 2 ezogabine phase 3 trials included only 359 (Brodie et al. 2010) and 153 (French et al. 2011) treated patients.

Other Adverse Effects

Ezogabine also has a REMS (risk evaluation and mitigation strategy) that provides warnings about urinary retention, neuropsychiatric symptoms, dizziness and somnolence, QT prolongation, suicidal thoughts or behavior, withdrawal seizures, adverse reactions, drug abuse and dependence, and dosing considerations. Ezogabine is a controlled substance, rated as schedule V, as are 2 other antiepileptic drugs for partial seizures, lacosamide and pregabalin.

Recommendations

Jacqueline French, MD, Professor of Neurology at New York University School of Medicine, New York, New York, and lead investigator of one of the phase 3 trials for ezogabine (French et al. 2011), responded in an email that she has not detected any pigment changes in her patients. Professor Martin Brodie, Director of the Epilepsy Unit, Western Infirmary, Glasgow, Scotland, and lead investigator of the other ezogabine phase 3 trial (Brodie et al. 2010), communicated in an email that he has treated 65 patients with ezogabine but has not seen any pigment problems. He plans to continue treatment and carefully monitor those currently on the drug but not start any new patients on ezogabine "until the situation is clarified."

The FDA advised that all patients have a "baseline eye exam, followed by periodic eye exams." According to the FDA, eye examinations should include "visual acuity, dilated fundus photography, and may include fluorescein angiograms, ocular coherence tomography, perimetry and electroretinograms." Risk factors for skin and pigment changes such as dose, duration or idiosyncratic susceptibility have not yet been determined. The FDA advised that all patients with ophthalmologic changes discontinue the drug unless there are no other treatment options, and that patients with skin changes seriously consider a substitute. For asymptomatic patients, the advisory did not mandate stopping the drug, nor is GlaxoSmithKline advising that all patients discontinue ezogabine (personal communication, GlaxoSmithKline Medical Affairs, April 2013).

Summary

A striking new adverse event of ezogabine, characterized by pigment changes of the skin, nails, and retina has been recognized. Although blue lips and nail beds traditionally signal hypoxia, when induced by ezogabine, they indicate actual pigment change. Whether other body systems are affected, the nature of the clinical consequences, and whether these changes can be reversed are all still unknown. The mechanism of action producing these pigment changes has not been determined.

Ezogabine is approved as adjunctive therapy with other antiepileptic drugs. Given vigabatrin's risk for retinal toxicity, it would seem prudent to avoid using ezogabine in conjunction with vigabatrin.

For many patients with partial seizures currently taking ezogabine, other treatment options are available. A switch to an alternative drug may be the most pragmatic solution while clinicians await further details about ezogabine-induced somatic pigment changes. As with all antiepileptic drugs, ezogabine should not be stopped abruptly, which could precipitate seizure recurrence or life-threatening status epilepticus. Physicians who encounter patients with adverse reactions to ezogabine should notify GlaxoSmithKline (1-888-825-5249) and the FDA MedWatch program (1-800-FDA-1088) or report it online at https://www.accessdata.fda.gov/scripts/medwatch/medwatch-online.htm.

References

US Food and Drug Administration. FDA Drug Safety Communication: Anti-seizure drug Potiga (ezogabine) linked to retinal abnormalities and blue skin discoloration, http://www.fda.gov/Drugs/DrugSafety/ucm349538.htm, April 26, 2013.

Gunthorpe MJ, Large CH, Sankar R. The mechanism of action of retigabine (ezogabine), a first-in-class K+ channel opener for the treatment of epilepsy. Epilepsia 2012;53:412-424.

Wilner AN. Ezogabine: a new drug for seizure control. Medscape Neurology, http://www.medscape.com/viewarticle745271, June 30, 2011.

Ben-Menachem E. Vigabatrin's complicated journey-to be or not to be? Epilepsy Curr 2009;9:130-132.

Brodie MJ, Lerche H, Gil-Nagel A et al. Efficacy and safety of adjunctive ezogabine (retigabine) in refractory partial epilepsy. Neurology 2010;75:1817-1824.

French JA, Abou-Khalil BW, Leroy RF et al. Randomized, double-blind, placebo-controlled trial of ezogabine (retigabine) in partial epilepsy. Neurology 2011;76:1555-1563.

Chapter 48

A NEW EPILEPSY ETIOLOGY

January 15, 2013

Introduction
Autoimmune epilepsy is a newly recognized treatable cause of uncontrolled seizures. A retrospective review of patients who presented with uncontrolled seizures to both the epilepsy and neuroimmunology clinics of the Mayo Clinic between 2005 and 2010 identified 32 patients (19 females, 13 males) with probable autoimmune epilepsy (Quek et al. 2012). Patients presented either exclusively with seizures (n=11) or with seizures as their predominant symptom (n=21). After immunotherapy, 67% became seizure free.

Clinical Profile
A history of autoimmune disease was present in 50% of the patients and a family history of autoimmune disease was present in 53%. Most of the patients presented with simple partial seizures and/or auras, 27/32 (84%), complex partial seizures, 26/32 (81%), and secondary generalized tonic-clonic seizures, 17/32 (53%). Twenty-six (81%) had daily seizures. Findings on electroencephalography (EEG) included interictal epileptiform discharges (n=20), electrographic seizures (n=15), focal slowing (n=13), and generalized slowing (n=12). Three patients had normal EEGs. Probable inflammatory changes were noted in 29 (63%) of MRIs. Cerebrospinal fluid revealed elevated protein in 17

(57%), elevated leukocytes in 5 (17%), oligoclonal bands in 5 (19%) and was normal in 11 (38%). Neural autoantibodies were present in 29 (91%) of patients. These included voltage-gated potassium channel (VGKC complex) (N=18, 56%), glutamic acid decarboxylase (GAD65) (N=7, 22%), collapsin response-mediator protein (CRMP-5) (N=2, 6%), Ma2 (N=1, 3%), N-methyl-D-aspartate receptor (NMDAR) (N=1, 3%), and ganglionic acetylcholine receptor (AChR) (N=1, 3%). Two patients with VGKC neural autoantibodies had malignancies (thyroid or prostate) and 1 patient with CRMP-5 had recurrent bladder cancer. Eight-one percent of patients had already tried 2 or more antiepileptic drugs. Two (6%) patients failed epilepsy surgery.

Therapy

Immunotherapy included intravenous (IV) methylprednisolone (n=12), IVIg (N=3), and combinations of IV methylprednisolone, IVIg, cyclophosphamide, or plasmapheresis (N=12). Patients were followed for 3-72 months (median, 17 months). Eighteen patients (67%) became seizure free and 27 (81%) improved.

Making the Diagnosis

Among the many possible causes for epilepsy, autoimmune epilepsy should be added to the list. Although an autoimmune cause may account for relatively few cases of epilepsy of previously "unknown" origin, recognition is particularly important because effective treatment may be instituted. Clinical clues include a patient or family history of autoimmune disease (i.e., celiac sprue, diabetes mellitus, lupus, Sjogren syndrome, rheumatoid arthritis, thyroid disease), a history of malignancy, relatively late age of onset without another obvious explanation for seizures, such as brain tumor or stroke, frequent (daily) seizures, multifocal or variable seizure types within 1 patient, and lack of control with antiepileptic drugs.

Associated neuropsychiatric symptoms may be present, such as anxiety, depression, cognitive difficulties, memory loss, or personality changes (Bergey 2012). However, one third of the patients in a study by Quek and colleagues (Quek et al. 2012) did not have memory impairment or affective changes to suggest the better-known neural autoantibody-mediated syndrome of limbic encephalitis.

To make the diagnosis of autoimmune epilepsy, patients should be screened for neural autoantibodies, and MRI and cerebrospinal fluid examined for inflammatory changes. The presence of neural autoantibodies accompanied by seizures suggests the possibility of a paraneoplastic syndrome, and patients should be evaluated for possible malignancies. In this study, only 3 patients had associated malignancies. Whether neural autoantibodies are directly pathogenic or merely markers of an autoimmune process is not yet known. Our increasing ability to detect neural autoantibodies and to conduct further bench and clinical research will ultimately clarify their role.

If there is a high degree of suspicion for autoimmune epilepsy, a trial of immunotherapy such as IV methylprednisolone or IVIg should be considered. The results may be gratifying.

References

Quek AML, Britton JQW, McKeon A et al. Autoimmune epilepsy. Clinical characteristics and response to immunotherapy. Arch Neurol 2012;69:582-593.

Bergey GK. Autoantibodies in the patient with drug-resistant epilepsy. Are we missing a treatable etiology? Arch Neurol 2012;69:565-566.

Chapter 49

ORPHAN DRUG PROGRAM BENEFITS PEOPLE WITH EPILEPSY

October 17, 2012

Introduction

Epilepsy affects approximately 1 in 100 people, but many specific epilepsy syndromes are rare. For example, Lennox-Gastaut syndrome accounts for only 4% of children with epilepsy, but this triad of intractable epilepsy, developmental delay, and slow spike and wave is notoriously difficult to treat. Two new medications for Lennox-Gastaut syndrome, clobazam (Onfi) and rufinamide (Banzel), recently received US Food and Drug Administration (FDA) approval and designation as orphan drugs under the Orphan Drug Act. Diastat, a rectal preparation of diazepam indicated for patients taking antiepileptic drugs who have breakthrough seizures, was also approved under the Orphan Drug Act. Another orphan drug of interest to people with epilepsy is everolimus, which received FDA approval in 2009 for the treatment of subependymal giant cell astrocytomas in people with tuberous sclerosis complex, a rare genetic disorder associated with tumor growth and seizures.

Orphan Drug Act

Passed in 1983, the Orphan Drug Act facilitates the development of treatments for disorders that affect less than 200,000 people. There are approximately 7,000 rare disorders that fall into this category, many of which are life threatening. Because the relatively small number of people with these disorders represents fewer customers, potential profits are reduced compared with drugs for more common health problems such as diabetes, high blood pressure, or hyperlipidemia. To encourage the development of medications for less common disorders, the US government provides incentives such as 7 years of market exclusivity post-FDA approval, 50% tax credit for clinical development costs, grant funding, FDA guidance in protocol design, an application fee waiver, expedited review and other assistance. Since passage of the Orphan Drug Act, more than 350 drugs have come to market under this program. The largest disease category for which orphan drugs have been approved is cancer, constituting about 30% of all orphan drug approvals.

Orphan Drug Research in Epilepsy

The investigational drug carisbamate received orphan drug designation on April 19, 2012, for infantile spasms, a severe epilepsy syndrome. Only 2,500 children per year are affected by infantile spasms in the United States, but these unfortunate children may experience multiple seizure clusters per day and long-term cognitive and behavioral morbidity. Infantile spasms often lead to Lennox-Gastaut syndrome later in life. The treatment of infantile spasms remains unsatisfactory and was the topic of a recent American Academy of Neurology Guideline.

Another drug, stiripentol, used for the treatment of severe myoclonic epilepsy in infancy (Dravet syndrome), received orphan drug designation in 2008. Neither caris-bamate nor stiripentol are FDA approved for the treatment of epilepsy.

Specialized Centers Advancing Research

The Center for Orphan Drug Research (CODR) at the College of Pharmacy, University of Minnesota, Minneapolis, Minnesota, was created in 2005. Directed by James Cloyd, PharmD, Professor and Lawrence C. Weaver Endowed Chair-Orphan Drug Development, the center's stated mission is to "improve the care of individuals suffering from rare diseases through research on new drug therapies; education of health professionals and health profession students; and contributions to the discussion and formulation of public policy relating to rare diseases and orphan drugs." Researchers at CODR include laboratory scientists, a research associate, a postdoctoral fellow, graduate students, residents and undergraduate students. To speed development, CODR partners with pharmaceutical and biotechnology companies. Its primary research focus is rare pediatric neurologic disorders.

Several projects are currently under way at CODR that may potentially help people with epilepsy. These include:

1. Use of topiramate for neuroprotection and seizure control in neonates

2. Development of responsive pharmacotherapy in canine partial epilepsy

3. Intranasal benzodiazepines for seizure emergencies

4. Development of water-soluble benzodiazepine prodrugs to treat seizure emergencies

Dr. Cloyd commented,

"These 4 projects address our interest in treating seizure emergencies in a vulnerable population. Neonatal seizures are a type of seizure emergency, and we are developing an injectable form of topiramate for that. We plan to determine whether it is safe and effective in neonatal seizures and whether it has the potential for neuroprotection in those babies.

"The other 3 projects are directed at finding a better way of treating seizure emergencies outside the hospital. At the moment, Diastat, another orphan drug, is the only alternative. Although Diastat is effective, because it must be administered rectally, there are problems with patient and caregiver acceptance. We think that the nasal delivery of diazepam would be at least as effective and far more practical. At least one other company is working on nasal diazepam and another company on nasal midazolam. Intramuscular benzodiazepines are another option under development for controlling breakthrough seizures outside the hospital."

Dr. Cloyd explained that the orphan drug designation can be applied to a new molecule or to an old drug that is repurposed for an orphan indication. In either case, patients with rare diseases could benefit. Projects at CODR include collaborations with the FDA, Mayo Clinic, and University of Pennsylvania as well as companies such as NeuroVista, which is developing seizure prediction software; Ligand Pharmaceuticals, which is participating in the development of intravenous topiramate, and Neurelis, which is supporting the development of intranasal diazepam.

Dr. Cloyd continued, "At CODR, we are trying to act like a small drug company and leverage resources across the University of Minnesota and elsewhere to get this work done in a way that is responsible and rigorous. We are filling a niche that really isn't being filled by anyone else. Our goal is to get new products out so that clinicians can prescribe them and patients can use them. Alternatively, we want to generate high quality information about old drugs so that they can be used safely and effectively for rare disorders."

In addition to CODR, other centers that focus on orphan drug research include The Center for Rare and Neglected Diseases at the University of Notre Dame, Notre Dame, Indiana; The Manton Center for Orphan Disease Research at Children's Hospital in Boston, Massachusetts; The Center for Rare Disease Therapies at the Keck Graduate Institute of Applied Life Sciences, Claremont, California; and The Raymond and Ruth Perelman School of Medicine at the University of Pennsylvania, Philadelphia, Pennsylvania.

Conclusions

The Orphan Drug Act of 1983 recognized the reality of the marketplace as an important factor influencing the development of new medications. Since 1983, hundreds of orphan compounds have been "adopted" by pharmaceutical developers and shepherded to FDA approval. Specialized centers such as CODR have emerged to address the unmet needs of orphan diseases, often in collaboration with private industry. As the Orphan Drug Act approaches its 30th anniversary, it continues to help people with epilepsy and many other rare disorders.

For more information, a recent book, *Orphan Drugs in Epilepsy*, addresses this topic as well.

References

Coles LD, Cloyd JC. The role of academic institutions in the development of drugs for rare and neglected diseases. Clin Pharmacol Ther 2012;92:193-202.

Epilepsy Foundation. Incidence and prevalence of epilepsy. http://epilepsyfoundation.org/aboutepilepsy/whatisepilepsy/.

Gandey A. FDA approves clobazam add-on for Lennox syndrome. http://www.medscape.com/viewarticle/752080, October 24, 2011.

Nevarez AK. Orphan drugs. http://www.ice-epilepsy.org/orphan-drugs.html, May 26, 2009.

US Food and Drug Administration. FDA approves new drug to treat severe form of epilepsy. http://www.fda.gov/NewsEvents/Newsroom/, November 20, 2008.

PressAnnouncements/2008/ucm116980.htm.

Chapter 50

CHANNELOPATHIES-ANOTHER CAUSE FOR EPILEPSY

September 5, 2012

Introduction: A Look at Channelopathies

In a recent study, genetic mutations of the KCNQ2 potassium ion channel were identified in 8/80 (10%) of children with early infantile seizures and associated psychomotor retardation (Avanzini 2010). Seizures started in all of the children before they were 3 months old. Six children had *de novo* mutations, while 1 child had a parent with epilepsy who was a mosaic for the mutation. For 1 child, DNA from the father was unavailable. Although most of the children ultimately became seizure free, all had persistent motor impairment and moderate to severe intellectual disability.

Discussion

Although the cause of epilepsy is often readily apparent, such as encephalitis, stroke, or traumatic brain injury, the cause of seizures remains unknown in approximately 50% of people with epilepsy. This is frustrating for families and offers no direction for the development of targeted therapies. Children with seizures and static encephalopathy constitute an important subset of this category of patients with "idiopathic" or "cryptogenic" epilepsy.

The finding by Weckhuysen and colleagues that heterozygous missense KCNQ2 mutations may be responsible for infantile seizures with associated psychomotor retardation removes these children from the taxonomic wastebasket of "epilepsy of unknown etiology" to the more precise category of "channelopathy" (Weckhuysen et al. 2012).

A channelopathy may be defined as a genetically determined alteration in ion channels resulting in acute and transient symptomatology in subjects who otherwise seem to be perfectly normal. Ion channels, located on the cell membrane, control the intracellular and extracellular concentrations of ions such as calcium, chloride, potassium, and sodium, which affect the cell membrane potential.

The first 2 epilepsy syndromes identified as channelopathies were autosomal dominant nocturnal frontal lobe epilepsy (ADNFLE), due to gene mutations in the acetylcholine nicotinic receptor, and benign familial neonatal convulsions (BFNC), due to mutations in KCNQ2 or KCNQ3 channels. Both of these syndromes had previously been considered to be "idiopathic" epilepsies. Approximately two thirds of cases of BFNC have been associated with mutations of KCNQ2 and KCNQ3, which encode the voltage-gated potassium channels Kv7.2 and Kv7.3, respectively. In this study, none of the children had KCNQ3 mutations (Avanzini 2010).

Other epilepsy syndromes with ion channel gene mutations include generalized epilepsy with febrile seizures (sodium channel or GABA receptor), severe myoclonic epilepsy of infancy, also known as Dravet syndrome (sodium channel), childhood absence epilepsy (calcium channel), and idiopathic generalized epilepsies (chloride channel).

Conclusions

The identification of KCNQ2 as the cause of 8 cases of early infantile seizures and associated psychomotor retardation helps chip away at the massive mountain of "idiopathic" epilepsies. For these 8 severely affected children and their families, the mystery of "why do I have epilepsy?" has been solved. But this successful classification delivers more than mere taxonomic satisfaction. Although most of the children in this study had *de novo* mutations, one had a father with epilepsy who was a mosaic for the mutation, demonstrating that this type of epilepsy may be inherited. While not directly affecting treatment, this additional information may influence family planning. Genetic screening for KCNQ2 may be appropriate for this population of children and their family members with epilepsy.

In addition, the identification of an abnormal potassium channel may lead to the development of antiepileptic drugs that target this specific genetic defect. Among the growing roster of new antiepileptic drugs, the latest is ezogabine (Potiga, Valeant Pharmaceuticals, North America, LLC), recently approved by the US Food and Drug Administration and soon to be commercially available (see Chapters 46 and 47). Ezogabine has a novel mechanism of action; it acts by opening voltage-gated potassium channels. As Weckhuysen and colleagues point out, perhaps ezogabine will be effective in epilepsies caused by KCNQ2 ion channel mutations.

Continued advances in genetic testing coupled with improved understanding of the pathophysiology of epilepsy promise to uncover additional causes of epilepsy that will lead to improved diagnosis, prognosis, and ultimately, freedom from seizures.

References

Avanzini G. Epileptogenic channelopathies. In: Panayiotopoulos CP, ed. Atlas of Epilepsies. Springer-Verlag, London, 2010.

Weckhuysen S, Mandelstam S, Suls A et al. KCNQ2 encephalopathy: Emerging phenotype of a neonatal epileptic encephalopathy. Ann Neurol 2012;71:15-25.

Chapter 51

SEIZURE FREEDOM: HOW MANY EPILEPSY DRUGS TO TRY?

July 30, 2012

Introduction: Seizure Freedom

For some people with epilepsy, seizure control comes with the first antiepileptic drug (AED). Others never succeed. A middle group eventually conquers their seizures with trials of 2, 3, or more AEDs. Outcomes vary depending on adherence to treatment, adverse events of medications, epilepsy syndrome, cause, seizure type, and other factors. Approximately 30% of patients do not achieve seizure remission with AED therapy. Focal seizures are the most common type in adults and are often difficult to control (Kwan et al. 2010, Kwan and Brodie 2000).

Focal Epilepsies

A new retrospective analysis offers some guidance on managing people with focal epilepsy (Gilioli et al. 2012). The authors reviewed a database containing records of 1,155 adults with focal epilepsy from 2 epilepsy centers, the Carlo Besta Foundation Neurological Institute and San Paolo University Hospital, both in Milan, Italy. Patients were classified as either seizure-free or AED-resistant. They also graded patients on whether 1, 2, 3, or more AEDs had failed. Noncompliant patients, those who had epilepsy surgery, or those whose treatment was unchanged for particular reasons were excluded.

Results

Of the 1,155 patients (584 female, 571 male), 588 (50.9%) were AED-resistant and 567 (49.1%) were seizure-free. Age and sex were similar in the 2 groups. Patients who were AED-resistant tried more antiepileptic drugs (3.7 ± 3.4) than those who became seizure free 1.5 ± 1.8) (p<0.001).

Patients were classified as having "symptomatic" (N=729) and "probably symptomatic" (N=426) episodes of epilepsy. Symptomatic episodes were defined as those with specific causes and/or signs of brain injury, such as mesial temporal sclerosis. All others were included in the probably symptomatic group, except for 5 patients with autosomal dominant genetic epilepsy.

In a multivariate analysis, statistically significant risk factors for AED resistance in the symptomatic group included tonic-akinetic seizures (odds ratio (OR) 2.44), a pathologic electroencephalogram (EEG) (OR 2.2), seizures with early impairment of consciousness (OR 1.61), and more than 1 seizure type (OR 1.48). In the probably symptomatic group, risk factors for AED resistance included a pathologic EEG (OR 2.36) and psychiatric symptoms (OR 1.97). Conversely, a family history of epilepsy was associated with decreased risk for AED resistance in the probably symptomatic group (OR 0.51). The only risk factor for AED resistance present in both the symptomatic and probably symptomatic groups was a "pathologic EEG."

In the entire population, 21% became seizure-free on their first AED, 12.2% on their second, 8.4% on their third, and 7.3% on their fourth. Of those who became seizure-free, 43% responded to their first AED, 24.9% to their second, 17.2% to their third, and 14.9% to their fourth.

Of interest, 43.2% of the 97 patients in whom a combination of 2 AEDs had failed became seizure-free with one of the newer AEDs, as did 50% of the 84 patients who had tried a combination of 3 AEDs.

Discussion

The ad hoc Task Force of the International League Against Epilepsy Commission on Therapeutic Strategies recently proposed a definition of "drug-resistant epilepsy" as "failure of adequate trials of two tolerated, appropriately chosen and used antiepileptic drug schedules (whether as monotherapies or in combination) to achieve sustained seizure freedom." Patients who fit the definition can now be classified as "drug-resistant," providing consistency for recruitment in clinical studies. In addition, identification of "drug-resistant" patients should trigger inquiry into other treatment options, such as epilepsy surgery, the vagus nerve stimulator, and the ketogenic or modified Atkins diets. However, according to the Task Force, classification of a patient as "drug-resistant" does not necessarily mean that he or she will never respond to pharmacologic therapy, only that the probability is "modest."

In this study by Gilioli and colleagues, two thirds of the patients who became seizure-free did so with their first or second AED, confirming the common clinical observation that patients who become seizure-free generally do so early and easily (Gilioli et al. 2012). However, the remaining one third became seizure free after a third or fourth drug trial.

Consequently, although "drug-resistant epilepsy" is currently defined as failure of 2 AEDs, it may be fruitful to persist with additional trials, at least up to 4 AEDs, before referring patients for nondrug treatment. If this strategy is followed, the trials should be done expeditiously so that patients in whom 4 drugs fail are not excessively delayed for referral for a potentially curative surgical resection, enrollment in a clinical study, neurostimulation or other therapy.

References

Kwan P, Arzimanoglou A, Bert AT et al. Definition of drug resistant epilepsy: Consensus proposal by the ad hoc Task Force of the ILAE Commission on Therapeutic Strategies. Epilepsia 2010;51:1069-1077.

Kwan P, Brodie MJ. Early identification of refractory epilepsy. NEJM 2000;342:314-319.

Gilioli I, Vignoli A, Visani E et al. Focal epilepsies in adult patients attending two epilepsy centers: Classification of drug-resistance, assessment of risk factors, and usefulness of "new" antiepileptic drugs. Epilepsia 2012;53:733-740.

Chapter 52

NEW EPILEPSY JOURNAL!

July 2, 2012

Introduction

The first issue of the *North African and Middle East Journal of Epilepsy* was published at the start of 2012. It focuses on 20 countries in Northern Africa and the Middle East, ranging from Mauritania in the West to Pakistan in the East. Articles are published in French or English. The editor-in-chief is Najib Kissani, a neurologist at the Faculty of Medicine and Pharmacy, University Cadi Ayyad of Marrakech, Marrakech, Morocco.

The new journal addresses several unmet regional needs. In his editorial, Dr. Kissani recognizes significant disparities in neurologic care among the countries of North Africa and the Middle East. For example, Egypt has 400 neurologists, whereas Mauritania has 3. Even the wealthiest countries, such as Algeria, the Gulf countries, Lebanon, and Tunisia, have only 1 neurologist for 35,000 residents, and poorer countries, such as Mauritania, Somalia, and Yemen, have less than 1 neurologist per 2 million persons. Many causes of epilepsy are potentially preventable, such as central nervous system tuberculosis, meningitis, and neonatal hypoxic encephalopathy, if only better care and more resources were available. Stigmatization of epilepsy still exists, and more education is needed. In addition, there are only 3 regional neuroscience journals. *Neurosciences* (Saudi Arabia),

Current Alzheimer Research (United Arab Emirates), and *CNS & Neurological Disorders Drug Targets* (United Arab Emirates), none of which are devoted to epilepsy. This new journal intends to become a platform for publication of clinical and research articles by regional physicians and researchers, although submissions from all countries are welcome. In addition to scientific articles, the journal welcomes "stories experienced by patients with epilepsy, physicians or other professionals involved in epilepsy" and news from regional societies, leagues, and associations against epilepsy. Articles may be submitted in French or English. The journal is not yet indexed in Medline.

The premier issue included an editorial on the state of epilepsy in the North African and Middle East region in light of the Arab Spring, a case report of polymicrogyria, a history of the Tunisian Association Against Epilepsy, and articles on epilepsy in Mali and Gambia. Six issues and 2 supplements per year are planned.

National Leagues or Associations represented by the journal include the Algerian League Against Epilepsy, Egyptian Society Against Epilepsy, Jordanian League Against Epilepsy, Kuwait League Against Epilepsy, Lebanese League Against Epilepsy, Qatar League Against Epilepsy, Moroccan Association Against Epilepsy, Moroccan League Against Epilepsy, Tunisian Association Against Epilepsy, Saudi Chapter of Epilepsy, Sudanese League Against Epilepsy, and Syrian League Against Epilepsy.

Journal sponsors include the University Cadi Ayyad of Marrakech, Moroccan Association Against Epilepsy, Moroccan League Against Epilepsy, and the Watania Press. The staff includes 12 associate editors, 2 editorial assistants, and 45 reviewers from multiple countries.* There are both print and electronic editions. Subscriptions are available for a fee. The editorial office is in Marrakech, Morocco.

Articles, case reports, and book reviews are invited. The secretary can be contacted at: secretariat.je@gmail.com.

*Disclosure: Dr. Wilner is one of many volunteer reviewers for this new journal.

Chapter 53

INTRAMUSCULAR MIDAZOLAM: A SHOT IN THE ARM FOR STATUS EPILEPTICUS

June 19, 2012

Introduction

Intramuscular midazolam is at least as effective as intravenous lorazepam for the initial treatment of status epilepticus, according to the results of the RAMPART study published in the *New England Journal of Medicine* (Silbergleit et al. 2012).

Status epilepticus is a medical emergency associated with significant morbidity and mortality. It is defined as "a single epileptic seizure of >30-min duration or a series of epileptic seizures during which function is not regained between ictal events in a >30-min period" (Guidelines 1993). Currently, epileptologists advise that seizures lasting longer than 5 minutes may not be self-limited and should be treated as status epilepticus.

Epidemiology

Approximately 200,000 episodes of status epilepticus occur in the United States each year, and 3 million worldwide. Status epilepticus is more common in children and elderly persons (Roth 2011). It is the presenting seizure type in approximately one third of new cases of epilepsy in elderly persons (Mauricio and Freeman 2011). Status epilepticus stems from many causes, including acute metabolic disturbances, such as electrolyte imbalance, hyperglycemia, hypoglycemia and hypocalcemia, alcohol and drug abuse, cerebral anoxia, central nervous system infection, cerebral tumor, low levels of antiepileptic drug, stroke, or traumatic brain injury.

Morbidity and Mortality
Overall mortality from status epilepticus is 15-22%, but varies depending on the etiology and quality of treatment for the condition (Hirsch 2012). Refractory status epilepticus results in approximately 40,000 deaths per year (Seif-Eddeine and Treiman 2011).

Treatment Overview
Initial treatment typically consists of benzodiazepines followed by phenobarbital, phenytoin, valproate or other antiepileptic drugs. In refractory cases, intubation and general anesthesia with midazolam, pentobarbital, propofol or other drugs may be required.

One of the most important factors affecting treatment outcome is the duration of status epilepticus; longer episodes are associated with treatment resistance and higher morbidity and mortality (Seif-Eddeine and Treiman 2011). Consequently, there is a strong rationale for emergency medical personnel to initiate treatment in the field as soon as possible, rather than waiting for patients to arrive at the hospital.

Intramuscular Midazolam vs. Intravenous Lorazepam
In RAMPART, 893 persons who had convulsions lasting more than 5 minutes that were still ongoing when emergency

medical personnel arrived were randomly assigned to receive either intramuscular midazolam plus intravenous placebo or intravenous lorazepam plus intramuscular placebo (Silbergleit et al. 2012). Participants included 4,313 paramedics, 33 emergency medical services agencies, and 79 receiving hospitals in the United States. Intramuscular midazolam was administered with an autoinjector.

Upon arrival in the emergency department, 329 (73.4%) of the 448 midazolam-treated patients vs. 282 (63.4%) of the 445 lorazepam-treated patients were seizure free, demonstrating both the noninferiority and superiority of midazolam ($p<0.001$). In addition, the proportion of patients who required hospital admission was significantly lower in the midazolam group than the lorazepam group (57.6% vs. 65.6%, p=0.01). Adverse event rates were similar in both groups.

Analysis of Results

The results emphasize the importance of rapid administration of an active drug in treating status epilepticus. Median times to treatment were 4 times longer with intravenous lorazepam (4.8 minutes) vs. intramuscular midazolam (1.2 minutes). The ease of administration of midazolam more than made up for the fact that it was slower-acting (3.3 minutes) than lorazepam (1.6 minutes). Consequently, the median time to seizure control was slightly longer with lorazepam (4.8 + 1.6 =6.4 minutes) than with midazolam (1.2 + 3.3 =4.5 minutes) (P values not significant).

Furthermore, 31 patients in the lorazepam group did not receive the active drug because of difficulty with intravenous access, whereas only 5 patients in the midazolam group did not receive drug owing to autoinjector failure. These results highlight the difficulty of establishing intravenous access in an actively convulsing patient.

Other routes of benzodiazepine administration, such as buccal, intranasal, and rectal, may also be effective in controlling seizures, but intramuscular administration by autoinjector offers more predictable dosing (Hirsch 2012).

Conclusions

The benefit of intramuscular midazolam for status epilepticus demonstrated by the double blind RAMPART study highlights the practical considerations of treating patients who are actively seizing. Although lorazepam had a faster onset of action, the fact that intramuscular midazolam could be administered more quickly resulted in similar times to effectiveness for the 2 drugs. More midazolam-treated patients were seizure-free upon hospital arrival (73.4% for midazolam vs. 63.4% for lorazepam)-a difference of 10 percentage points, which demonstrated the noninferiority and superiority of midazolam.

Because prompt treatment of status epilepticus strongly influences morbidity and mortality, it is likely that the results of this study will translate into US Food and Drug Administration approval of intramuscular midazolam for status epilepticus in the near future.

References
Silbergleit R, Durkalski V, Lowenstein D et al. NETT Investigators. Intramuscular versus intravenous therapy for prehospital status epilepticus. NEJM 2012;366:591-600.

Guidelines for epidemiologic studies on epilepsy. Commission on Epidemiology and Prognosis, International League Against Epilepsy. Epilepsia 1993;34:592-596.

Roth JL. Status Epilepticus. http://emedicine.medscape. com/article/1164462-overview, May 26, 2011.

Mauricio EA, Freeman WD. Status epilepticus in the elderly: differential diagnosis and treatment. Neuropsychiatr Dis Treat 2011;7:161-166.

Hirsch LJ. Intramuscular versus intravenous benzodiazepines for prehospital treatment of status epilepticus. NEJM 2012;366:659-660.

Seif-Eddeine H, Treiman DM. Problems and controversies in status epilepticus. A review and recommendations. http://www.medscape.com/viewarticle/754309, December 6, 2011.

Chapter 54

A BIG STEP FORWARD FOR EPILEPSY TRIALS

February 21, 2012

Introduction

The Epilepsy Study Consortium is helping to bring better seizure control to people with epilepsy. Despite the introduction of 13 new antiepileptic drugs (AEDs) since 1993, approximately 30% of people with epilepsy continue to have seizures (Kwan and Brodie 2000). Many others achieve seizure control at the expense of disagreeable side effects. The National Institute of Neurological Disorders and Stroke has screened more than 28,000 chemicals with maximal electroshock, subcutaneous pentylenetetrazole, 6-Hz, and other tests, but a universally effective AED remains elusive (Brodie 2010).

The challenge of providing more effective AEDs to people with epilepsy is further complicated by the difficulty of designing and carrying out clinical trials. Clinical trials are often lengthy and expensive, and they must be carefully planned and completed to yield meaningful results.

Testing New Treatments

To accelerate drug development and enhance the capabilities of epilepsy researchers through formal collaboration, The Epilepsy Study Consortium, a nonprofit 503(c) corporation, was formed in 2007. The Consortium began with 11 core regional centers and expanded to 25 US centers and 25 European affiliates. Affiliates in Australia will soon join the list. Such a large number of epilepsy centers facilitates participation of experienced investigators who can readily identify patients with the appropriate epilepsy syndrome, seizure type, number of seizures, and other inclusion and exclusion criteria of a new trial.

Prompt and careful recruitment is crucial to the success of clinical trials. Consortium goals include early identification of promising drugs and early elimination of those less likely to deliver efficacy and tolerability. The Consortium handles administrative and other functions with 2 full-time and 1 part-time employee.

Progress So Far

According to Jacqueline French, MD, President of The Epilepsy Study Consortium and Director of Translational Research and Clinical Trials Epilepsy, Department of Neurology, New York University Comprehensive Epilepsy Center, New York, New York, the Consortium has completed 2 trials, provided the bulk of investigators for 2 others, written 4 protocols, and had major input into several others. The Consortium helps identify appropriate patients, trains investigators, and interacts with the US Food and Drug Administration to explore novel trial designs. For example, innovative therapies, such as intranasal AEDs and anti-inflammatories, may benefit from customized protocols. The Consortium is also examining trial designs that improve patient safety by reducing exposure to prolonged placebo periods.

Last year, the Consortium reported that older trials may suffer from patient misclassification, which may confuse results. Such misclassification could be prevented by additional expert oversight. Recently, the Consortium assisted with a proof of concept study for a potential new AED, VX-765, developed by Vertex Pharmaceuticals (Cambridge, Massachusetts). Data from this study were presented at the annual meeting of the American Epilepsy Society, December 2-6, 2011, Baltimore, Maryland. A single-dose proof-of-concept study of a new AED for patients with photosensitive epilepsy is currently recruiting.

A Greater Voice for Investigators

Dr. French observed, "Ultimately, it is the responsibility of the epilepsy community to ensure that clinical trials in the epilepsy space are performed appropriately, and that drugs which are ultimately capable of helping our patients arrive at the clinic accompanied by the most accurate clinical trial data acquired through trials that have been performed efficiently and ethically. Because the consortium represents a resource of capable investigators, we now have a much greater voice in trial design and methodology."

Dr. French added, "The response from the pharmaceutical industry has been very positive. They appreciate the fact that there is a knowledgeable source of information, and since we are a nonprofit, they have a certain trust that our ultimate motivation is to improve trials and help people with epilepsy."

Conclusions

The Epilepsy Study Consortium has filled an important niche by providing a reliable and capable resource of academicians and clinical investigators to assist with the design and execution of clinical trials of AEDs. Their concerted efforts promise to speed the process of AED approval from discovery in the chemistry laboratory to a little tablet that makes seizures go away.

Additional information
www.epilepsyconsortium.org

References

Kwan P, Brodie MJ. Early identification of refractory epilepsy. NEJM 2000;342:314-319.

Brodie MJ. Antiepileptic drug therapy the story so far. Seizure 2010;19:650-655.

Update May 23, 2013

The Epilepsy Study Consortium continues its work. The proof of concept photosensitive epilepsy trial has been completed and is being submitted for publication. Results for VX-765 are also forthcoming. The consortium has addressed suicidal ideation and behavior screening in intractable focal epilepsy in a recent paper. The consortium is also developing white papers to present to the FDA regarding new approaches for epilepsy drug approval. The Australian Epilepsy Clinical Trials Network (AECTN) is now aligned with the Epilepsy Study Consortium.

The Consortium recently co-sponsored the Antiepileptic Drug and Device Trials XII symposium, May 15-17, 2013, held in Aventura, Florida. Other co-sponsors were the Epilepsy Therapy Project and the University of Pennsylvania. At the conference, Steven Schachter, MD, Professor of Neurology, Harvard Medical School and Utkan Demirci, PhD, Assistant Professor of Medicine Brigham and Women's Hospital, Harvard Medical School and Harvard-MIT Division of Health Sciences and Technology, received a $100,000 "Shark Tank" award to accelerate their research on a disposable microfluidic chip that can detect antiepileptic drug concentrations at the point of care inexpensively and with only a drop of blood from a finger prick.

Chapter 55

CLOBAZAM: A WELCOME NEW OPTION IN EPILEPSY THERAPY

January 5, 2012

Introduction

On October 21, 2011, the US Food and Drug Administration (FDA) approved clobazam (Onfi)* as adjunctive treatment for seizures associated with Lennox-Gastaut syndrome in adults and children aged 2 and older (Gandey 2011). This is good news for people with Lennox-Gastaut syndrome, and their families and physicians, because successful treatment of seizures associated with Lennox-Gastaut syndrome has been an elusive goal.

Lennox-Gastaut Syndrome

People with Lennox-Gastaut syndrome typically have mixed seizure types, developmental delay, and a specific pattern of slow spike and wave (≤ 2.5 Hz) on the electroencephalogram (EEG). Seizures usually begin in childhood before the age of 8 years and may follow infantile spasms. In Lennox-Gastaut syndrome, multiple seizure types such as atypical absence seizures, drop attacks, and nocturnal tonic seizures are often accompanied by disabilities such as blindness, cerebral palsy, hearing impairment and mental retardation, culminating in its designation as a "catastrophic epilepsy." Many etiologies may be responsible, including anoxic, cryptogenic, infectious, malformations of cortical development, metabolic, and post-traumatic. Although Lennox-Gastaut syndrome accounts for only about 4% of cases of childhood epilepsy, affected children are overrepresented in neurology clinics because of treatment-resistant seizures, behavioral problems, and multiple comorbidities. Drop attacks, which occur in at least 50% of patients, are particularly problematic because the sudden falls may result in facial and head injuries, often requiring the child to wear a protective, but stigmatizing helmet (Camfield 2011). Episodes of status epilepticus require frequent visits to the emergency department.

A Look at Clobazam
Clobazam, a 1,5-benzodiazepine, was approved for adjunctive therapy of epilepsy in children over 3 years old in Europe in 1975 (Camfield and Camfield 2010) and is available in over 100 countries (Gandey 2011). Clobazam is a benzodiazepine, the same family that includes familiar drugs used for acute seizure control such as diazepam (Valium) and lorazepam (Ativan). Clobazam acts as a gamma-aminobutyric acid alpha ($GABA_A$) receptor agonist. It is primarily metabolized in the liver by cytochrome P450 (CYP)3A4, which produces an active metabolite, N-desmethylclobazam. N-desmethylclobazam has a long half-life of 30-65 hours and is metabolized by CYP2C19 (Camfield and Camfield 2010).

Clinical Trials and Clinical Role
The FDA approval of clobazam was based on 2 recent studies (Conry et al. 2009 and Ng et al. 2011). In the first study, 68 patients (2-26 years) with Lennox-Gastaut syndrome received open-label low dose (0.25 mg/kg/day) or high dose

(1.0 mg/kg/day) clobazam for a 3-week titration, 4-week maintenance, and 3-week taper in addition to their usual treatment (Conry et al. 2009). Both doses significantly reduced the frequency of drop attacks, the low dose (p=0.01) and the high dose (p<0.0001). The high dose also significantly reduced nondrop seizures (p<0.0001).

The second study was a phase III, multicenter, randomized, double blind, placebo controlled, parallel group trial of 238 patients (aged 2-60 years) with childhood onset of Lennox-Gastaut syndrome (Ng et al. 2011). After a 4-week baseline, patients were titrated for 3 weeks and maintained on treatment for 12 weeks with either placebo, low dose (0.25 mg/kg/day), medium dose (0.5 mg/kg/day) or high dose (1.0 mg/kg/day) clobazam. Patients were then tapered off treatment over 2-3 weeks or entered into the extension phase. The mean percentage decrease in average weekly drop seizures from baseline to the maintenance period was 12.1% for placebo vs. 41.2% for low dose (p=0.01), 49.4% for medium dose (p=0.0015), and 68.3% for high dose (p<0.0001), demonstrating increasing efficacy with dose. Decreases in nondrop seizures were not significant. Adverse events that occurred notably more often with clobazam than placebo were somnolence, pyrexia, lethargy, drooling, and constipation.

Conclusions

Clobazam joins 5 other FDA-approved antiepileptic drugs for the treatment of Lennox-Gastaut syndrome: clonazepam, felbamate, lamotrigine, topiramate, and more recently, rufinamide. Valproate is traditionally used as well. However, despite multiple medications and attempts at seizure control with the ketogenic diet, vagus nerve stimulator, and epilepsy surgery, patients rarely become seizure free (Conry et al. 2009, Kanner et al. 2011). The long experience of clobazam use outside the United States suggests that this drug harbors no unpleasant surprises regarding safety or side effects. The FDA approval of clobazam represents a valuable additional tool for physicians to decrease drop attacks in their patients with Lennox-Gastaut syndrome. Clobazam is now available at retail pharmacies in the US.

*Manufactured by Catalent Pharma Solutions, Winchester, KY, and distributed by Lundbeck, Inc.

References

Gandey A. FDA approves clobazam add-on for Lennox Syndrome. http://www.medscape.com/viewarticle/752080, October 24, 2011.

Camfield PR. Definition and natural history of Lennox-Gastaut syndrome. Epilepsia 2011;52(Suppl 5):3-9.

Camfield CS, Camfield PR. Clobazam. In: Panayiotopoulos CP, ed. Atlas of Epilepsies. Springer-Verlag, London, 2010.

Conry JA, Ng YT, Paolicchi JM et al. Clobazam in the treatment of Lennox-Gastaut syndrome. Epilepsia 2009;50:1158-1166.

Ng YT, Conry JA, Drummond R et al. Randomized, phase III study results of clobazam in Lennox-Gastaut syndrome. Neurology 2011;77:1473-1481.

Kanner AM, Sankar R, Wilner A. Individualizing care of patients with Lennox-Gastaut syndrome: Current and emerging approaches to treatment. CME program, http://www.medscape.org/viewprogram/32149?src=0_mp_cment_0, 9/19/2011.

Chapter 56

"SMARTWATCH"-A NEW SEIZURE DETECTION DEVICE

December 7, 2011

Introduction

Wristwatch gadgets are no longer limited to imaginary characters like Dick Tracy and James Bond. A new device, dubbed the "SmartWatch," combines the new, commercially available technologies of Bluetooth, GPS, and 3-D accelerometers in order to detect shaking movements consistent with a convulsion and transmit a location signal to an Android cell phone.

The SmartWatch is an example of many advanced technologies displayed in the Exhibit Hall at the American Epilepsy Society meeting in Baltimore, MD, December 2-6, 2011. According to Anoo Nathan, President of Smart Monitor, Inc., the company behind SmartWatch, the new device is meant to be an "early warning system for a generalized tonic clonic seizure." When the watch detects a rapid rhythmic, repetitive motion that fits its programmed algorithm, it can send a text message, email, or even call a prespecified phone number. Another movement monitor at the Exhibit, made by EMFIT, is a sensor placed under a patient's mattress that can detect convulsions and set off an audible alarm.

Tool for Worried Parents

The SmartWatch can alert a parent or other caregiver of a child with epilepsy as soon as a seizure starts. GPS coordinates can also be sent, so that the location of the watch (and the child) can be viewed on the recipient's cell phone. These alerts can make caregivers aware of all convulsions, even those that are unwitnessed because the child is alone, perhaps in bed, in the bathroom, or playing outside. In addition, if the wearer feels an aura coming on, an "emergency button" can be pressed that transmits an alert. When an alert is sent, the SmartWatch also vibrates. If the alert was accidental, the wearer can cancel it.

"Snooze Mode"

If the wearer is going to engage in an activity that might inadvertently trigger the device, such as climbing or running, the SmartWatch can be put in "snooze" mode, where it is temporarily disabled for 10 minutes. It automatically resumes functioning when the "snooze" period is over.

Programmable

Seizure detection parameters such as duration and sensitivity are programmed into the SmartWatch's algorithm via an Android cell phone using Bluetooth. Sensitivity is adjusted to prevent normal activities such as walking or climbing from setting off an alert. Data from seizure alerts can be archived and shared later with the patient's physician. The rechargeable battery lasts about 2 days.

Testing

The SmartWatch was tested in the inpatient epilepsy monitoring unit at Stanford University, where its seizure detection correlated well with standard EEG/video monitoring (Lockman et al. 2011). Studies at the University of California, San Francisco, CA, are ongoing.

Robert Fisher, MD, Professor of Neurology and Neurological Sciences, Stanford University Medical Center, Stanford, CA, has assisted in the development of the SmartWatch as a paid consultant. Dr. Fisher cautioned, "The Smart Watch doesn't pick up partial complex seizures. It might conceivably be used to prevent SUDEP, but there is no experience with the watch in SUDEP."

Funding

Research grants that contributed to the development of the SmartWatch came from the Danny Did Foundation, which has a particular interest in SUDEP, as well as the Epilepsy Therapy Project.

Still in Development

The company expects to make SmartWatch available as a "movement monitor" in the first quarter of 2012. They will also seek Food and Drug Administration (FDA) approval as a seizure detector specifically for generalized tonic clonic seizures. The anticipated price is less than $1,000. In addition to telling time, other features such as temperature and weather forecasts may be added to the display.

Conclusions

The SmartWatch joins a growing number of home health biomonitoring devices made possible by the miniaturization of electronics and Internet connectivity. Once the parameters are set, the SmartWatch functions automatically, although it can be triggered by the wearer as well. While the price is not trivial, parents may find that the SmartWatch pays off in piece of mind regarding their awareness of unwitnessed convulsions. While some patients might find the GPS monitoring of their whereabouts intrusive, others may feel that the SmartWatch permits greater freedom from direct caregiver supervision. James Bond might not embrace the SmartWatch's close surveillance of his personal activities, but his mother would probably make him wear it.

References

Lockman J, Fisher RS, Olson DM. Detection of seizure-like movements using a wrist accelerometer. Epilepsy & Behavior 2011;20:638-641.

Update May 23, 2013

The SmartWatch is currently for sale in "standard" and "premium" versions. More information and an explanatory video appear on the company's product page: http://www.smart-monitor.com/products/.

Chapter 57

OPTIMAL CONTRACEPTION IN WOMEN WITH EPILEPSY: ENTER FACEBOOK

November 16, 2011

Introduction: Epilepsy Birth Control Registry

Imagine how helpful it would be if there were a Website dedicated to education and research about birth control for women with epilepsy. The Website would collect information from women with epilepsy regarding their personal experiences with different types of birth control, effectiveness, and side effects as well as provide education regarding the advantages and disadvantages of specific types of contraception.

Thanks to the efforts of Andrew Herzog, MD, MSc, Anne David, MD, MPH, W. Allen Hauser, MD, the Epilepsy Foundation and other collaborators, the Epilepsy Birth Control Registry (www.epilepsybirthcontrolregistry.com) is up and running. Dr. Herzog, Professor of Neurology, Harvard Medical School, directs the Neuroendocrine Unit at Beth Israel Deaconess Medical Center, Boston, Massachusetts. Anne Davis, MD, MPH, Assistant Clinical Professor of Obstetrics and Gynecology at Columbia University, New York, New York, specializes in gynecology, family planning, and contraception. W. Allen Hauser, MD, Professor of Neurology and Epidemiology, Columbia

University, New York, New York, has published extensively on the epidemiology of epilepsy.

Origins and Goals

Dr. Herzog explained the origins of the Epilepsy Birth Control Registry, "One of the frequent questions that I am asked in my practice is, 'What is safe and effective birth control for women with epilepsy?' While there is some evidence-based information, the information remains sparse and does not cover the wide range of demographic, epilepsy, antiepileptic drug (AED) and birth control method variables...The ultimate goal of the project is to develop evidence-based guidelines for safe and effective practices for women with epilepsy, identify disparities in the availability and use of optimal contraceptive methods related to demographic factors, and develop educational interventions based on information from the registry."

Initial Research Results

The Epilepsy Birth Control Registry has leveraged the power of the Internet and social media to collect its surveys and disseminate epilepsy information by establishing a presence on Facebook and Epilepsy.com. Data have already been collected from 300 women who completed a 15 minute, 30 question survey. Here are some highlights of the findings so far:

Highly effective contraceptive methods were used by 68% of the 178 (59%) sexually active women at risk. Types of birth control included oral contraception (32.6%), intrauterine device (IUD) (15.8%), depo-medroxyprogesterone (DMPA) (7.3%), tubal ligation (4.5%), vasectomy (3.9%), ring (2.2%), and contraceptive implant (1.7%). Highly effective contraceptive methods were also used by 68% of the control population, but women with epilepsy were more likely to use oral contraceptives (32.6% vs. 25%) and IUDs (15.8% vs. 5%), while tubal ligation was more common in controls (24% vs. 4.5%).

When asked the top 3 reasons for selecting a particular birth control method, the women responded: 1) AED interaction (56.9%), 2) efficacy (52.6%), and 3) convenience (44.9%). These results indicate that many women with epilepsy are informed about the potential failure of hormonal birth control when combined with enzyme-inducing antiepileptic drugs. One reason for the increase in IUD use in women with epilepsy may be the lack of AED interaction with this form of birth control. Women taking enzyme-inducing AEDs were also less likely to use hormonal contraception than those taking nonenzyme-inducing AEDs or glucuronidated AEDs.

Additional Questions
Data collected by the Website will allow investigators to stratify responders by age, race, ethnicity, education, income, region of country, seizure type and other factors. The frequency of folic acid use will also be documented, as well as regional or socioeconomic disparities regarding types of contraception. Whether contraceptives affect seizure control or neuropsychiatric symptoms will also be explored. Because the registry is open to women all over the world, cultural and geographic differences regarding birth control will also be assessed.

Academic researchers may propose other research topics to the Epilepsy Birth Control Registry. If accepted, they will have the possibility to share the Website's database.

Confidentiality
The Website protects the confidentiality of women who participate. No identifiers are used except for the email address, which is used to contact the women for updates.

Education
Survey participants gain access to the Website's education materials designed for women with epilepsy.

Future Research and Conclusions
Approximately 100 women who participated in the initial survey will also complete quarterly 5-minute surveys to track their seizure control, report unplanned pregnancies, and contribute additional information regarding birth control. Women who participate in a follow-up survey will receive a $10 gift certificate from Amazon.com.

Conclusions
The long-term, Web-based epilepsy research pioneered by the Epilepsy Birth Control Registry has already provided interesting information and may prove to be a cost-effective and valuable approach for additional types of epilepsy research as well. Neurologists and others who care for women with epilepsy should encourage their patients to participate. More detail regarding research results from the Epilepsy Birth Control Registry can be found on Facebook. Dr. Herzog and his colleagues will also formally present their findings at this year's American Epilepsy Society annual meeting in Baltimore, Maryland, on December 4, 2011.

More Information
Epilepsy Birth Control Registry
www.epilepsybirthcontrolregistry.com
1-800-562-4789
EBCRinfo@gmail.com

Update May 23, 2013

The Epilepsy Birth Control Registry is still active on Facebook. More than 650 women have completed the birth control survey. Check out the site for more details: https://www.facebook.com/EpilepsyBirthControlRegistry.

Chapter 58

WHICH ANTIEPILEPTIC DRUGS WORK BEST?

October 17, 2011

Introduction: Which Antiepileptic Drugs Are Best for Seizures?

A wide range of antiepileptic drugs (AEDs) is available for the treatment of epilepsy (Table 1):

Table 1. Currently Available Antiepileptic Drugs

Old Drugs (since 1912)	New Drugs (since 1993)
Carbamazepine (Tegretol)	Ezogabine (Potiga)
Divalproex sodium (Depakote)	Felbamate (Felbatol)
Ethosuximide (Zarontin)	Gabapentin (Neurontin)
Phenobarbital (Luminal)	Lacosamide (Vimpat)
Phenytoin (Dilantin)	Lamotrigine (Lamictal)
Primidone (Mysoline)	Levetiracetam (Keppra)
Valproic acid (Depakene)	Oxcarbazepine (Trileptal)
	Pregabalin (Lyrica)
	Rufinamide (Banzel)
	Tiagabine (Gabitril)
	Topiramate (Topamax)
	Vigabatrin (Sabril)
	Zonisamide (Zonegran)

Since 1993, the US Food and Drug Administration (FDA) has approved 13 new AEDs, with more in the pipeline. As the number of therapeutic options has increased, choosing the best AED for a particular patient has become more challenging. With the exception of rufinamide, which is indicated uniquely for seizures associated with Lennox Gastaut syndrome, all of the new drugs are approved for the treatment of partial seizures.

Choosing an Antiepileptic Drug

Many factors must be considered when prescribing an AED for a particular patient including the patient's seizure type, epilepsy syndrome, history of allergies, medical and psychiatric comorbidities, potential drug-drug interactions, renal function, hepatic function, protein binding, possibility of pregnancy, dosing schedule, availability of liquid, parenteral and extended release formulations, pharmacogenetics, and cost. When AEDs are similar in efficacy, differences in tolerability often guide medication selection.

The growing science of pharmacogenetics has not yet provided new tools to predict drug efficacy in an individual patient (Johnson et al. 2011). However, pharmacogenetics does enable identification of Asian patients more likely to suffer carbamazepine-induced Stevens-Johnson syndrome and toxic epidermal necrolysis (Chen et al. 2011). These potentially life-threatening adverse reactions may be avoided by prospectively testing patients for the human leukocyte antigen-B*1502 allele.

Overall, only about 50% of patients with newly diagnosed seizures become seizure free with their first AED (Kwan and Brodie 2003). This sobering statistic emphasizes the importance of trying the drug most likely to succeed the first time around to prevent further seizures and their related medical and psychosocial morbidity.

Head-to-Head Trials

Additional information that would help physicians select the best AED for a given patient is data from head-to-head trials. This new study that compares pregabalin with lamotrigine is one of a growing list of valuable such trials (Kwan et al. 2011). A landmark head-to-head study that has strongly influenced epilepsy care is the Veterans Administration (VA) multicenter, monotherapy trial that compared the most widely used AEDs at the time: carbamazepine, phenobarbital, phenytoin, and primidone (Mattson et al. 1985). The VA study revealed that carbamazepine and phenytoin offer better total control of partial seizures, but that all 4 drugs had similar efficacy for secondarily generalized tonic clonic seizures.

A subsequent VA study concluded that carbamazepine had greater efficacy and fewer persistent side effects when treating complex partial seizures than valproate, but both were comparable for the treatment of secondarily generalized tonic clonic seizures (Mattson et al. 1992).

A prospective, multicenter, double blind, parallel group trial compared an older drug (controlled release carbamazepine) with a newer drug (levetiracetam) in patients with newly diagnosed epilepsy and determined "noninferiority" of levetiracetam (Brodie et al. 2007). Both drugs produced similar seizure free rates and incidence of adverse reactions. Side effect profiles differed, with more back pain in patients treated with controlled release carbamazepine and more depression and insomnia in patients taking levetiracetam.

Examples of other head-to-head trials include an open label comparison of lamotrigine and carbamazepine as monotherapy in patients with newly diagnosed or recurrent epilepsy, which concluded that both were equally effective, but lamotrigine was better tolerated (Reunanen et al. 1996). A study of elderly patients revealed that carbamazepine had the highest seizure-free rates, but patients treated with gabapentin or lamotrigine were more likely to remain in the study at 12 months (Rowan et al. 2005).

None of the newer drugs has been shown to control seizures better than any of the older drugs in a head-to-head trial (Kwan and Brodie 2003). However, new drugs offer different side effect profiles that affect tolerability. Comparative trials yield important information, but not necessarily the last word on drug choice. Factors such as dose selection, dose escalation schedules, use of immediate or controlled release preparations, and other variables in trial design may bias the results toward 1 drug or the other (Kwan et al. 2011).

Pregabalin vs. Lamotrigine

The authors of the aforementioned study comparing pregabalin with lamotrigine randomly assigned patients with newly diagnosed partial seizures to pregabalin (N=330) or lamotrigine (N=330) in a phase 3, double blind, multicenter study (Kwan et al. 2011). Patients began dosing with pregabalin 150 mg/day, which could be increased to 300 mg/day, 450 mg/day, or 600 mg/day. Lamotrigine was started at 100 mg/day, which could be increased to 200 mg/day, 400 mg/day, or 500 mg/day. More patients receiving lamotrigine (68%) reached the primary endpoint of seizure freedom for 6 or more months than patients on pregabalin (52%). The 5 most common adverse events were headache, dizziness, somnolence, fatigue, and weight increase, and were all more common in subjects on pregabalin than lamotrigine, although these differences were not statistically significant.

Pharmaceutical Sponsorship

Parenthetically, this Pfizer-sponsored study disproves the cynical notion professed by some that all comparative studies sponsored by pharmaceutical companies can be summarily dismissed because they always conclude that their drug is superior. Pfizer manufactures pregabalin.

Conclusions

Choosing an AED for a patient with epilepsy is a complex decision that must be individualized for each patient based on numerous factors including seizure type, epilepsy syndrome, comorbidities, and many other variables. An increasing number of head-to-head trials, although imperfect, offer guidance for the practitioner. The most recent study comparing pregabalin and lamotrigine in patients with newly diagnosed partial seizures suggests that while both AEDs have similar tolerability, lamotrigine provides better seizure control.

References

Johnson MR, Tan KCK, Kwan P, Brodie MJ. Newly diagnosed epilepsy and pharmacogenomics research: A step in the right direction. Epilepsy Behav 2011;22:3-8.

Chen P, Lin JJ, Lu CS et al. Carbamazepine-induced toxic effects and HLA-B*1502 screening in Taiwan. NEJM 2011;364:1126-1133.

Kwan P, Brodie MJ. Clinical trials of antiepileptic medications in newly diagnosed patients with epilepsy. Neurology 2003;60:S2-S12.

Kwan P, Brodie MJ, Kalviainen R et al. Efficacy and safety of pregabalin versus lamotrigine in patients with newly diagnosed partial seizures: a phase 3, double-blind, randomised, parallel-group trial. Lancet Neurol. 2011;10:881-890.

Mattson RH, Cramer JA, Collins JF et al. Comparison of carbamazepine, phenobarbital, phenytoin, and primidone in partial and secondarily generalized tonic-clonic seizures. NEJM 1985;313:145-151.

Mattson RH, Cramer JA, Collins JF and the Department of Veterans Affairs Epilepsy Cooperative Study No. 264 Group. A comparison of valproate with carbamazepine for the treatment of complex partial seizures and secondarily generalized tonic-clonic seizures in adults. NEJM 1992;327:765-771.

Brodie MJ, Perucca E, Ryvlin P et al. Comparison of levetiracetam and controlled-release carbamazepine in newly diagnosed epilepsy. Neurology 2007;68:402-408.

Reunanen M, Dam M, Yuen AWC. A randomized open multicenter comparative trial of lamotrigine and carbamazepine as monotherapy in patients with newly diagnosed or recurrent epilepsy. Epilepsy Res. 1996;23:149-155.

Rowan AJ, Ramsay RE, Collins JF et al. New onset geriatric epilepsy. A randomized study of gabapentin, lamotrigine, and carbamazepine. Neurology 2005;64:1868-1873.

Update May 23, 2013

Treatment options continue to multiply. Since this article was published, clobazam (Onfi) received FDA approval on October 21, 2011 (see Chapter 55) and perampanel (Fycompa) on October 23, 2012.

Chapter 59

VALPROIC ACID: A HAPPY ACCIDENT, AGAIN?

September 29, 2011

Introduction

A recent study suggested that patients with glioblastoma treated with radiation and temozolomide lived a few months longer if they were taking valproic acid for seizure control rather than an enzyme-inducing antiepileptic drug (AED) or no AED at all (Weller et al. 2011).

All of the patients had newly diagnosed glioblastoma and participated in a large randomized clinical trial of initial radiotherapy or radiotherapy with adjuvant temozolomide chemotherapy. Overall survival was 17.35 months in patients on valproic acid (N=49), 14.42 months on an enzyme-inducing AED (N=113), and 13.96 months on no AED (N=103). Benefits in the valproic acid group could not be explained by an increased number of patients with the O^6-methylguanine methyltransferase gene, which is associated with better response to temozolomide.

An Abundance of Serendipity

Could it be? Has valproate been discovered by accident as an anti-brain tumor drug?

If so, it would be at least the second time that valproic acid has accidentally been discovered as a useful drug for neurologic disease. In 1962, Pierre Eymard observed that valproic acid had potent anticonvulsant properties while using it as an organic solvent in rat epilepsy experiments (Sidhu and Cooper 2010). Valproic acid has a broad spectrum of activity and is now widely used for both partial and generalized seizures (Sidhu and Cooper 2010).

Or could it be the third time, because headache specialists noted that valproic acid could prevent migraine?

Of the fourth, because psychiatrists found that it also acts as a mood stabilizer in bipolar disorder?

A Devastating Disease
Glioblastoma multiforme has proven remarkably resistant to effective therapy, despite decades of oncologic research. The clinical course of my most recent patient with glioblastoma multiforme, an active businesswoman and mother in her 40s, was typically discouraging. She presented with partial seizures (initially believed to be panic attacks until she had a full-blown convulsion on her living room couch). Over the next few months, her seizures were well controlled with levetiracetam. However, despite aggressive medical and surgical therapy for her brain tumor, she was dead within 6 months.

How Does It Work?
Valproic acid has many mechanisms of action. The authors suggest that valproic acid may prolong survival because of its histone deacetylase-inhibiting property, thought to induce cell differentiation, growth arrest, and apoptosis (Weller et al. 2011). Valproic acid also enhances gamma-aminobutyric acid activity, binds to voltage-gated sodium channels, and inhibits low-voltage-activated (T-type) calcium channels. It

increases dopaminergic and serotonergic neurotransmission, which may be responsible for its mood-stabilizing effects. Other, as yet undefined, mechanisms including neuroprotection may exist as well (Sidhu and Cooper 2010). The possibility that valproic acid can prevent neurodegeneration in retinitis pigmentosa is currently being explored in a randomized, double blind, placebo controlled trial.

Downside

In the brain tumor study, patients taking valproic acid were more likely to develop thrombocytopenia (p=0.002), neutropenia (p=0.004), and leukopenia (p=0.03) than patients taking either an enzyme-inducing AED or no AED. In addition, valproic acid patients were nearly twice as likely to experience a delay of their adjuvant treatment compared with the other patient groups.

Valproic acid is associated with potentially fatal adverse reactions such as hepatitis and pancreatitis, as well as many other adverse effects including alopecia, gastrointestinal symptoms, tremor, and weight gain (Sidhu and Cooper 2010). Valproic acid also appears more teratogenic than other AEDs (Meador et al. 2006) and causes developmental delay (Meador et al. 2009). However, none of these adverse events would categorically preclude the use of valproic acid in glioblastoma if the upside were improved survival.

Need for Confirmation

An editorial accompanying the study urged caution before clinicians embrace the results of this unplanned retrospective analysis of an underpowered and nonrandomized study, particularly given the increased hematologic toxicity of valproic acid compared with other AEDs (Wen and Schiff 2011).

Of note, patients in the radiation treatment group without temozolomide had the opposite effects; overall survival with valproate was only 10.09 months (N=48), compared with patients on no AED who lived 11.96 months (N=72), and those on an enzyme-inducing AED who lived 12.48 months (N=139).

Additional information that discourages early acceptance of these findings comes from another study that concluded that enzyme-inducing AEDs were associated with "superior outcome of patients with glioblastoma" compared with patients receiving a nonenzyme-inducing AED (like valproate) or no AED (Jaeckle et al. 2009). However, in that study, 72% of the patients were treated with an enzyme-inducing AED, 26% were not taking AEDs, and only 2% were taking nonenzyme-inducing AEDs, which would have likely missed any beneficial effect of valproic acid.

Conclusions

Seizures occur in 30-50% of patients with glioblastoma, usually necessitating treatment with an AED. The study by Weller and colleagues provides an argument for the preferential selection of valproic acid for seizure control. If the superior survival of valproic acid-treated patients is borne out, one could even propose adding valproic acid as adjuvant therapy in patients with glioblastoma treated with temozolomide and radiation who did not require an AED for seizure control.

These provocative results require confirmation from future studies and set the stage for investigation into the mechanisms of action potentially responsible for any anti-tumor activity of valproic acid. Such research could lead to a novel approach to brain tumor treatment.

Valproic acid has proven effective in the treatment of seizures, migraine, and bipolar disorder. It would be yet another wonderful, serendipitous discovery if valproic acid improves survival from glioblastoma.

References

Weller M, Gorlia T, Caimcross JG et al. Prolonged survival with valproic acid use in the EORTC/NCIC temozolomide trial for glioblastoma. Neurology 2011;77:1156-1164.

Sidhu MK, Cooper PN. Valproate. In: CP Panayiotopoulos ed. Atlas of Epilepsies. Springer Verlag, London, 2010.

Meador KJ, Baker GA, Finnell RH et al. In utero antiepileptic drug exposure. Fetal death and malformations. Neurology 2006;67:407-412.

Meador KJ, Baker GA, Browning N et al. Cognitive function at 3 years of age after fetal exposure to antiepileptic drugs. NEJM 2009;360:1597-1605.

Wen PY, Schiff D. Valproic acid as the AED of choice for patients with glioblastoma? The jury is out. Neurology 2011;77:1114-1115.

Jaeckle KA, Ballman K, Furth A, Buckner JC. Correlation of enzyme-inducing anticonvulsant use with outcome of patients with glioblastoma. Neurology 2009;73:1207-1213.

Update May 24, 2013

A retrospective study of 31 patients with retinitis pigmentosa who received valproic acid suggested that the drug was primarily associated with *decline* in visual acuity and visual fields, not improvement. (This is contrary to initial findings that valproate was helpful for patients with retinitis pigmentosa.) In addition, more than a third of the patients suffered adverse effects related to valproic acid treatment (Bhalla et al. 2013). A Phase 2, randomized, controlled trial of oral valproic acid for retinitis pigmentosa, initiated in 2010, is still recruiting patients. The results of this trial should be more definitive regarding whether valproate is helpful or harmful in treating retinitis pigmentosa.

The experience with retinitis pigmentosa exemplifies the need for randomized, controlled studies before initial optimistic results, such as those reported for glioblastoma patients with valproate, should be adopted as standard of care.

Additional References
Bhalla S, Joshi D, Bhulla S et al. Long-term follow-up for efficacy and safety of treatment of retinitis pigmentosa with valproic acid. British Journal of Ophthalmology 2013;00:1-5, doi:10.1136/bjophthalmol-2013-303084.

Chapter 60

ANTIEPILEPTIC DRUGS AND BIRTH DEFECTS

August 31, 2011

Introduction

A recently published epidemiologic study suggests that prenatal exposure to any of 5 new antiepileptic drugs (AEDs) in the first trimester of pregnancy is not associated with major congenital malformations (Molgaard-Nielsen and Hviid 2011). This population-based cohort study compared the incidence of major congenital anomalies among 1,532 infants exposed to gabapentin, lamotrigine, levetiracetam, oxcarbazepine, or topiramate during the first trimester with the incidence of major anomalies in 836,263 control infants. Data came from the Danish Medical Birth Registry and included all Danish births from January 1, 1996, through September 30, 2008.

Major Congenital Malformations

The study included women who took antiepileptic drugs for epilepsy (N=1,164), migraine (N=34), mood disorders (N=28) and other conditions. Of the 1,532 infants exposed to one of the new AEDs during the first trimester, 49 had a major birth defect (3.2%). Of the 836,263 controls, 19,911 had a major birth defect (2.4%). After correction for confounding factors such as concomitant use of older-generation AEDs and the maternal diagnosis of epilepsy, these differences were not statistically significant.

Major congenital anomalies were defined in accordance with the European Surveillance of Congenital Anomalies (EUROCAT) registry and included abnormalities such as anophthalmos, bilateral renal agenesis, congenital heart disease, limb reduction, neural tube defects, oral-facial clefts and many others (EUROCAT 2011). Minor abnormalities (EUROCAT 2011) were not included. Infants with chromosomal aberrations, genetic disorders, birth defects with known causes such as the fetal alcohol syndrome, or aborted fetuses were also excluded.

New AEDs

The most commonly prescribed antiepileptic drugs were lamotrigine (N=1,019) and oxcarbazepine (N=393), followed by topiramate (N=108), gabapentin (N=59), and levetiracetam (N=58). When the drugs were examined individually, there were 4 instances of eye abnormality in fetuses exposed to lamotrigine, with an elevated adjusted prevalence odds ratio of 4.11. Each eye defect was etiologically different, prompting the authors to argue against a causal association.

An American Academy of Neurology Practice Parameter comprehensively addressed the issue of teratogenicity and AEDs (Harden et al. 2009)*. Overall, the panel concluded that AEDs taken during the first trimester "probably" increased the risk for major congenital malformations. Data were available to individually assess the risks of carbamazepine and valproate. Valproate monotherapy was "possibly" responsible and valproate polytherapy "probably" responsible for major congenital malformations. Conversely, carbamazepine "probably" did not substantially increase the risk. Further, valproate was "probably" associated with poor cognitive outcomes while carbamazepine "probably" was not. The panel recommended avoiding valproate during pregnancy. A subsequent prospective, multicenter, observational study revealed that fetal exposure to valproate resulted in significantly lower IQ at age 3 compared to carbamazepine, lamotrigine or phenytoin (Meador et al. 2009). The effect of valproate on lowering fetal IQ was dose dependent (Meador et al. 2009).

Study Limitations

Although the Danish study is the largest single analytic cohort to date, the numbers of exposures to individual drugs are too small to conclude that they are not associated with major malformations. (The association between eye abnormalities and lamotrigine appears to be significant, but was dismissed by the authors as "likely a chance finding.") The Danish data are also in conflict with the FDA's recent conclusion that topiramate is associated with an increased risk for oral clefts and warrants "category D" status, indicating "positive evidence of human fetal risk" (FDA News Release 2011).

Further, minor malformations were not included in this study, nor were cognitive problems such as developmental delay. Data regarding medication adherence and serum levels of the respective AEDs were not reviewed. Abortion information was also excluded, which could mask severe drug-induced congenital malformations that resulted in accidental or intentional pregnancy termination.

Conclusions

The Danish population-based study suggests that the new AEDs are not associated with major congenital malformations. Although these data are reassuring, there are multiple limitations. Indeed, the authors confess that they "cannot exclude teratogenic effects with certainty."

Regardless of whether an AED is "new" or "old," each drug should be evaluated individually, as suggested by the findings of the AAN Practice Parameter. The evidence-based practice parameter found conflicting results for 2 "old" drugs. Valproate was identified as a drug to avoid because of an increased risk for congenital malformations and developmental cognitive deficits, while carbamazepine (an even older drug) was not.

Women who are planning pregnancy or who are already pregnant should not take AEDs unless the benefits outweigh the risks. As is good general practice, physicians should reassess the need for AEDs in women of childbearing potential on a regular basis, and particularly in cases where the woman is considering pregnancy. The number of different AEDs should be decreased when possible, as polytherapy appears more teratogenic than monotherapy. For monotherapy, a lower dose is preferable to a higher dose, assuming that seizure control can be maintained. Close monitoring of adherence, dosage, and serum levels during pregnancy may improve seizure control and avoid excessive fetal exposure to AEDs. If seizures have been well controlled for a significant period of time, a trial without AEDs *before* the woman becomes pregnant may be indicated.

Continued accumulation of data from the ongoing pregnancy registries and more research on teratogenicity will assist physicians in choosing the safest AEDs for women of childbearing potential.

*I was one of the many co-authors of this AAN Practice Parameter.

References

Molgaard-Nielsen D, Hviid A. Newer-generation antiepileptic drugs and the risk of major birth defects. JAMA 2011;305:1996-2002.

EUROCAT. Coding of EUROCAT subgroups of congenital anomalies. http://www.eurocat-network.eu/content/EUROCAT-Definition-New-Subgroups-Feb-2007.pdf.

EUROCAT. Minor anomalies for exclusion. http://www.eurocat-network.eu/content/EUROCAT-Guide-1.3-Chapter-3.2.pdf.

Harden CL, Meador KJ, Pennell PB et al. Practice Parameter update: management issues for women with epilepsy-focus on pregnancy (an evidence-based review): teratogenesis and perinatal outcomes. Neurology 2009;73:133-141.

Meador KJ, Baker GA, Browning N et al. Cognitive function at 3 years of age after fetal exposure to antiepileptic drugs. NEJM 2009;360:1597-1605.

FDA News Release. Risk of oral birth defects in children born to mothers taking topiramate. http://www.fda.gov/NewsEvents/Newsroom/PressAnnouncements/ucm245594.htm, March 4, 2011.

Chapter 61

A NEW EPILEPSY THERAPY?

March 15, 2013

Introduction
The first double blind, randomized study of trigeminal nerve stimulation for the treatment of drug-resistant epilepsy was recently reported in the journal *Neurology* (Degiorgio et al. 2013). Although the results failed to meet any of the prespecified primary outcomes, there was a hint that this novel modality might have some promise for the treatment of both epilepsy and depression.

Unmet Need
Although the vast majority of people with epilepsy achieve seizure control with antiepileptic medications, approximately one quarter continue to have seizures that predispose them to injury, psychosocial problems, and premature death (Kwan et al. 2011). In addition to medications, several neuromodulatory approaches have been applied to the treatment of epilepsy, including deep-brain stimulation of the anterior nucleus of the thalamus (and other targets), responsive cortical neurostimulation with an implanted intracranial stimulator, transcranial magnetic stimulation, and vagus nerve stimulation (VNS). Of these neuromodulatory approaches, only VNS has received approval by the US Food and Drug Administration (FDA) for the treatment of

intractable epilepsy. VNS is also indicated for the treatment of refractory depression.

Theory

The trigeminal nerve is the largest cranial nerve, with 3 facial branches. It projects to the nucleus of the tractus solitarius in the brainstem, as does the vagus nerve. Projections of the nucleus tractus solitarius include the amygdala, hypothalamus, insula, lateral prefrontal cortex, and other regions. Both the trigeminal and vagus nerves also connect to the locus coeruleus and can influence the cortex through the ascending reticular activating system and other pathways. Consequently, exogenous trigeminal nerve stimulation may function similarly to VNS with respect to an antiepileptic effect.

Unlike the vagus nerve, the trigeminal nerve may be easily accessed on the skin of the face. This anatomical accessibility invites investigation of the trigeminal nerve as an alternative to VNS because the latter requires a surgical procedure in order to attach an electrode to the vagus nerve in the neck.

Methods

The study randomly assigned 50 patients with drug-resistant epilepsy to a treatment or an active-control group (Degiorgio et al. 2013). The treatment group received high-intensity trigeminal nerve stimulation (120 Hz and pulse duration <250 μsec) for at least 12 hours daily. The control group received stimulation at 2 Hz and a pulse duration of 50 μsec, 2 seconds on and 90 seconds off. External gel-based electrodes stimulated the right and left branches of the ophthalmic and supratrochlear branches of the trigeminal nerve.

Investigators assessed the patients at 6, 12, and 18 weeks. The active control paradigm insured that all participants had the experience of stimulation, with electrical parameters modeled after those of key VNS trials.

Overall, 84% of the patients completed the study. This included 23/25 (92%) patients in the treatment group and 19/25 (76%) in the control group.

Results

There were 3 primary outcome measures; change in seizure frequency, responder rate, and time to fourth seizure. With respect to seizure frequency, the median change in seizures per month was -1.4 in the treatment group and -0.5 in control participants. The responder rate, defined as at least 50% reduction in seizures, was 30.2% for the treatment group and 21% for control participants. Lastly, time to the fourth seizure increased by 2.5 days in the treatment group and decreased by 5 days in the control group. None of these differences between the study groups achieved statistical significance.

One possible sign of success was an increase in responder rate in the treatment group from 17.8% at 6 weeks to 40.5% at 18 weeks. The responder rate of the active control group showed an initial increase from 16% at 6 weeks to 31.5% at 12 weeks, but reverted to 15.6% at 18 weeks.

Scores on the Beck Depression Inventory improved significantly more in the treatment group, with a decline of 8.13 points vs. 3.95 points for the control group (p=0.002).

Adverse Events

The most common adverse events were skin irritation (14%), anxiety (4%) and headache (4%). There were no significant effects on heart rate or blood pressure, and no serious complications.

Study Limitations

Perhaps the most troubling limitation was a vast difference in seizure frequency at baseline between the treatment and control groups; a median frequency of 8.7 seizures per month in the treatment group vs. 4.8 in the control group. Although this was not statistically different, there is the possibility that these 2 groups would respond differently to treatment.

Blinding was also an issue. It is possible that patients talked with each other in the waiting room regarding their various experiences with stimulation, or that loss of blinding occurred through other mechanisms. However, such breaches would have been more likely to strengthen the study results, which still remained weak.

With respect to the statistically significant result of an improvement on the Beck Depression Inventory score, even this finding is suspect because the baseline scores were much higher in the treatment group (16.7) than the control group (12). This difference approached statistical significance at the onset (p=0.07).

Potential Missteps

Following the path of VNS in epilepsy treatment may not be without its drawbacks. Despite the implantation of more than 60,000 vagus nerve stimulators for the treatment of epilepsy since FDA approval in 1997, exactly how VNS works still remains under investigation. Indeed, there are those who question whether it works at all (Hoppe 2013).

Nonetheless, VNS effects on the central nervous system seem to be widespread. In addition to affecting the locus coeruleus, tractus solitarius, and reticular activating system, VNS may alter the activity of the thalamus, cortex and other structures (Schrader et al 2011). Ultimately, VNS may exert is antiepileptic effect by destabilizing hypersynchronous neuronal discharges that lead to epileptic seizures (Faught and Tatum 2013).

Conclusions

The results of this first double blind, randomized study of trigeminal nerve stimulation are disappointing. The study suffered from multiple limitations, including a small number of participants, a large difference in seizure frequency between the treatment and control groups at baseline, and near statistical difference in baseline Beck Depression Inventory scores. In addition, a certain leap of faith is required to accept that treatment and active control groups were truly blinded.

The effectiveness of VNS tends to improve over many months, and it may be that the study duration of 18 weeks was too short to demonstrate benefit from trigeminal nerve stimulation. The importance of a longer study can also be seen in the high variability in responder rates for the active control group; 16% at 6 weeks, 31.5% at 12 weeks (nearly doubled), and 15.6% at 18 weeks (back to baseline). Had the study concluded at 12 weeks, it would have demonstrated a dramatic placebo effect. To help compensate for the imperfect nature of the "active control" paradigm, a third control group, with no stimulation at all, would serve as an additional check against the natural variability of epileptic seizure frequency.

Although all participants had drug-resistant epilepsy, the information provided does not allow further analysis of whether some seizure etiologies, such as temporal lobe epilepsy, were more or less responsive to the intervention. It may be that a larger study would be required to see a differential effect regarding epilepsy type. Also, none of the patients had a vagus nerve stimulator. It would be of interest to discover whether the addition of trigeminal nerve stimulation to VNS had a positive or negative effect on seizure control or mood modulation. These observations could inform investigations into potential mechanisms of action as well.

Consequently, a larger and longer study would provide more information and help ascertain whether this study just missed demonstrating efficacy for seizure control. In addition, multiple neuropsychological measures should be included in future clinical trials in order to fully explore initial observations that trigeminal nerve stimulation alleviates depression in people with epilepsy. If trigeminal stimulation could improve seizure control or depression, or both, this new alternative to antiepileptic drug treatment would help improve the quality of life of many people with epilepsy.

References

Degiorgio CM, Soss J, Cook IA et al. Randomized controlled trial of trigeminal nerve stimulation for drug-resistant epilepsy. Neurology 2013;80:786-791.

Kwan P, Schachter SC, Brodie MJ. Drug-resistant epilepsy. NEJM 2011;365:919-926.

Hoppe C. Vagus nerve stimulation: urgent need for the critical reappraisal of clinical effectiveness. Seizure 2013;22:83-84.

Schrader LM, Cook IA, Miller PR et al. Trigeminal nerve stimulation in major depressive disorder: first proof of concept in an open pilot trial. Epilepsy Behav 2011;22:475-478.

Faught E, Tatum W. Trigeminal stimulation: a superhighway to the brain? Neurology 2013;80:780-781.

Chapter 62

MARIJUANA: A VIABLE EPILEPSY THERAPY?

June 9, 2011

Introduction: Epilepsy and Marijuana

During a recent TV episode of Dr. Oz, a woman stood up and claimed that "medicinal marijuana" had stopped her seizures. She had been unable to tolerate the "horrible medicine" her doctor had prescribed, but thanks to marijuana she was now a "productive member of society," able to take care of her 6 children and drive a car (Dr. Oz 2011). Following this TV episode, the American Epilepsy Society (AES) received a number of telephone inquiries regarding the treatment of epilepsy with marijuana (American Epilepsy Society 2011).

A Medicine for Epilepsy?

Marijuana (*Cannabis sativa*) is a hemp plant that has been used for making rope for 300 years (Girling and Fraser 2011). Marijuana is not approved by the US Food and Drug Administration (FDA) for the treatment of epilepsy or any other medical condition. However, 15 states (Alaska, Arizona, California, Colorado, Hawaii, Maine, Michigan, Montana, Nevada, New Jersey, New Mexico, Oregon, Rhode Island, Vermont, and Washington) now permit its medicinal use (Susman 2011). This is an increase from 10 states in 2004 (Sirven and Berg 2004).

In Canada, the Marijuana Medical Access Regulations allow the prescription of marijuana for specific conditions including arthritis, cancer, epilepsy, HIV, multiple sclerosis, spinal cord injury and disease, and terminal illness (Sirven and Berg 2004). A telephone survey and chart review of patients in the University of Alberta Epilepsy Clinic database revealed that 21% of patients had used marijuana the prior year (Gross et al. 2004). More than half (54%) reported a decrease in seizure frequency, while 46% found no effect. Sixty-eight percent reported improvement in seizure severity and 32% reported no effect. There were no reports that marijuana worsened either seizure frequency or severity. Overall, 24% believed it was an effective therapy. Four subjects (3%) met DSM-IV criteria for marijuana dependence.

Schedule I and the DEA

The FDA considers marijuana a Schedule I drug under the Controlled Substances Act (FDA 2004). Other Schedule I drugs include gamma hydroxybutyric acid (GHB), lysergic acid diethylamide (LSD), methylfentanyl (China White), methylenedioxymethamphetamine (Ecstasy), phencyclohexylpyrrolidine (PCP), and many others (US Drug Enforcement Administration-Orange Book). Schedule I drugs have a high potential for abuse, no accepted medical use in the United States, and suffer from a lack of safety data (FDA 2004). The primary responsibility for enforcing the Controlled Substances Act rests with the US Drug Enforcement Administration (DEA). The FDA has concluded that there is "sound evidence that smoked marijuana is harmful" (FDA 2006). Further, the FDA argues that there are other alternatives (i.e., more than 15 FDA-approved antiepileptic drugs) that can be used while awaiting more data on marijuana for medicinal purposes (FDA 2006).

What Does the Research Show?

Research on medical uses of marijuana has been limited, in part because it was considered a political "hot potato," according to comments posted on the American Epilepsy Society Blog by Harvey Kupferberg, PhD, a retired researcher at the Epilepsy Branch, National Institute of Neurological Disorders and Stroke, National Institutes of Health (Kupferberg 2011). Dr. Kupferberg participated in the development of epilepsy drugs, including lacosamide (FDA approved) and retigabine (FDA approved as ezogabine).

Medical research can be performed on Schedule I drugs but faces more restrictions (FDA 2004). Research-grade marijuana can be obtained from the federal government under a specific protocol (FDA 2004). Despite these limitations, a search of www.clinicaltrials.gov lists 354 studies involving marijuana. None of them are for epilepsy.

Before the FDA will approve a drug for medicinal use, it must be shown to be "safe and effective." To achieve FDA approval, animal experiments, basic safety and dosing research in humans, and at least 2 scientifically controlled, large clinical trials that clearly document the drug's efficacy for a particular indication, such as epilepsy, as well as its side-effect profile are typically required. To date, there is no research on smoked marijuana that fulfills these requirements for epilepsy or any other medical condition.

Research on smoked marijuana for medicinal purposes is further complicated by the inherent variability in potency of the active ingredient, which tends to vary from plant to plant. In addition, smoked marijuana exposes the user to multiple harmful substances (FDA 2004).

However, these problems can be circumvented. In 1985, the FDA approved Marinol Capsules for chemotherapy-related nausea and vomiting. In 1992, the FDA added anorexia associated with weight loss in AIDS patients as another approved indication. The active ingredient of Marinol Capsules is dronabinol, a synthetic delta-9-tetrahydrocannabinol (THC), considered to be the major psychoactive ingredient of marijuana (FDA 2004). The synthetic dronabinol allows for dose standardization and the capsule eliminates the problem of smoke and associated toxin inhalation.

With respect to the treatment of epilepsy, animal studies have suggested both anticonvulsant and proconvulsant properties of THC (Sirven and Berg 2004). A recent article described the development of seizures and other medical complications in 3 green iguanas that ingested a large amount of cannabis (Girling and Fraser 2011). Clinical evidence for efficacy of marijuana for seizure control is sparse and contradictory. For example, an early case report described a 24 year old man with intractable epilepsy who controlled his seizures when he began smoking marijuana in addition to taking phenytoin and phenobarbital (Consroe et al. 1975). The marijuana alone was not effective, as he had breakthrough seizures several days after running out of his prescribed medicines. Conversely, an earlier case report described an exacerbation of grand mal convulsions in a 20 year old man who smoked marijuana (Consroe et al. 1975).

Conclusions

An evidence-based medicine approach to therapeutics requires scientific demonstration of a drug's efficacy as well as knowledge of short- and long-term adverse events that must be balanced against the drug's potential benefits. All of this information is lacking regarding the effects of smoking marijuana in the treatment of epilepsy. More research is needed before patients should consider marijuana for seizure relief, particularly because this represents criminal activity under US federal law and may be accompanied by adverse medical (and legal) events.

References

Dr. Oz. Medical marijuana: Why it's prescribed, Part II. http://www.doctoroz.com/videos/marijuana-why-it-s prescribed-pt-2.

American Epilepsy Society. Marijuana and epilepsy. eNews, April 13, 2011.

Girling SJ, Fraser MA. Cannabis intoxication in three green iguanas (Iguana iguana). J Small Animal Practice 2011;52:113-116.

Susman E. Docs get advice on medical marijuana. http://www.medpagetoday.com/MeetingCoverage/ AAPM/25601, March 29, 2011.

Sirven JI, Berg AT. Marijuana as a treatment for epilepsy and multiple sclerosis? Neurology 2004;62:1924-1925.

Gross DW, Hamm J, Ashworth NL, Quigley D. Marijuana use and epilepsy. Prevalence in patients of a tertiary care epilepsy center. Neurology 2004;62:2095-2097.

US Food and Drug Administration. Potential merits of cannabinoids for medical uses. http://www.fda.gov/NewsEvents/Testimony/ucm114741.htm, April 1, 2004.

US Drug Enforcement Administration. Drug Scheduling. http://www.deadiversion.usdoj.gov/schedules/orange-book/orangebook.pdf.

US Food and Drug Administration. Inter-agency advisory regarding claims that smoked marijuana is a medicine. http://www.fda.gov/NewsEvents/Newsroom/PressAnnouncements/2006/ucm108643.htm, April 20, 2006.

Kupferberg H. Comments. http://connect.aesnet.org/AESNET/AESNET/Blogs/BlogViewer/Default.aspx?BlogKey=4a223123-66e6-42d5-9416-3f91abfb98b3, April 13, 2011.

Consroe PF, Wood GC, Buchsbaum H. Anticonvulsant nature of marihuana smoking. JAMA 1975;234:306-307.

Chapter 63

DANGERS OF EPILEPSY: A POPULATION STUDY

April 15, 2011

Introduction

A new study reveals that people with epilepsy are at higher risk for motor vehicle accidents, attempted or completed suicides, and injuries inflicted by others (Kwon et al. 2011). Kwon and coworkers compared the medical records of 10,240 people with epilepsy with the records of 40,960 age- and sex-matched controls who lived in the Alberta Health Services Calgary Zone in Alberta, Canada.

The 1-year incidence of motor vehicle accidents, attempted or completed suicides, and injuries inflicted by others was increased for people with epilepsy compared with the control population ($p<0.001$ for all). The odds ratio (OR) for motor vehicle accidents was 1.83, for attempted or completed suicides, 4.32, and for injuries inflicted by others, the OR was 3.54. However, after adjusting for comorbidities, including psychiatric conditions, only inflicted injuries remained significantly elevated in the epilepsy population, with an OR of 1.46.

Mortality and Morbidity

It is well known that people with epilepsy face increased mortality, estimated between 1.6-9.3 times higher than that of the general population (Nouri and Balish 2011, Ottman et al. 2011). Causes of mortality include the underlying neurologic cause of epilepsy, sudden unexpected death in epilepsy (SUDEP), accidents during an epileptic attack, status epilepticus, suicide, and iatrogenic death (Ottman et al. 2011). Physicians routinely counsel people with uncontrolled seizures to avoid driving, climbing, swimming, working with dangerous machinery and other activities that place the patient at risk for injury or death should an ill-timed seizure occur. People with epilepsy have a higher prevalence of comorbidities, particularly neuropsychiatric disorders such as anxiety, depression and pain (Sillanpaa and Shinnar 2010). These comorbidities may be responsible for some of the increased morbidity and mortality associated with epilepsy.

Violence

The finding that people with epilepsy are more likely to be victims of violence, even after controlling for multiple comorbidities, exposes a hidden aspect of the trials and tribulations of living with epilepsy (Drazkowski and Sirven 2011). Why are people with epilepsy more likely to suffer from violence? Is it because they are defenseless after a seizure? To what extent is stigma responsible (Wilner 2010) (see Chapter 70)? Are caregivers or family members abusive toward the individual with epilepsy? Is their behavior somehow more aggressive (or perceived that way) and likely to engender violence? Is low socioeconomic status a contributing factor?

Study Limitations

Although the researchers carefully matched patients and controls for age and sex, they did not control for socioeconomic disparities. This is an important omission, because low socioeconomic status is associated with an increase in violence (American Psychological Association). People with epilepsy may have lower income (Ottman et al. 2011) and higher rates of unemployment (Jennum et al. 2011). Consequently, it is still unclear whether epilepsy, low socioeconomic status, or some other factor or combination of factors is responsible for the increased number of violent assaults detected in the epilepsy population.

Implications for Practice and Research
In the univariate analysis, this study demonstrated a significantly increased risk for motor vehicle accidents, suicide attempts and suicides, and violence against people with epilepsy. Further analysis indicated that motor vehicle accidents as well as suicide attempts and suicides were related to comorbidities rather than the epilepsy itself. However, patients cannot separate their index disease (i.e., epilepsy) from their comorbidities and must live with both. Consequently, in addition to trying to control seizures, physicians should aggressively treat comorbidities, including psychiatric disease. Routine screening for mental illness, more referrals to psychiatrists, and increased psychiatric training for neurologists and others who care for people with epilepsy are indicated (Boro and Haut 2003).

The researchers concluded that comorbidities were not responsible for injuries inflicted by others on people with epilepsy. This finding needs confirmation in additional populations with an exploration of the contribution of socioeconomic and other variables. Regardless of the etiology, the observation of increased violent assaults against people with epilepsy highlights the need for violence prevention and psychosocial support for this vulnerable population.

References

Kwon C, Liu M, Quan H et al. Motor vehicle accidents, suicides, and assaults in epilepsy. A population based study. Neurology 2011;76:801-806.

Nouri S, Balish M. Sudden unexpected death in epilepsy. eMedicine. http://emedicine.medscape.com/article/1187111-overview, updated January 21, 2011.

Ottman R, Lipton RB, Ettinger AB et al. Comorbidities of epilepsy: results from the epilepsy comorbidities and health (EPIC) survey. Epilepsia 2011;52:308-315.

Sillanpaa M and Shinnar S. Long-term mortality in childhood-onset epilepsy. NEJM 2010;363:2522-2529.

Drazkowski JF, Sirven JI. Motor vehicle crashes, suicides, and assaults. The dangers of epilepsy? Neurology 2011;76:770-771.

Wilner AN. Epilepsy in 2010: does stigma still exist? Medscape Neurology & Neurosurgery. http://www.medscape.com/viewarticle/725720, July 29, 2010.

American Psychological Association. Violence and socio-economic status. Fact sheet. http://www.apa.org/pi/ses/resources/publications/factsheet-violence.pdf.

Jennum P, Gyllenborg J, Kjellberg J. The social and economic consequences of epilepsy: a controlled national study. Epilepsia 2011, January 28 (Epub ahead of print).

Boro A, Haut S. Medical comorbidities in the treatment of epilepsy. Epilepsy Behav 2003;4:2-12.

Chapter 64

MANAGING NONCONVULSIVE SEIZURES IN THE PICU

March 28, 2011

Introduction: How Common Are Nonconvulsive Seizures in Children?

In a recent study by Abend and colleagues, 100 children (52 girls, 48 boys, median age 2.9 years) with encephalopathy were monitored with continuous electroencephalographic (EEG)/video in the pediatric intensive care unit (PICU) (Abend et al. 2011). Nearly half (46/100) of the children were found to have nonconvulsive epileptic seizures.

Indications for Continuous EEG

In this study, indications for continuous EEG/video monitoring were "persisting altered mental status after a convulsion, altered mental status without a preceding convulsion that either had an unclear etiology or was disproportionate to the known medical condition, and the presence of abnormal movements or vital sign fluctuations." Diagnoses included hypoxic-ischemic encephalopathy (N=31), epilepsy (N=24), central nervous system infection (N=10), traumatic brain injury (N=7), stroke (N=7), neurosurgery (N=5) and other (N=16).

Silent Seizures

The key finding of this study was that electrographic seizures occurred in 46 children and electrographic status epilepticus occurred in 19 children.

It could be argued that if a patient has both convulsive and nonconvulsive ("subclinical," "electrographic") seizures, the nonconvulsive variety is relatively unimportant, because treatment would probably be instituted for clinical seizures anyway. However, of the 19 patients with nonconvulsive status epilepticus, 12 (63%) had exclusively nonconvulsive seizures. Of the 27 patients with nonconvulsive seizures (but not status), 20 (74%) had exclusively nonconvulsive seizures. Overall, 32/46 (70%) of children had exclusively nonconvulsive seizures, which by definition would not have been recognized without EEG monitoring.

Iatrogenic paralysis can mask clinical seizures. However, only 4 patients with seizures received paralyzing agents (2 children with exclusively nonconvulsive seizures and 2 with both nonconvulsive and clinical seizures) Consequently, iatrogenic paralysis could only account for missing 2/32 (6%) of the patients with exclusively nonconvulsive seizures.

The Nonconvulsive Seizure

According to Abend and associates, epileptic activity without clinical accompaniment had to last at least 10 seconds on the EEG to be considered a "nonconvulsive seizure" and at least 30 minutes to be considered "nonconvulsive status epilepticus." Frequent electrographic seizures that amounted to more than 30 minutes of seizure activity within an hour were also counted as nonconvulsive status epilepticus. The high percentage of children with nonconvulsive seizures does not appear attributable to "EEG overreading," as periodic lateralized epileptiform discharges were specifically excluded.

Duration of Monitoring

Because only 52% of the patients had seizures detected during the first hour of monitoring, a routine 30 minute EEG would have missed many children with nonconvulsive seizures. However, most (87%) of the convulsive and non-convulsive seizures occurred during the first 24 hours of monitoring, suggesting that a single day of monitoring might be a practical compromise if resources are limited. Specific clinical situations, such as an increase in seizures during the rewarming phase of children treated with therapeutic hypo-thermia, may require an extended monitoring protocol.

Practicality

Arguments in favor of continuous EEG monitoring include the fact that it is noninvasive and poses no risk for harm to the patient. Current digital server-based EEG systems al-low local and distant record review over the Internet, im-proving the practicality of continuous EEG monitoring. However, monitoring is labor intensive, requiring skilled technicians for the application and maintenance of elec-trode contacts (Hahn 2011). Proper interpretation of these records requires significant training, can be time consum-ing, and must be done promptly for the recordings to have clinical value.

Risk Factors

The only risk factor for seizures in this study was younger age. Seizures occurred in 56% of children younger than 1 year old, 43% of children 1-5 years old, and 40% of children older than 5 years. Surprisingly, a history of epilepsy did not prove to be a risk factor for seizures in the PICU. Of the

20/100 (20%) patients with a history of seizures, 10 (50%) had seizures and 10 (50%) did not.

Outcomes
The key question is whether detection and subsequent treatment of nonconvulsive seizures change the outcome of critically ill children with encephalopathy (Hahn 2011). In adults, ICU mortality has been associated with delay to diagnosis and duration of nonconvulsive status epilepticus (Young et al. 1996). However, the attractive hypothesis that suppression of nonconvulsive seizures in critically ill patients is neuroprotective has not been proven.

A Window Into the Brain
In this prospective study, nonconvulsive epileptic seizures commonly occurred in children with encephalopathy who were hospitalized in the pediatric intensive care unit. More than two-thirds of these children had exclusively nonconvulsive seizures. These data demonstrate that EEG monitoring provides a window into brain function that is far superior for seizure detection than routine clinical observation.

Why younger children were at greater risk for seizures should be investigated. What is different about their pathophysiology? Could the answer to this question lead to more effective antiepileptic treatments?

"Common sense" dictates that suppressing abnormal electrical activity, particularly nonconvulsive status epilepticus, to limit brain injury is the correct therapeutic approach. However, further research on outcomes is necessary to support a blanket recommendation for continuous EEG/video monitoring of children (or adults) with encephalopathy in the ICU. Clinical trials to produce such data are possible, but will not be easy to perform. Until such data become available, physicians must rely on their training and instincts with respect to the diagnosis and treatment of nonconvulsive seizures in the ICU.

References

Abend NS, Gutierrez-Colina AM, Topjan AA. Nonconvulsive seizures are common in critically ill children. Neurology 2011; February 9 (Epub ahead of print).

Hahn CD. Nonconvulsive seizures among critically ill children. Look and you shall find. Neurology 2011; February 9 (Epub ahead of print).

Young GB, Jordan KG, Doig GS. An assessment of nonconvulsive seizures in the intensive care unit using continuous EEG monitoring: An investigation of variables associated with mortality. Neurology 1996;47:83-89.

Chapter 65

CHILDHOOD-ONSET EPILEPSY TRIPLES RISK FOR DEATH

March 17, 2011

Introduction

Epilepsy has been defined as a "condition characterized by recurrent unprovoked seizures" (Hauser et al. 1993), but it is really much more than that. People with epilepsy may experience significant economic, medical, personal and societal burdens (Fountain et al. 2011). Even children with absence epilepsy, previously thought to be a "benign" condition, have an increased risk for poor psychosocial outcome, including alcohol abuse, inadvertent pregnancy, low employment skills, school failure and psychiatric disorders (Camfield and Camfield 2005). In addition, new data emphasize that epilepsy is a condition with increased mortality (Sillanpaa and Shinnar 2010).

New High-Quality Data

A recent long-term population-based, prospective study revealed that the death rate for children with epilepsy was triple that expected for the general population (Sillanpaa and Shinnar 2010). This study's 40 year follow-up and high autopsy rate (70%-80%) offer extraordinarily high-quality information. Nearly half (48%) of the patients with uncontrolled seizures died. Children with symptomatic epilepsy had significantly higher mortality rates (11.1/1,000 person years) compared with those who had idiopathic or crypto-genic epilepsy (3.2/1,000 person years, p<0.001). Children whose epilepsy was in 5 year remission on medications had lower mortality (5/35, 14%), and children with controlled seizures who were off medications for 5 years fared even better-only 4/103 (4%) in this category died.

Although some children with epilepsy do indeed "out-grow" their seizures, those who do not face continued risks to their health. This study emphasizes the potential lethality of childhood epilepsy, which is perhaps underappreciated by many physicians and others who provide care for people with epilepsy.

Importance of Seizure Freedom

In the study by Sillanpaa and Shinnar, patients who did not achieve 5 year terminal remission of their seizures experi-enced a significantly higher risk for death, whether cate-gorized as "all deaths," "epilepsy-related deaths," or "sud-den unexplained deaths" (Sillanpaa and Shinnar 2010). As if the consequences of continued seizures-injury, loss of driving privileges, and social embarrassment from uncon-trolled seizures-were not sufficient motivating factors, the increased risk for death in those with uncontrolled seizures provides more ammunition for physicians and caregivers to insist on 100% adherence with therapy. In addition, this elevated risk emphasizes that people with drug-resistant epilepsy who are appropriate candidates should consider epilepsy surgery, which offers the potential for seizure free-dom and a decreased risk for premature death (Sperling et al. 2010).

Mystery of Sudden Unexplained Death in Epilepsy

The possibility of sudden unexplained death in epilepsy (SUDEP) has been known for more than 200 years (Nouri and Balish 2011), but recently awareness of and research into this devastating problem have increased. SUDEP is responsible for 8%-17% of deaths in people with epilepsy (Nouri and Balish 2011). One reassuring note for parents from the findings of Sillanpaa and Shinnar is that SUDEP did not occur in children younger than 14 years old who had cryptogenic or idiopathic epilepsy.

The observation that SUDEP tended to occur in older individuals raises critical questions about the essential nature of SUDEP. Is it the duration of seizures that predisposes to SUDEP? Does childhood have some protective effect, or conversely, are hormonal changes associated with puberty essential for the development of the syndrome? Does progressive autonomic dysfunction related to recurrent seizures ultimately result in lethal asystole or apnea? An understanding of the pathophysiology of SUDEP may lead to other preventive strategies besides the obvious one of seizure control. Recent research in mice has identified KCNQ1 potassium channel mutations that may play a role in SUDEP and sudden death from the long QT syndrome (Goldman et al. 2009).

Research and Practice Implications
People with epilepsy face an increased risk of death from status epilepticus, accidents such as burns, drowning and head injury, exacerbation of comorbid heart and lung disease, from suicide, and SUDEP. The data collected by Sillanpaa and Shinar demonstrate that the best protection against premature death for people with epilepsy is seizure

freedom. This observation should raise the bar on the definition of "effective" epilepsy treatments. To date, none of the new antiepileptic drugs have offered seizure freedom to a significant number of people with drug-resistant epilepsy. For the many patients who have encephalitis, head trauma, or stroke, no treatments have yet been found to successfully limit epileptogenesis and reduce the risk for acquired epilepsy. Patient education on the increased mortality of epilepsy should be individualized according to the patient's risk and other factors, but this information should buttress arguments for improved medication adherence. Future research must continue to investigate the pathophysiology of epilepsy to develop interventions that will prevent epileptogenesis in patients at risk and achieve seizure freedom in those with epilepsy.

References

Hauser WA, Annegers JF, Kurland LT. Incidence of epilepsy and unprovoked seizures in Rochester, Minnesota: 1935-1984. Epilepsia 1993;34:453-468.

Fountain NB, Van Ness PC, Swain-Eng R et al. American Academy of Neurology Epilepsy Measure Development Panel and the American Medical Association-Convened Physician Consortium for Performance Improvement Independent Measure Development Process. Quality improvement in neurology: AAN epilepsy quality measures. Neurology 2011;76:94-99.

Camfield C, Camfield P. Management guidelines for children with idiopathic generalized epilepsy. Epilepsia 2005;46(Suppl 9):112-116.

Sillanpaa M, Shinnar S. Long-term mortality in childhood-onset epilepsy. NEJM 2010;363:2522-2529.

Sperling M, Durbhakula S, Stott L et al. Mortality after epilepsy surgery. Program and abstracts of the American Epilepsy Society 64th Annual Meeting, San Antonio, Texas, Abstract 2.320, December 3-7, 2010.

Nouri S, Balish M. Sudden unexpected death in epilepsy. eMedicine. http://emedicine.medscape.com/article/1187111-overview, January 21, 2011.

Goldman AM, Glasscock E, Yoo J et al. Arrhythmia in heart and brain: KCNQ1 mutations link epilepsy and sudden unexplained death. Sci Transl Med 2009;1:2ra6.

Chapter 66

FOLLOW THE PATH TO PROGRESS-WALK FOR EPILEPSY!

March 7, 2011

Introduction
The Epilepsy Foundation's 5th Annual Walk for Epilepsy will be held Sunday, March 27, 2011, at the National Mall in Washington, DC. This fundraising endeavor will raise money for advocacy, education, services, and research in epilepsy. The Annual Walk is the largest awareness event sponsored by the Epilepsy Foundation. Over the last 4 years, 25,000 people have participated in Annual Walks for Epilepsy and raised more than $4 million. A video with highlights of the 2008 Epilepsy walk can be viewed on the Epilepsy Foundation Website. Volunteers are needed to ensure the Walk's continued success, as well as sponsors and individual donations.

Global Campaign Against Epilepsy
In addition to its role as a fundraiser, the Annual Walk for Epilepsy supports the theme of the Global Campaign Against Epilepsy, a joint initiative of the World Health Organization, the International Bureau for Epilepsy, and the International League Against Epilepsy (ILAE) that intends to bring epilepsy "out of the shadows" by improving diagnosis, prevention, social acceptability and treatment. A walk in view of the nation's capitol brings the cause of epilepsy into broad daylight. The Global Campaign Against Epilepsy was launched

in 1997 with goals of "increasing public and professional awareness of epilepsy as a universal treatable brain disorder." The Campaign continued with a second phase beginning in 2001 "devoted primarily to activities that promote public and professional education about epilepsy, identify the needs of people with epilepsy on a national and regional basis, and encourage governments and departments of health to address the needs of people with epilepsy."

Improving quality of care is a priority for the Epilepsy Foundation, which has partnered with the Centers for Disease Control and Prevention and developed research programs such as the Managing Epilepsy Well Network. Other programs, such as "Get Seizure Smart," which was launched during last November's Epilepsy Month, strive to educate the public.

Battling the Stigma of Epilepsy
Like many other fundraising events, participants will have the option to wear commemorative t-shirts. In accordance with the "out of the shadows" theme, registrants may choose to indicate that they have epilepsy. If so, they will be issued a purple shirt instead of a white shirt, allowing them to announce that they have epilepsy and "are not ashamed." Although the battle against stigma has not been won, such frank openness about epilepsy is testimony to recent progress. Greg Grunberg, star of *Heroes* and *Love Bites*, is also the father of a child with epilepsy and has been the chair of the National Epilepsy Walk for the last 4 years. Grunberg has championed the cause of epilepsy by recruiting other celebrities such as Harrison Ford, Jeff Goldblum, and others, raising money with his "Band From TV" and contributing to public awareness with his Website "TalkAboutIt."

New Treatments, New Hope

Recent advances in epilepsy treatment include new drugs (i.e., lacosamide (Vimpat), rufinamide (Banzel), vigabatrin (Sabril)), improved predictors of seizure surgery success, research on brain stimulation (responsive neurostimulation and deep brain stimulation), an increased focus on psychiatric issues including depression and suicide, and a recommendation to avoid valproate in pregnancy because of teratogenicity and adverse cognitive outcomes (Rudzinski and Meador 2011). In a recent article, Steven Schachter, MD, Editor-in-Chief of the journal *Epilepsy & Behavior*, outlined goals for clinical and social management and research for the next 60 years (Schachter 2010). These include:

- Empowering people with epilepsy to become partners in managing their health
- Developing new biomarkers for diagnosis and treatment response
- Expanding access to surgery
- Finding ways to terminate seizures
- Avoiding the development of behavioral problems such as anxiety and depression
- Preventing death from status epilepticus, sudden unexpected death in epilepsy (SUDEP), and suicide
- Establishing affordable therapies for the global epilepsy population
- Increasing public knowledge about epilepsy

Dr. Schachter advocated expanding the current goal of "no seizures, no side effects," to "no seizures, no side effects, no comorbidities, no stigma."

Events like the National Epilepsy Walk and the continued efforts to inform healthcare providers, educators, social workers, as well as people with epilepsy and their families will continue to decrease stigma, raise money for research, and improve the physical, psychological, and social lives of people with epilepsy.

References

Rudzinski LA, Meador KJ. Epilepsy: five new things. Neurology 2011;76(7 Suppl 2):S20-S25.

Schachter S. What needs to change: goals for clinical and social management and research in the next 60 years. Seizure 2010;19:686-689.

Update May 25, 2013

The Epilepsy Foundation held its 7th National Walk for Epilepsy on April 20th, 2013. Photos are posted on the Epilepsy Foundation website. The next walk will be held on March 22, 2014.

Chapter 67

NEW EPILEPSY GUIDELINES: ARE THEY NECESSARY?

January 27, 2011

Introduction

The American Academy of Neurology (AAN) recently published eight epilepsy quality measures that were developed through the American Medical Association-convened Physician Consortium for Performance Improvement (PCPI) (Fountain et al. 2011). The guidelines were derived from literature published from 1998-2008 that included 160 recommendation statements from 19 sets of guidelines and 2 consensus papers. The 40 member expert panel concluded that, "It is anticipated that implementation of these performance measures will improve care for patients with epilepsy if adopted by providers." These performance benchmarks are listed below:

AAN and PCPI Approved Quality Measures

1. Document seizure type and frequency

2. Document epilepsy etiology or syndrome

3. Review EEG

4. Review CT or MRI

5. Discuss antiepileptic drug side effects

6. Refer patients with drug-resistant epilepsy for surgery

7. Counsel about safety from seizures

8. Counsel women of childbearing potential

Physicians, physician assistants, nurse practitioners, nurses and other healthcare providers all desire the best care for their patients. What "best care" entails depends upon the provider's best judgment. The AAN, promoter of the new epilepsy quality measures, agrees. "The AAN recognizes that specific patient care decisions are the prerogative of the patient and the physician caring for the patient, based on all of the circumstances involved" (Harden et al. 2009).

A Solution Searching for a Problem

Whether formal guidelines are needed for "quality improvement" in epilepsy care has not been demonstrated. The eight recommendations approved by the AAN and the PCPI are fundamental to the care of people with epilepsy. It is unimaginable that any epileptologist does not already follow these eight recommendations, which begs the question: why are recommendations needed in the first place?

Part of the AAN's justification is that these quality measures fulfill the American Board of Psychiatry and Neurology's performance in practice maintenance of certification requirement for neurologists. The implication is that some neurologists are not following these basic tenets of care. Are there actually neurologists caring for epilepsy patients without following these guidelines? If so, who are they, which guidelines are not being followed, and why? If there is no evidence that neurologists are *not* providing good epilepsy practice, why should they have to prove the contrary for a "maintenance of certification" requirement? Aren't they already licensed? Aren't they already board eligible or certified as neurologists? Is some flaw assumed in their training? If the problem is the latter, efforts should be made to improve residency training, not encumber practitioners with more documentation requirements for imaginary deficiencies. If their training was adequate, does the AAN postulate that neurologists, after treating hundreds if not thousands of people with epilepsy since their certification years earlier, forgot these basic principles of care? Do these quality measures attempt to solve a problem that doesn't exist?

Practicality and Impact
Guideline #6 requires that patients with intractable epilepsy be considered for epilepsy surgery, and that this question be revisited and its outcome documented every 3 years. Although the recommendation may seem reasonable, I cannot imagine how physicians in private practice could possibly remember when they last had this discussion with each intractable epilepsy patient without a laborious chart review. One solution to fulfill this requirement would be to address the question, and document it, at every visit, largely a waste of time. Perhaps in some future world with sophisticated electronic medical records, such a requirement could be "flagged" to appear every 3 years, but this is not the state-of-the-art for most of us in 2011.

Even if new epilepsy guidelines are needed, it is not clear that they would significantly influence physician behavior. The 2003 American Academy of Neurology Practice

Parameter on surgery for intractable epilepsy (Engel et al. 2003) has so far failed to achieve its goal of getting patients referred earlier for surgery (Haneef et al. 2010). Why would this new guideline be any more effective?

Specialty Guidelines in Primary Care

Perhaps the Quality Measurement and Reporting Subcommittee of the AAN identified a need for these guidelines because many patients with epilepsy are cared for by primary care physicians who have little neurologic training. For this group, easily referenced "quality measures" may serve as valuable benchmarks to basic care. As mentioned above, most patients with drug-resistant epilepsy are not promptly referred for an epilepsy surgery evaluation (Haneef et al. 2010). Practice measure #6 addresses this deficiency. Recent data on teratogenicity of various antiepileptic drugs, their effects on hormonal contraception, and antiepileptic blood levels during pregnancy should be shared with women with epilepsy of childbearing potential, as recommended in practice measure #8.

Conclusions

Integration of the eight quality guidelines into medical school and residency curricula should be the next step to ensure that all providers have at least the basic tools to care for patients with epilepsy. For those who have already completed their training, CME programs that address these fundamental quality measures should be made available to primary care and other clinicians. New "quality improvement" guidelines for neurologists should be practical and reflect documented deficiencies in patient care, not hypothetical ones.

References

Fountain NB, Van Ness PC, Swain-Eng R et al. Quality improvement in neurology: AAN epilepsy quality measures: Report of the Quality Measurement and Reporting Subcommittee of the American Academy of Neurology. Neurology 2011;76:94-99.

Harden CL, Pennell PB, Koppel BS et al. Practice parameter update: management issues for women with epilepsy-focus on pregnancy (an evidence-based review): Vitamin K, folic acid, blood levels, and breastfeeding: report of the Quality Standards Subcommittee and Therapeutics and Technology Assessment Subcommittee of the American Academy of Neurology and American Epilepsy Society. Neurology 2009;73:142-149.

Engel J, Wiebe S, French J et al. Practice parameter: Temporal lobe and localized neocortical resections for epilepsy. Report of the Quality Standards Subcommittee of the American Academy of Neurology, in Association with the American Epilepsy Society and the American Association of Neurological Surgeons. Neurology 2003;60:538-547.

Haneef Z, Stern J, Dewar S, Engel J. Referral pattern for epilepsy surgery after evidence-based recommendations. A retrospective study. Neurology 2010;75:699-704.

Chapter 68

A GOLD MINE OF EPILEPSY RESOURCES

November 22, 2010

Introduction

Imagine a disorder that suddenly impairs your ability to speak, talk, think or walk. At any time, without warning, you could have a seizure, fall, and hurt yourself. To add insult to injury, you might suffer the indignity of urinary or fecal incontinence. When it's all over, you wake up not knowing where you are, with sore muscles and a throbbing headache. A seizure can occur when you are home alone or, possibly worse, when you are out in public with your friends or strangers. If uncontrolled, seizures probably prevent you from driving, working, and limit your ability to socialize. Anxiety, depression, and suicidal ideation may be part of the picture. Add to this grim scenario the problem of stigma (See Chapter 70), and it would be next to impossible to lead what most people would call "a normal life."

This is the difficult circumstance faced by many people who live with uncontrolled epilepsy. According to a US Centers for Disease Control and Prevention (CDC) surveillance study, epilepsy affects approximately 1% of adults in the United States.

New Treatments

Pharmaceutical research has recently delivered 3 epilepsy drugs - lacosamide (Vimpat), rufinamide (Banzel) and vigabatrin (Sabril) - that offer additional alternatives for seizure control. Another new medication, ezogabine, received approval from the US Food and Drug Administration (FDA) advisory board and may soon be available (see Chapters 46 and 47). In addition, a novel approach to seizure control is thalamic stimulation, which was recently approved in Europe. Thalamic stimulation also received FDA advisory board recommendation and is pending approval in the United States. In addition, research continues on the neuroresponsive stimulator, which may provide yet another strategy for epilepsy treatment.

Impact on Quality of Life

Despite these advances, approximately one-third of people with epilepsy still have seizures. Even those with controlled seizures must take daily medication, attend doctor's visits, submit to blood tests, limit their activities, and otherwise modify their lives. If they do have a seizure, coworkers, friends, and family members may not know what to do. As a result, bystanders may fail to help or, even worse, hurt someone with epilepsy by misguided efforts - such as putting something in the person's mouth.

November is National Epilepsy Awareness Month!

As part of National Epilepsy Awareness Month, the Epilepsy Foundation has embarked on a special education campaign, "Get Seizure Smart." Get Seizure Smart intends to improve public education in regard to seizure recognition, seizure types, and seizure first aid. Flyers for doctors' offices and other locations are available free of charge. The flyer features a short quiz.

Partners in Epilepsy Education
As part of its ongoing endeavor to improve epilepsy care and public education, the Epilepsy Foundation has formed a co-operative agreement with the CDC "to develop and implement programs to enhance epilepsy public awareness and promote partnerships, education, and communication at local and national levels." One such project is the Managing Epilepsy Well (MEW) Network, an alliance of the Epilepsy Foundation and four of the CDC's Prevention Research Centers (Emory University, Atlanta, Georgia; University of Texas Health Science Center, Houston, Texas; University of Washington, Seattle; and University of Michigan, Ann Arbor). According to the CDC, MEW's mission is "to advance the science related to epilepsy self-management by facilitating and implementing research, conducting research in collaboration with network and community stakeholders, and broadly disseminating the findings of research." MEW recently sponsored a Webinar on New Community-based Programs and e-tools for Depression Treatment and Epilepsy Self-management. Information presented in this recent Webinar is available in the November issue of *Epilepsy & Behavior.*

The Epilepsy Foundation and the CDC have also developed two online training programs, one for law enforcement and the other for fire and emergency medical service personnel. These education programs teach first responders to recognize seizures and provide first aid. They are available at the Public Health Foundation training network.

Conclusions and Resources

National Epilepsy Awareness Month highlights public education by the Epilepsy Foundation, CDC, physicians, healthcare workers, and others to combat ignorance and improve the safety and quality of life for people with epilepsy.

Centers for Disease Control and Prevention (www.cdc.gov)

Epilepsy Foundation (www.epilepsyfoundation.org)

La Epilepsia (Spanish) (www.epilepsyfoundation.org/epilepsia)

Epilepsy.com

www.drwilner.org

Update May 25, 2013

Thalamic stimulation and responsive neurostimulation have not yet received FDA approval.

Chapter 69

ASEPTIC MENINGITIS FROM LAMOTRIGINE-A NEW HEADACHE FOR PEOPLE WITH EPILEPSY?

September 8, 2010

Introduction: FDA Warning

On August 12, 2010, the US Food and Drug Administration (FDA) warned that lamotrigine (Lamictal) may cause aseptic meningitis. Updated prescribing information and patient medication guides from the manufacturer, GlaxoSmithKline, will soon be available.

According to Yolanda Fultz-Morris, from the FDA's Center for Drug Evaluation and Research, "Aseptic meningitis is a rare but serious side effect of Lamictal."

Clinical Presentation

Aseptic meningitis typically presents with symptoms of meningeal infection (i.e., fever, headache, stiff neck, lethargy, confusion, photophobia) resembling bacterial meningitis but with negative spinal fluid bacterial cultures. The cause is usually a virus, most commonly enterovirus. Other etiologies include mycobacteria, fungi, spirochetes, autoimmune disease, parameningeal infections, malignancies and medications (Up-to-Date 2010).

Medications are usually last on the list when considering possible etiologies for aseptic meningitis and remain a diagnosis of exclusion. Nonsteroidal anti-inflammatory drugs

(NSAIDs) such as ibuprofen are the most common medication causes (Nettis et al. 2003). Other offenders include antimicrobials such as trimethoprim-sulfamethoxazole, intravenous immunoglobulins, monoclonal antibodies, and vaccines (Nettis et al. 2003). Among antiepileptic drugs, carbamazepine has also been associated with aseptic meningitis (Simon et al. 1990).

There is no confirmatory test for lamotrigine-induced aseptic meningitis. A lamotrigine re-challenge is probably ill-advised, as symptoms may be more severe after re-exposure. Possible risk factors include systemic lupus erythematosis or other autoimmune diseases. The pathophysiology of lamotrigine-induced or other drug-induced aseptic meningitis is presumed to be an allergic or nonallergic hypersensitivity mechanism (Nettis et al. 2003).

In the Clinic

People with epilepsy often complain of headache, which may be due to comorbid migraine, postictal headache, or other causes (Haut et al. 2006). For many patients, particularly women of childbearing age, lamotrigine has become an appealing substitute for divalproex sodium (Depakote), which has recently received its own FDA warning regarding teratogenicity. The likelihood of aseptic meningitis in these patients is exceedingly rare, but it should be considered in the differential diagnosis when other symptoms of meningitis are present.

Lamictal is available in multiple preparations including immediate and extended release tablets. The FDA specifically cited the brand name Lamictal in its warning, but it is likely that the same rare, adverse effect will occur in newly available generic preparations as well. (This will be an interesting test of "generic bioequivalence.")

How Rare Is It?

Very, very rare. Between December 1994, when lamotrigine was approved, and November 2009, 40 cases of lamotrigine-induced aseptic meningitis were reported. During this time, 46 million prescriptions were dispensed, resulting in an estimated incidence of 0.87/1,000,000. To put this in perspective, it's less than half the odds of being struck by lightning in a given year.

All cases of lamotrigine-induced aseptic meningitis occurred within 42 days of starting the drug. Most patients required hospitalization, and symptoms usually resolved after the drug was discontinued. One patient died of possibly unrelated causes. Cerebrospinal fluid results were similar to other cases of drug-induced aseptic meningitis; mild to moderate pleocytosis, normal glucose, mild to moderate protein increase, and neutrophilic rather than lymphocytic predominance (Nettis et al. 2003).

Now that physicians have been alerted to the association between lamotrigine and aseptic meningitis, perhaps more cases will turn up. Physicians should not hesitate to report suspected cases to the FDA via Medwatch.

Reassurance

Physicians should reassure patients that the risk of developing aseptic meningitis from lamotrigine is literally less than 1 in a million. For those who have been taking lamotrigine for longer than 2 months, no increased risk for aseptic meningitis has been identified. While the FDA has informed physicians of this newly identified serious adverse event, issuing a "warning" for such an uncommon occurrence may create public hysteria when none is needed. Perhaps a footnote discussing adverse events might have been more appropriate. Whether every patient prescribed lamotrigine should be routinely informed of such a rare adverse reaction remains a judgment call. Physicians who feel obligated to share this warning with their already worried patients should advise evasive action for lightning strikes as well.

References

Up-To-Date Online, Last literature review version 18.2 May 2010. This topic last updated: February 5, 2010.

Nettis E, Calogiuri G, Colanardi MC et al. Drug-induced aseptic meningitis. Curr Drug Targets Immune Endocr Metabol Disord 2003;3:143-149.

Simon LT, Hsu B, Adomato BT. Carbamazepine-induced aseptic meningitis. Ann Intern Med 1990;112:627-628.

Haut SR, Bigal ME, Lipton RB. Chronic disorders with episodic manifestations: focus on epilepsy and migraine. Lancet Neurol 2006;5:148-157.

Update May 25, 2013

Shortly after I wrote this article I diagnosed a case of lamotrigine-induced meningitis that required hospitalization.

Chapter 70

EPILEPSY IN 2010-DOES STIGMA STILL EXIST?

July 29, 2010

Introduction

"My friend had it. My mommy told me to stay away from her because I could get it. I'm glad I don't have it."

Fourth-grader's response when asked, "What is epilepsy?"

The stigmatization of people with epilepsy dates back thousands of years (Kale 1997). While stigma literally means a "mark," in social terms it may be defined as "a distinguishing personal trait that is perceived as or actually is physically, socially, or psychologically disadvantageous" (Valeta and de Boer 2010). In an effort to clarify whether the problem of stigma still exists in the world of epilepsy, I queried several colleagues regarding their experience and viewpoints. A child neurologist referred me to one of his patients with epilepsy, who expressed yet another side of the story. Here is a brief summary of what I learned:

A Social Worker's Perspective

Patricia Gibson, MSSW, ACSW, Associate Professor, Wake Forest University School of Medicine, Winston-Salem, North Carolina, has been the Director of the Epilepsy Information Service since 1979. (I had the opportunity to work with Ms. Gibson for a number of years when I directed the Carolinas

Epilepsy Center in Charlotte, North Carolina.) I asked Pat for her perspective regarding stigma and epilepsy:

"When I first got out of school and started working with the state health department of Virginia, it was the children with epilepsy who touched me most and it was the stigma involved that made me want to do something about the unfairness of how people perceived their condition. Stigma basically just reflects ignorance of the disorder. Stigma continues to be alive and well, I am sorry to report, and it is my opinion that as long as we have human beings, there will probably be stigma. I have to say that from my observations, stigma is much reduced in comparison to when I first started working in the field of epilepsy in 1976. I seldom hear stories that can begin to compare with those of years ago. However, recently I got a call from an upset mother whose son was not allowed to go to the school prom because 'he might have a seizure there,' and from the distraught mother of a 4 year old who had been expelled from her church-sponsored daycare because 'we are not equipped to handle epilepsy,' even though the girl had yet to have a seizure in class! These are the kinds of situations we try and correct by providing information and training programs with educational materials. My program doesn't just teach about seizures, or first-aid, but also the importance of emotionally supporting and caring for others."

Evidence for Progress
Chrysostomos Panayiotopoulos, MD, PhD, FRCP, Consultant Emeritus, Department of Clinical Neurophysiology and Epilepsies, St. Thomas Hospital, London, United Kingdom, and Locum Consultant Neurologist in Epilepsies, John

Radcliffe Hospital, Oxford, United Kingdom, is the editor of a new epilepsy textbook, which includes an erudite chapter on stigma and discrimination. Dr. Panayiotopoulos commented:

"Despite some progress made mainly in developed countries, enacted and felt stigmata for people with epilepsy are still prominent in our society. Fear, misunderstanding, and the resulting social stigma and discrimination surrounding epilepsy often force people with this disorder into the shadows. Of course, today, we do not have any more eugenic sterilization programmes such as in Sweden (until 1975) and many states of the USA (until 1956) and laws that people with epilepsy are not allowed to marry (in the UK until 1970). However, in Europe and USA there is still a large number of people believing that epilepsy is a mental or untreated disorder and object to their children marrying a person with epilepsy. In many poor-resource countries, it is still believed that epilepsy is related to witchcraft, evil spirits, or sorcery, and the disease is contagious. The Global Campaign Against Epilepsy of the World Health Organization and Epilepsy Associations are raising the profile of epilepsies with governments and health system providers for better services and less discrimination."

Dr. Panayiotopoulos added, "Another aspect of the problem of stigma is that epilepsy is not one condition. Epilepsies are many syndromes and diseases of multitude and disparate causes, manifestations, prognoses and management. Individuals and their families are entitled to diagnosis, prognosis, and management that are specific and precise."

Where are the Celebrities?

Selim Benbadis, MD, Professor and Director, Comprehensive Epilepsy Program and Clinical Neurophysiology Laboratory, University of South Florida and Tampa General Hospital, Tampa, Florida, observed:

"There is definitely some stigma still going on. Certainly it is difficult to identify high profile celebrities to contribute to epilepsy research and care. Alzheimer's disease has Ronald Reagan, Parkinson's has Michael J. Fox, Progressive Supranuclear Palsy has Dudley Moore, etc. Yet, epilepsy is much more common than those disorders. It seems that people with epilepsy are less likely to talk about it. The few spokespersons that there are speak on behalf of their children. So there must still be a stigma."

(Note: Greg Grunberg of the TV show, "Heroes," has become an outspoken epilepsy advocate, no doubt motivated by his son Jake's struggle with epilepsy.)

Fear of Stigma May Perpetuate It

A college student with epilepsy since sixth grade offered her insights:

"My own grandparents went to the grave referring to the disease that had affected their son (my dad) as a toddler and me a teen as 'that disease,' refusing to even say the word, 'epilepsy.' In my generation, however, things are different. The stigma is perpetuated by ignorance among others and the overwhelming fear of stigma that people with epilepsy have. If our doctors are telling people not to say that they have epilepsy, instead calling it a 'seizure disorder,' and we avoid telling people of our mysterious condition at all costs, we are the ones creating the stigma. Most people who live unaffected by epilepsy don't know what to think about it. They take their cues from us. If we are open and honest about it, offering to educate them about the disease, we can easily dispel any trace of stigma surrounding epilepsy. After I had 3 tonic-clonic seizures during class, I decided that it was my responsibility to help my classmates understand that my seizures were not something they needed to fear. I explained the different types of seizures and went through seizure first aid. After that, everyone in my class took a genuine interest in how I was doing, and none of them ever teased me again. Everyone else I have met has acted the same way. If they understand what epilepsy is and how to respond to a seizure, they realize that it is nothing to be afraid of, especially when they see that people with epilepsy are real people, not just something to skim over in a health textbook."

Conclusions: Where Do We Stand on Stigma?

While the stigma of epilepsy still exists, reports from those who have been fighting this battle for decades suggest a definite decline. Persistent and increased education efforts have yielded encouraging results. Celebrities have been slow to embrace the cause of epilepsy, but this is starting to change. The Internet has allowed for wide distribution of information about epilepsy. The National Institute of Neurological Disorders and Stroke provides information about epilepsy on their Website, as well as links to many other organizations and resources such as Epilepsy.com. Organizations such as the Epilepsy Foundation, International Bureau for Epilepsy, and International League Against Epilepsy officially confront the barriers of stigma. Many healthcare professionals take on the task of epilepsy education in their day-to-day exchanges with patients, colleagues and the public.

The euphemism of "seizure disorder," long used to avoid the stigma of epilepsy, may well be counterproductive as suggested by the college student who has lived much of her life with epilepsy. As health professionals, we should carefully consider the merits of always using the medical term, "epilepsy."

Dr. Panayiotopoulos titled his new epilepsy textbook, *Atlas of Epilepsies*, because, as he rightly points out, "epilepsy" is not a single disease. This distinction is not merely semantics. As we refine our knowledge of this group of disorders and develop more specific treatments, the benefits of "splitting" will more clearly outweigh the ease of "lumping." Perhaps as we become more knowledgeable regarding the medical aspects of the epilepsies, including etiologies, pathophysiology, and prognosis, the veil of stigma through which many people with epilepsy are viewed will eventually fall away.

Incontrovertible evidence for the effectiveness of epilepsy education appears below in an eloquent letter by a fourth-grader who took Ms. Gibson's class a number of years ago.

"Dear Ms. Gibson,

I have learned a lot about epilepsy. Before you came, I did not know much about seizures. Now, I know what to do and what not to do. Your film and magazines helped me, too. I met someone a few days ago who is now my friend and when I found out she had epilepsy, I told her it wouldn't change our friendship. Thanks for helping me make a new friend!"

References

Kale R. Bringing epilepsy out of the shadows. BMJ 1997;315:2-3.

Valeta T, de Boer H. Stigma and discrimination in epilepsy. In: Panayiotopoulos CP, ed. Atlas of Epilepsies. Springer-Verlag, London, 2010.

Chapter 71

PROGRESS IN EPILEPSY: AN EXPERT INTERVIEW WITH CHRYSOSTOMOS P. PANAYIOTOPOULOS, MD

July 14, 2010

Introduction

Chrysostomos P. Panayiotopoulos, MD, is one of the world's leading experts on epilepsy. Over the past few decades he has witnessed-and participated in-great advances in epilepsy bench science, diagnosis, and management.

For the last 2 years, I have had the pleasure of volunteering as a section editor in the development of a formidable new 3-volume, 2,000 page book, *Atlas of Epilepsies*, conceived and edited by Dr. Tomis Panayiotopoulos.

Dr. Panayiotopoulos is also the editor of *A Clinical Guide to Epileptic Syndromes and Their Treatment*, as well as the author of more than 180 articles published in prestigious medical journals. He has described not one, but two epilepsy syndromes. The first is the eponymous "Panayiotopoulos Syndrome," an autonomic epilepsy specific to childhood. The second is "idiopathic generalized epilepsy with phantom absences," which is characterized by a triad of phantom absences, generalized tonic-clonic seizures, and absence status epilepticus.

Although Dr. Panayiotopoulos and I have never met in person, we have exchanged hundreds of emails. I have been awed by his encyclopedic knowledge of epilepsy, his clarity of thought, and unfailing graciousness. Now in his early 70s, Dr. Panayiotopoulos continues to treat people with epilepsy. I could not think of anyone better qualified to provide some perspective on the progress of epilepsy care. I interviewed him by email, and a selection of his responses are summarized below.

AW: How is it that you became a specialist in epilepsy?

Dr. Panayiotopoulos: From the early stages of my medical career, I was impressed by the kindness, loyalty, patience, and unmet needs of children and patients with epileptic seizures. I was also adversely impressed, frustrated, and sometimes angry that traditional medical teaching and attitudes to the diagnosis and management of epilepsies often differed from those applied in other medical conditions. The fundamental rules of diagnosis that apply in all other physical diseases were often ignored in epilepsies, resulting in avoidable morbidity and sometimes mortality.

AW: What has changed over the last 45 years in the treatment of epilepsy?

Dr. Panayiotopoulos: There have been spectacular advances in all fields of epilepsy, from basic research to clinical diagnosis, investigative procedures, epidemiology, etiology, genetics, comorbidities, psychosocial implications, and therapeutic options. The diagnosis of epilepsies has become more specific with the identification of epileptic syndromes, and the treatment has expanded beyond the control of seizures to include improvement of quality of life. The epilepsies have become an important part of pediatric and adult medicine, properly assessed and managed with the same rules as other medical diseases. Precise syndromic diagnosis, prognosis, and management for every patient are the ultimate and often achievable goal.

AW: How has neuroimaging such as computed tomography (CT) and magnetic resonance imaging (MRI) changed the practice of treating patients with epilepsy?

Dr. Panayiotopoulos: Modern structural and functional brain imaging methodologies have made a colossal impact on the diagnosis and management of epilepsies. The combination of appropriate new imaging techniques has led to greater insights into the pathophysiology underlying symptomatic epilepsy and has advanced our knowledge both to the cause and effect of epilepsies. In clinical practice, optimal brain imaging allows *in vivo* visualization of structural causes of epilepsies. MRI abnormalities are identified in 80% of patients with refractory focal seizures and 20% of patients with single unprovoked seizures or epilepsy in remission. MRI often adds new and important data in terms of characterizing the nature and extent of the underlying pathology and of identifying other lesions. Identification of a structural lesion often indicates the site of seizure onset. Hippocampal sclerosis may be reliably identified, whereas quantitative studies are useful for research and, in equivocal cases, clinical purposes. A range of malformations of cortical development may be determined. The proportion of cryptogenic cases of epilepsy has decreased with improvements in MRI hardware, signal acquisition techniques, and post-processing methodologies. Automated voxel-based analysis can identify subtle changes in the neocortex over time that are not evident on visual inspection. White matter tracts, including connections of eloquent areas, can be visualized with tractography and thus reduce the risks for surgery.

AW: Is electroencephalography (EEG) still important, even though it is a very old test?

Dr. Panayiotopoulos: The EEG, which is entirely harmless and relatively inexpensive, is the most important investigative tool in the diagnosis and management of epilepsies. The EEG is an integral part of the diagnostic process in epilepsies, and particularly the type of epileptic seizure or syndrome. It is mandatory for all patients with epileptic seizures, and there is more than enough justification for performing an EEG after the first seizure or in patients suspected of having epilepsy. However, for the EEG to provide accurate assessments, it must be properly performed by experienced technologists and carefully studied and interpreted in the context of a well-described clinical setting by experienced physicians.

AW: What work needs to be done to improve the care of people with epilepsy?

Dr. Panayiotopoulos: Heightening medical and social education about epilepsies is crucial. Inappropriate generalizations on epilepsies is the single most important factor of errors and failures in diagnosis and management. The practice parameter guidelines of the American Academy of Neurology are the best examples of how this can be achieved.

There are currently over 20 antiepileptic drugs and more are being developed, but there are still around 20% of patients with epilepsies that fail to achieve acceptable seizure control. Also, epileptic encephalopathies are largely pharmacoresistant, and adverse drug reactions are another major problem. The ultimate aim of drugs that prevent epileptogenesis and drugs that cure has not been satisfied.

Until then, and this may be a long way off, we depend on prophylactic antiepileptic drugs, which to be ideal (or near ideal), should be highly efficacious with little if any direct or indirect, acute or chronic, adverse drug reactions.

Chapter 72

EARTHQUAKE HIGHLIGHTS PROBLEM OF GLOBAL EPILEPSY

March 2, 2010

Introduction

On Monday, December 7, 2009, the Presidential Symposium at the 63rd American Epilepsy Society's Annual Meeting in Boston, Massachusetts, addressed the treatment of epilepsy worldwide, especially in developing countries.

Solomon Moshe, MD, incoming President of the International League Against Epilepsy (ILAE), observed that many millions of people with epilepsy around the world do not receive appropriate treatment, or any treatment at all, "This may be the biggest challenge and the biggest opportunity in the field of epilepsy today."

Pete Engel, MD, PhD, Past President of the American Epilepsy Society and ILAE, and author of *Global Issues for the Practicing Neurologist*, explained that people may receive suboptimal healthcare due to limited resources, paucity of physicians, poor transportation, unreliable drug supplies, tropical conditions, disease, lack of refrigeration, social unrest, and cultural beliefs that may be in conflict with Western medicine.

If ever there was a country that fits this description, it is Haiti.

On the afternoon of Tuesday, January 12, 2010, a 7.3 magnitude earthquake shattered the city of Port-au-Prince,

Haiti, leaving thousands of dead and wounded in the city's rubble. Even before the earthquake, many people in Haiti lived without shelter, plumbing, electricity, jobs, or schools. In what has been called the worst natural disaster to strike the Western Hemisphere in the past century, teams from around the world have come to Haiti to help, including Doctors Without Borders and Project Hope's floating hospital ship, the *USNS Comfort.* Volunteers from my own hospital, Lawrence and Memorial, In New London, Connecticut, also raised funds and flew down to assist.

There was one epilepsy clinic in the country, La Clinique d'Epilepsie de Port-au-Prince, and after the earthquake, it closed.

In addition to first aid, immediate needs for people with epilepsy include antiepileptic medications. Prior to the earthquake, many people had difficulty affording these medications. After the earthquake, with many pharmacies destroyed and money even more scarce, people with epilepsy are likely to have more seizures. Another developing problem is the occurrence of posttraumatic epilepsy due to head injuries in survivors.

Grass Technologies, a subsidiary of Astro-Med, Inc., has stepped in to donate a $20,000 portable EEG machine that can be used in the field and the hospital to help evaluate people with head injuries and altered states of consciousness. (The hospital has no EEG machine due to the risk for theft.)

The Port-au-Prince Epilepsy Clinic reopened on January 25, 2010. Lionel Carmant, MD, Director of the Epilepsy Clinic and Epilepsy Research at Saint Justine Hospital in Montreal, Canada, coordinates the international effort supporting the Port-au-Prince clinic.

Dr. Carmant, a pediatric neurologist and native of Haiti, explained that the epilepsy clinic opened in June, 2008, thanks to a $6,000 grant from the North American Commission of the ILAE, matched by the Canadian Federation for Neurological Sciences Foundation, as well as a $10,000 grant from the Savoy Foundation for Epilepsy. Alix Elie, MD, one of only 2 neurosurgeons in Haiti, directs the epilepsy clinic, as Haiti has no full-time neurologist. The clinic has one EEG machine, donated by Stellate Systems, Montreal, Canada. Prior to the earthquake, the epilepsy clinic had been very successful, treating over 1,000 patients in its first 18 months.

Miraculously, although only 5 minutes away from the pulverized Presidential Palace, the clinic building escaped harm from the earthquake. Fully operational, the clinic has transformed into an acute-care center for people with head trauma and mental disabilities as well as epilepsy. More than 600 patients received treatment at the clinic last week.

Other assistance for earthquake victims includes the near instant creation of digital street maps that include hospitals and refugee camps.

Long-term efforts to improve the plight of people with epilepsy in Haiti include $25,000 donated by the ILAE via its North American Commission to a sustainability project to help ensure continued local epilepsy care. Dr. Carmant has initiated the Hispaniola Project, which will combine resources with the Dominican Republic to treat Haitians who require epilepsy surgery. In addition, there are plans to develop a neurology program at the Faculty of Medicine in Haiti to train local neurologists. Information and education to reduce stigma are also essential, as ignorance about epilepsy remains a "huge barrier to our efforts," according to Dr. Carmant. Dr. Carmant plans to return to the Port-au-Prince clinic later this month.

Multiple global efforts to improve the care of people with epilepsy are ongoing. These range from the "Epilepsy Out of the Shadows Global Campaign," sponsored by the ILAE, International Bureau for Epilepsy, and the World Health Organization, research in cerebral malaria and epilepsy in Zambia, Africa, by Gretchen Birbeck, MD, to a textbook written for neurologists practicing in countries with limited resources and published by the World Federation of Neurology.

Conclusions

The earthquake in Haiti has created a national healthcare crisis and highlights the vulnerability of people with disabilities. The worldwide response to this natural disaster has been amazing. If these efforts can be sustained longer than the earthquake's aftershocks, the long-term health of people in Haiti will benefit for years to come.

Although additional help is needed, Dr. Carmant was reluctant to encourage more doctors to come to Haiti because safe accommodations are not yet available. Hopefully, these can be provided in the near future. Contributions to the Port-au-Prince Epilepsy Clinic can be made through the American Epilepsy Society, at https://www.aesnet.org/go/haiti.

For an update, see Chapter 73.

Chapter 73

EPILEPSY IN HAITI AFTER THE EARTHQUAKE: AN UPDATE

June 14, 2010

Introduction

It's been more than four months since an earthquake registering 7.3 on the Richter scale left 200,000 people dead and countless more injured in Haiti. A worldwide humanitarian relief effort ensued, with multiple aid organizations and volunteers struggling to help survivors. Since then, the dust has settled over the capital city of Port-au-Prince, the American hospital ship *USNS Comfort* has left, and the government and its people face the monumental task of rebuilding Haiti's healthcare infrastructure.

A couple of months ago, I reported on the fate of Haiti's epilepsy clinic after the earthquake. One of my sources was Lionel Carmant, MD, a pediatric neurologist and Director of the Epilepsy Clinic and Epilepsy Research at Saint Justine Hospital in Montreal, Canada, who helped start the Port-au-Prince epilepsy clinic in 2008 and coordinates its international support. In March 2010, he traveled to Haiti to work at the clinic. Dr. Carmant is of Haitian origin and lives in Quebec, Canada.

Dr. Carmant was kind enough to give me a telephone interview from his office in Montreal, Canada, regarding the progress of rebuilding epilepsy services after the earthquake. During our discussion, Dr. Carmant had a sober tone. If anything, he observed, the situation for people with epilepsy in Haiti is worse than before the earthquake. But first, the good news.

Good News

Since the earthquake on January 12, 2010, the Port-au-Prince epilepsy clinic has become better known as a local healthcare resource. It is staffed primarily by Alix Elie, MD, a neurosurgeon, and Marcel Severe, MD, a pediatrician who trained for 6 months in electroencephalography (EEG) in Montreal, Canada. The clinic treats 30-40 people per week and runs 5-7 EEGs/day. The new portable EEG machine donated by Astro-Med (Grass Technologies, West Warwick, Rhode Island) after the earthquake allows EEGs to be done at the hospital on neonates and severely injured patients.

Approximately $150,000 of antiepileptic medication has been donated, which is distributed to patients for free. Whereas academic epileptologists often follow complex algorithms to decide on the best antiepileptic medication for a particular patient, the choices at the epilepsy clinic are governed by donated medications. Currently, 3 antiepileptic drugs are available; levetiracetam (Keppra), carbamazepine (Tegretol), and generic valproic acid sent from Karen Creighen, a pharmacist in Prince Edward island, Canada. Because levetiracetam may not be available in Haiti after the donated supplies run out, it is reserved for the more refractory cases.

Volunteers continue to express an interest in assisting at the clinic. Later this year, Joseph Kass, MD, JD, a French-speaking neurologist at Baylor College of Medicine in Houston, Texas, will spend one week working at the clinic. Dr. Carmant will also return in August or September.

The Dominican Republic, Haiti's wealthier neighbor, has been very supportive throughout this crisis. Nearly all the international aid that arrived by air has come through the Dominican Republic, which has also offered equipment to help clean up the rubble, sent physicians, and opened their hospitals to injured Haitians. In addition, the Hispaniola Project, a joint effort to provide epilepsy surgery to Dominicans and Haitians, is moving forward.

To date, more than $15,000 has been donated to the epilepsy clinic through the American Epilepsy Society Website, and $25,000 has been provided by the International League Against Epilepsy.

Bad News

Injuries resulting from the earthquake include approximately 60,000 neurologically impaired people with brain, spinal cord, and peripheral nerve damage. The epilepsy clinic has treated approximately 100 people with posttraumatic epilepsy caused by cerebral injuries sustained during the earthquake. Brain imaging is not available. Dr. Carmant expressed particular frustration at being unable to get a computed tomography (CT) scan on patients with seizures and hemiparesis.

Before the earthquake, the clinic provided care to everyone, attempting to balance finances by accepting payment from those who could pay and providing free care to those who could not. According to Dr. Carmant, because things have gotten so bad, people with the means to leave Haiti are exiting the country, leaving behind only those with no money. Consequently, there are few people left to subsidize the free care offered by the clinic.

The exodus applies to physicians as well. The schools for their children have closed, and the general hospital has been reduced to a collection of crowded tents assembled next to the crumbling remains of the hospital building. "The living conditions for the patients are unbearable," lamented Dr. Carmant. "I had to bring my own sanitizer gel, because there wasn't any."

New healthcare reforms in the United States are perceived to create job opportunities for primary care physicians. Consequently, doctors are fleeing Haiti for new jobs in the United States, and the doctor shortage in Haiti is getting worse. "There is no good reason for a doctor to stay in Haiti," observed Dr. Carmant.

Dr. Carmant also expressed concern regarding the staffing of the epilepsy clinic. Dr. Severe has worked for the last 6 months without any salary, and Dr. Carmant wonders how long he can continue.

Because Haiti was without a full-time neurologist, Dr. Carmant began a neurology training program at the Faculty of Medicine in Haiti. However, the medical facility was destroyed by the earthquake, taking with it all hopes for a neurology training program in the foreseeable future.

With respect to constructing new hospitals and other facilities, Dr. Carmant observed, "The government doesn't have the infrastructure to rebuild. They are totally dependent on outside help."

The Future
The international community has pledged nearly $10 billion dollars to rebuild Haiti. Former President Bill Clinton, United Nations special envoy to Haiti, is the co-chair of the

Interim Haiti Recovery Commission with Haitian Prime Minister Jean-Max Bellerive to ensure that the aid money is properly spent and does not fall prey to corruption. Private investment in Haiti will also be encouraged.

Although there is an urgent need for more physicians in Haiti, Dr. Carmant emphasized that proper accommodations for visiting volunteers are still not available. Volunteers should only come if they have contacts in Haiti who can provide lodging, he advised. Further, to be effective, volunteers should speak either French or Creole.

For those with epilepsy in Haiti, the Port-au-Prince epilepsy clinic remains an island of hope. Because of Dr. Carmant and others like him, the mountains of obstacles to adequate healthcare look a little less large. Dr. Carmant asserted, "The Haitian people deserve their medical care."

Donations

Those wishing to donate to the Port-au-Prince Epilepsy Clinic can do so through the American Epilepsy Foundation Website: https://www.aesnet.org/go/haiti.

Chapter 74

A GENETIC PANEL WITH THAT DILANTIN LEVEL, PLEASE?

March 5, 2010

Introduction

The International League Against Epilepsy (ILAE) recently published a review of genetic testing in epilepsy (Ottman et al. 2010). Because of the increasing use of genetic testing in epilepsy and other disorders, physicians and other health-care providers should be aware of advances in this field.

Genetic testing has four main functions; prenatal diagnosis, diagnosis, predictive testing, and carrier testing. Genetic testing may be carried out in research laboratories, ordered by clinicians, or obtained directly by the consumer, primarily through services marketed over the Internet. The ILAE report addresses both potential benefits and harms.

Genetic Abnormalities in Epilepsy

Epilepsy remains a clinical diagnosis, with no definitive diagnostic genetic, radiologic, electrophysiologic, or other test data. To date, more than 20 genes have been associated with genetic (idiopathic) epilepsies. In addition, seizures may be part of the clinical manifestations of other neurologic diseases, such as Tay-Sachs, for which genetic testing is available.

A variety of genetic epilepsy syndromes have been identified, such as those beginning in the first year of life, those with prominent febrile seizures, idiopathic generalized epilepsies, focal epilepsies, and epilepsies associated with other paroxysmal disorders. These may be associated with one or more abnormal gene products, which include sodium channels, potassium channels, gamma-aminobutyric acid-A receptors, calcium channels, aristaless-related homeobox protein, protocadherin, and others. The ILAE article provides a list of these, and more information is available on the publicly funded Gene Tests Website.

Techniques

Molecular methods for genetic testing include DNA sequencing, mutation scanning, targeted mutation analysis, fluorescent *in situ* hybridization, array-comparative genomic hybridization, single nucleotide polymorphism arrays, multiplex ligation-dependent probe amplification and others.

Potential Benefits of Genetic Testing

To assist in the care of people with epilepsy, genetic testing may be helpful in 5 fundamental ways.

1. Confirm a suspected genetic syndrome. This may help the patient by limiting further diagnostic studies, which may be time-consuming, anxiety-producing, and expensive. Examples include Ohtahara syndrome, X-linked infantile spasms, autosomal dominant frontal lobe epilepsy, and epilepsy with paroxysmal exercise-induced dyskinesia, which may be confirmed with highly accurate genetic tests.

2. Direct therapy. At present, most genetic testing does not help the clinical neurologist control seizures in individual patients. However, one notable exception

is severe myoclonic epilepsy in infancy (Dravet syndrome), an epileptic encephalopathy that presents with prolonged seizures in the first year of life. Dravet syndrome is characterized by status epilepticus, alternating hemiconvulsions, myoclonic seizures, and developmental regression, and can be confused with Lennox-Gastaut syndrome, myoclonic-astatic epilepsy, benign myoclonic epilepsy, and other childhood epilepsies. Specific mutations of the voltage-gated sodium channel alpha subunit Nav1.1 in the *SCN1A* gene are found in 67%-86% of children with Dravet syndrome (Millichap et al. 2009) and can be identified with commercially available tests. Diagnosis is important because valproate, topiramate, and levetiracetam (and stiripentol in Europe) are more likely to control seizures, while carbamazepine and lamotrigine tend to aggravate them (Millichap et al. 2009). Early seizure control may improve long-term developmental outcome, highlighting the need for prompt, effective therapy.

3. Prenatal screening. Genetic testing has already had a definite impact in the incidence of neurologic disease due to prenatal testing, and is becoming more accepted by physicians and the public. Thanks to the availability of prenatal genetic testing, inherited diseases such as familial dysautonomia may soon disappear (Lerner 2009).

4. Advance research. The knowledge of genetic mutations underlying specific seizure disorders may guide the development of more effective therapies.

For example, because the *SCN1A* gene mutation in Dravet syndrome affects the sodium channel, targeting therapies to overcome this defect may lead to innovative methods to control seizures. Increased understanding of genetic mutations underlying epileptic disorders may also lead to interventions that impede or stop epileptogenesis in patients at risk for the development of epilepsy due to inherited factors or acquired causes, such as head trauma or encephalitis.

5. Pharmacogenetic testing. Identifying genetic variations within individual patients may lead to the development of personalized medication therapy. Pharmacogenetic testing and treatment remain a largely unfulfilled promise of genetic testing. A related use is the identification of patients at risk from specific treatment. For example, testing for the HLA-B*1502 allele identifies patients more likely to develop a serious rash from carbamazepine.

Potential Harm of Genetic Testing
Psychological distress due to knowledge of a genetic defect, particularly one that leads to a disease without specific treatment, is a potential consequence of genetic testing. This drawback has been explored regarding other neurologic conditions such as Huntington's disease. People with known genetic disorders may perceive stigma related to their "bad genes." Needless to say, delivery of genetic information to patients and families must be done with sensitivity and confidentiality. Appropriate counseling services should be available regarding the wisdom of choosing genetic testing

in the first place, and in dealing with the results. Informed consent should be obtained before testing.

Discrimination regarding employment, health, and life insurance is a possible adverse consequence if the results of genetic testing are made public. The Genetic Information Nondiscrimination Act (GINA) of 2008 prohibits discrimination in health coverage and employment based on genetic information. This federal statute defines genetic tests "as an analysis of human DNA, RNA, chromosomes, proteins, or metabolites that detects genotypes, mutations, or chromosomal changes." However, GINA does not protect against discrimination regarding life, disability, or long-term care insurance.

Conclusion

For the moment, most physicians taking care of people with epilepsy rarely need to order genetic tests for diagnosis or clinical management. Dravet syndrome is a notable exception, where early confirmation of the diagnosis may direct treatment and potentially improve prognosis. Prenatal testing has already proven its merits in decreasing the incidence of devastating neurologic diseases such as Tay-Sachs and familial dysautonomia. As more epilepsy-associated genes are identified and genetic mechanisms of epilepsy are elucidated, genetic testing may soon join electroencephalography and magnetic resonance imaging as a useful diagnostic and management tool for the many disorders that constitute epilepsy.

References

Ottman R, Hirose S, Jain S et al. Genetic testing in the epilepsies-Report of the ILAE Genetics Commission. Epilepsia 2010, January 19 (Epub ahead of print).

Millichap JJ, Koh S, Laux LC, Nordli DR. Child Neurology: Dravet syndrome: when to suspect the diagnosis. Neurology 2009;73:e59-e62.

Lerner BH. When diseases disappear-the case of familial dysautonomia. NEJM 2009;361:1622-1625.

Chapter 75

THALAMIC STIMULATION: NEW APPROACH TO THE TREATMENT OF EPILEPSY

April 2, 2010

Introduction
The treatment of epilepsy relies primarily on antiepileptic medications, which control seizures in approximately two-thirds of patients. Other proven therapeutic modalities include epilepsy surgery, vagus nerve stimulation, and the ketogenic and modified Atkins diets. Scientific evidence for benefit from alternative therapies, such as Yoga, biofeedback, or herbal therapy remains minimal. The effectiveness of a dramatic new approach, bilateral stimulation of the anterior nucleus of the thalamus, has recently been reported (Fisher et al. 2010).

Thalamic Stimulation
A double-blind, randomized trial of bilateral stimulation of the anterior nucleus of the thalamus for epilepsy (SANTE) demonstrated a reduction in seizures among a majority of patients with medically refractory partial seizures (Fisher et al. 2010). The multicenter trial was sponsored by medical device manufacturer Medtronic.

Background
Wide experience in deep-brain stimulation (DBS) in the treatment of Parkinson's disease has paved the way for the

use of this technique for the treatment of refractory epilepsy. Advances in magnetic resonance imaging, stereotactic devices, and microelectrodes allow more precise targeting and electrode placement.

The authors selected the anterior nucleus of the thalamus for stimulation on the basis of the knowledge that it projects to the superior frontal and temporal lobes and previous observations that its stimulation can reduce seizures and produce changes on the electroencephalogram. Stimulation of a relatively small anatomic site in the thalamus can affect widespread areas of cortex (Kerrigan et al. 2004).

Results

The SANTE study, led by Robert Fisher, MD, PhD, Professor of Neurology and Director of the Stanford Comprehensive Epilepsy Center, Stanford, California, randomly assigned 110 adults with medically refractory partial seizures to 3 months of blinded stimulation or no stimulation, followed by unblinded stimulation for all participants. In all patients, at least 3 antiepileptic drugs had previously failed. Although seizures decreased in both groups, stimulated patients had an unadjusted median decline at the end of the blinded phase of 40.4% compared with a decrease of only 14.5% in the nonstimulated group. Stimulated patients with temporal lobe seizures improved compared with the control group, whereas those with extratemporal (i.e., frontal, parietal, occipital) seizures did not.

At the end of 2 years, 91 patients remained active in the study; 54% had a seizure reduction of at least 50%, and 14 patients were seizure free for at least 6 months. In addition, seizure-related injuries occurred in only 7% of the treatment group compared with 26% of the control group during the blinded phase (p=0.01).

Mechanism of Action

The thalamus has long been implicated in epilepsy (Kanner 2004) but is more often discussed in terms of idiopathic generalized epilepsy rather than localization-related epilepsy. The mechanism of action of seizure reduction by anterior thalamic DBS has not been elucidated but is under investigation.

Advantages

Unlike brain surgery, DBS is nondestructive. The stimulator can be turned off and removed if necessary, leaving the brain essentially intact.

Adverse Events

Device-related adverse events included paresthesias (18.2%), implant site infections (12.7%), and implant site pain (10.9%). Five hemorrhages (4.5%) were observed on neuroimaging but were not symptomatic. One patient had a meningeal reaction. Patients who received stimulation were significantly more likely to report depression or memory problems. Cognitive and mood scores from neuropsychological testing were similar between the groups. Eighteen patients (16.4%) withdrew from the study because of adverse events.

Conclusions

The SANTE study results are under review by the Food and Drug Administration for possible approval for the treatment of medically refractory partial seizures. It is too early to determine the role that DBS may have in the treatment of epilepsy. The risk/benefit ratio of this procedure needs to be further clarified, with more attention to the long-term effects of repeated stimulation on epileptic brain circuitry, depression, and memory. For patients who are not surgical candidates, DBS may become an additional alternative. Even for those who are candidates for surgery, a trial of DBS may be warranted before surgical resection. A comparison of DBS with the vagus nerve stimulator would be of interest. If approved, DBS will be a very important option for seizure control in people with refractory partial seizures.

References

Fisher R, Salanova V, Witt T et al. Electrical stimulation of the anterior nucleus of thalamus for treatment of refractory epilepsy. Epilepsia 2010;doi:10.111/j.1528-1167.2010.012536.x.

Kerrigan JF, Litt B, Fisher RS et al. Electrical stimulation of the anterior nucleus of the thalamus for the treatment of intractable epilepsy. Epilepsia 2004;45:346-354.

Kanner AM. Thalamic dysfunction in idiopathic generalized epilepsy: new findings of old news. Epilepsy Curr 2004;4:57-58.

Update May 27, 2013

Robert Fisher, MD, was kind enough to provide follow-up on the SANTE study, "The 5 year results were presented at the 2012 AES (American Epilepsy Society) and are being submitted for publication. Of the 110 implanted subjects, 83 were still using stimulation at 5 years. The median percent reduction from base line at one year was 41%, at 2 years was 56% and at 5 years was 69%. Even with a worst case assumption for drop outs, the treatment was still beneficial at 5 years. The SANTE DBS method was approved and is marketed in European nations, Canada and several Asian nations. The FDA is still considering whether to approve it in the US or to require further trials."

Chapter 76

VIGABATRIN (SABRIL): A NEW EPILEPSY DRUG-WITH STRINGS ATTACHED

December 31, 2009

Introduction

Another new antiepileptic drug, vigabatrin (Sabril), received US Food and Drug Administration (FDA) approval in 2009-good news for the 30% of patients with treatment-resistant epilepsy (Kwan and Brodie 2000). Vigabatrin joined the 11 antiepileptic drugs that have received FDA approval since 1993; felbamate (Felbatol), gabapentin (Neurontin), lacosamide (Vimpat), lamotrigine (Lamictal), levetiracetam (Keppra), oxcarbazepine (Trileptal), pregabalin (Lyrica), rufinamide (Banzel), tiagabine (Gabitril), topiramate (Topamax), and zonisamide (Zonegran). All of these drugs offer the potential for seizure control, which must be weighed against their risk for adverse effects. Physicians must be aware of each drug's idiosyncratic side effects, such as hyponatremia with oxcarbazepine, edema with pregabalin, and metabolic acidosis with topiramate. Felbamate was implicated in life-threatening anemia and hepatic failure, for which it received a black box warning. All of these antiepileptic drugs can be prescribed without enrolling patients in a drug surveillance program, except the newest one, vigabatrin.

Irreversible Visual Field Defects and the SHARE Program

Because of its substantial risk for permanent visual field defects (Willmore et al. 2009), vigabatrin can only be prescribed by physicians who participate in the SHARE (Support, Help and Resources for Epilepsy) program (1-800-45-SHARE). The purpose of SHARE is to monitor patients for the development of visual field defects, and to stop the drug as quickly as possible if these develop. The field defects are permanent, but stopping the drug may limit the damage. SHARE is a "risk mitigation program," developed jointly by the company (Lundbeck) and the FDA.

To prescribe vigabatrin, 4 different forms must be completed and returned to the company (www.lundbeck-SHARE.com). The first is a "Prescriber Enrollment and Agreement Form," which enlists the physician into the SHARE program. This form requires physicians to agree that they, "have experience in treating epilepsy," "know the risks of Sabril treatment, specifically vision loss," "must order and review visual assessment testing at baseline," "counsel patients," "report all serious adverse events" to the FDA and the manufacturer, and make other commitments.

A New Business Partner

Each patient must complete a "Treatment Initiation Form," which includes their personal information, the site of vigabatrin administration (home, hospital, or other facility), and their insurance information. The physician must also complete the form, which requires a National Provider Identifier (NPI) number. The physician must also authorize TheraCom as a "designated agent" and "business associate" for payment purposes.

Sign Here

If the prescription is for infantile spasms, a "Parent/Legal Guardian-Physician Agreement" must be completed, which requires the parent/legal guardian to sign twice and initial 12 points. If the prescription is for partial complex seizures, a "Patient/Parent/Legal Guardian-Physician Agreement" is required. The patient/parent/legal guardian must sign twice and initial 10 points. Physicians are also required to sign the form for each seizure type.

Not Available in Stores

After the patient is accepted into the program, all prescriptions must go through the SHARE Call Center. Then the drug is shipped from a specialty pharmacy. Only a 30-day supply is provided at a time. Vigabatrin is not available at community or hospital pharmacies. Patients receive a "Sabril Starter Kit," which includes the necessary forms, a patient diary, medication guide, instructions for mixing the oral solution, and other information.

After the first 30 days of treatment for infantile spasms, a "Treatment Maintenance Form" must be submitted to attest to the necessity of continuing therapy. For patients with infantile spasms, a treatment response should be evident by this time. If infants do not respond by 30 days, keeping them on the drug exposes them to the risk for visual loss with little potential benefit. Subsequently, ophthalmologic evaluations must be submitted every 3 months. Without evidence of these periodic examinations, the company will cease to provide the medication. For patients with refractory partial complex seizures, a treatment maintenance form must be submitted after 90 days.

There is no question that the risk for irreversible visual loss with vigabatrin treatment is substantial and significant. While the SHARE program provides heightened supervision regarding the potential complication of visual loss, it places an additional administrative burden on the physician. The company provides no compensation for the additional paperwork, there is no billing code for the process, and physicians may assume additional liability risk when treating patients with a known retinal toxin.

SHARE and TOUCH

The SHARE program is similar to the TOUCH (Tysabri Outreach Unified Commitment to Health) prescribing program for natalizumab (Tysabri), which requires physicians, pharmacies, and patients to register to monitor the incidence of progressive multifocal leukoencephalopathy in patients with multiple sclerosis, a life-threatening complication of natalizumab. A potential consequence of programs like SHARE and TOUCH may be to restrict the prescribing of new drugs with harmful idiosyncratic adverse events to relatively few doctors, probably those practicing at specialized centers. If these mandatory drug registries continue to proliferate, it is difficult to imagine how a general neurologist could keep up with the stringent bureaucratic requirements of multiple drug programs. One multiple sclerosis specialist told me that the extra physician time required by the TOUCH program is minimal, as long as he has a trained nurse to help. This solution may be practical, but begs the question of where the money will come from to support additional office staff.

More Referrals to Epilepsy Centers?

If general neurologists cannot manage the burdens of these registry programs, patients who require these treatments will be steered to tertiary centers for epilepsy, multiple sclerosis and other diseases as new potent, complex, and potentially toxic treatments evolve. Some neurologists may be reluctant to refer and too busy to participate in these programs, making it less likely that their patients will benefit from these new medications. Patients who live far from specialized centers may also be at a disadvantage. For other patients, their need for specialized drugs that require enrollment in a patient registry may spur their neurologists to refer them to a center of excellence.

Conclusions

For the 30% of patients with drug-resistant epilepsy, referral to an epilepsy center for vigabatrin will have the added benefit of a comprehensive evaluation and consideration for the ketogenic diet, vagus nerve stimulator, epilepsy surgery, and other specialized treatment. It will be important to assess how programs like SHARE and TOUCH affect the dynamics of neurologic practice and treatment outcomes.

References

Kwan P, Brodie MJ. Early identification of refractory epilepsy. NEJM 2000;342:314-319.

Willmore LJ, Abelson MB, Ben-Menachem E et al. Vigabatrin: 2008 Update. Epilepsia 2009;50:163-173.

Update June 18, 2013

As of August 22, 2012, 4,292 patients were enrolled in the SHARE program. Approximately 2/3 were taking vigabatrin for infantile spasms, and the other 1/3 for refractory epilepsy. More than half of the patients enrolled in the registry discontinued vigabatrin (2,339/4,292, 55%). Only 14 (0.6%) discontinued the drug because of visual field defects.

Chapter 77

SEIZURE CALENDARS FOR THE 21ST CENTURY

December 28, 2009

Introduction

A seizure calendar is an essential tool for the management of epilepsy (Wilner 2008). Whether patients are treated with antiepileptic medications, surgery, diet, or the vagus nerve stimulator, a written record saves time in the clinic and provides a rational basis for medication adjustment. Because patients with epilepsy often have memory difficulties, documentation of seizures is particularly important. Patients tend to remember their most recent or most severe seizure, often forgetting prior seizures or long periods of time when they were seizure free. A seizure calendar does not guarantee complete accuracy, as patients may not be aware of all their seizures, but a written record is better than no record at all.

State of the Art

A seizure calendar may be as simple as a blank calendar with an "X" to mark the occurrence of a seizure, or may have more sophisticated coding (e.g., "X" is a convulsion, "Y" a partial complex seizure, "Z" an aura). Seizure calendars may also include other important events besides seizures, such as intercurrent illness, symptoms of toxicity, sleep deprivation, stress, mood, or missed medication.

Close examination of a seizure calendar may reveal patterns susceptible to therapeutic intervention. For example, the calendar may reveal that seizures tend to cluster on the weekends, perhaps related to sleep deprivation or missed medication. Seizures may tend to be more frequent around the menstrual cycle, indicating a need for perimenstrual medication adjustment. Typically, patients keep a seizure calendar on a piece of paper, which they bring to clinic visits. However, countless times seizure calendars are "left on the refrigerator" or otherwise forgotten, and patients and physicians are forced to make clinical decisions without reliable information.

New Technology

A new generation of seizure calendars may improve patient care, particularly for patients and/or caregivers who are technologically inclined. These calendars range from simple downloadable forms that can be printed out to online seizure tracking systems. All of the seizure calendars described below are free of charge.

Seizure calendars, which can be downloaded and printed out, are available from many sources. For example, GlaxoSmithKline offers a downloadable "event calendar" that includes coding for seizure types, side effects, menstruation, and room for other notes. A calendar provided by the Minnesota Epilepsy Group is similar, and also includes space for medication information, as well as the response to important questions such as, "Were medications changed during the month?" or "Were you hospitalized this month?" and others. The Center for Epilepsy at Southern Illinois University School of Medicine provides a seizure calendar as part of its intake form for a clinic appointment. Other organizations offer seizure diaries as well, such as the National Society for Epilepsy and www.fromyourdoctor.com.

UCB Pharma also provides a simple, downloadable seizure calendar, but goes one step further. For patients who wish to record their seizures and other medical information on their personal computer, a downloadable, interactive calendar is provided. A Macintosh version is under development.

The Epilepsy Foundation provides a downloadable form that allows for recording considerable detail, including seizure type, date, time and seizure duration, postictal state, and possible triggers. A calendar available at www.seizure-tracker.com harnesses Internet technology by allowing patients to enter data online by computer or smartphone. This software keeps an electronic record of the patient's seizures, medications, and other information and can generate written and graphical reports. The software is simple to use and the reports are extremely clear.

Epilepsy.com offers a practical downloadable seizure calendar, as well as a sophisticated, interactive, online version. Similar to the seizure tracker, the Epilepsy.com online diary produces valuable tabular and graphical reports that can be printed out and brought to clinic visits. In addition, patients can download a browser icon to their computer or smartphone that provides a quick link to the calendar. The calendar can be programmed to generate reminders to take medications, refill prescriptions, keep a doctor's appointment, or other information, which can be sent to the patient by text message or email. Missed or extra doses can also be charted. Videos, documents, and other files can be appended to the diary. A downloadable, well-illustrated user's guide is available. Patient information is password protected at both the Epilepsy.com and seizuretracker.com online sites.

Conclusion

Managing seizures can be challenging for healthcare providers and patients. A reliable, accurate history of seizure type, frequency, adverse events, medication changes, hospitalizations, and other variables is essential to optimal care. The new generation of seizure calendars ranges from downloadable printable forms, calendars that can be used on a home computer, to Web-based tracking systems. Seizure calendars are important tools that truly embrace the concept of a physician/patient partnership. If a patient contributes regularly to the calendar, the results can save time in the clinic and enable a more scientific approach to seizure management. A well-kept seizure calendar streamlines this essential part of the history, allowing more time to address other issues, such as mood and quality of life.

These modern calendars are well designed and easy to use. Electronic seizure calendars may be particularly helpful for parents whose children with epilepsy may be too young or otherwise unable to use a calendar. Caregivers in a group home or other residential setting may also benefit. Formal studies to evaluate whether assiduous attention to keeping a seizure calendar improves medication adherence or otherwise enhances clinical outcomes would be valuable. Physicians and other healthcare providers should recommend electronic seizure calendars to their patients, parents of children with epilepsy, and caregivers who are motivated and able to use these 21st century healthcare tools.

References

Wilner AN. Epilepsy: 199 Answers, 3rd Edition. A Doctor Responds to His Patients' Questions. Demos Medical Publishing, New York, NY, 2008.

Update May 27, 2013

Seizure calendars are keeping pace with the growing acceptance of smartphone technology. For example, a seizure tracker "App" may be downloaded from iTunes for iPhone, iTouch, or iPad. "My Epilepsy Diary," available at Epilepsy.com, also has "Apps" downloadable from iTunes for the iPhone and iPod.

Section 11.

Physician Practice Issues

Chapter 78

WHAT DOES A NEUROHOSPITALIST DO? SHORT QUIZ!

January 15, 2011

Introduction

Last year I worked as a neurohospitalist in a 300 bed community hospital. According to a recent review, "Neurohospitalists are best defined as 'site-based' subspecialists dedicated to providing and improving inpatient neurologic care" (Barrett and Freeman 2010). In recognition of this growing subspecialty, a new journal, The *Neurohospitalist*, has recently been launched.

The development of the "neurohospitalist" has followed the widely successful "hospitalist" movement, which began in earnest in the 1990s. Approximately 40% of community hospitals have hospitalists, a number that increases to 70% in hospitals with more than 200 beds. There are at least 15,000 hospitalists, and the number is projected to top 30,000 by the time you read this (Annals of Neurology 2007). The number of neurohospitalists is expected to increase as well (Freeman et al. 2008).

According to Vanja Douglas, MD, editor-in-chief of *The Neurohospitalist*, neurohospitalists include all neurologists who provide acute care in the hospital setting, including neurointensivists and stroke neurologists (Douglas 2011). There is now a "community" for neurohospitalists on the American Academy of Neurology website.

Hospitalists are usually internal medicine physicians who care for hospitalized patients, often forsaking their outpatient practices. Similarly, neurohospitalists focus on inpatient care. While sacrificing outpatient practice might seem counterproductive, as the patients lose continuity with "their" physician, the advantages of 24/7 onsite coverage have proven even more important due to the fast pace of inpatient testing and abbreviated hospital stays.

The number of job openings for neurohospitalists has grown each year since 2005 (Barrett and Freeman 2010). In addition, neurohospitalist fellowship programs have been launched at the University of California, San Francisco, Duke, Harvard, and the Universities of Arizona, New Mexico, South Carolina, Washington, and others.

As a neurohospitalist, I worked closely with community neurologists, who would have to pick up the treatment plan where the acute hospitalization left off. The outpatient neurologist received a copy of the discharge summary, and we discussed the cases by phone when necessary.

My schedule was 7 days on, 7 days off. The "on" days lasted 10-12 hours, then I carried the beeper for the rest of the night, often receiving a preview from the emergency room of some of the next day's consults. My work included regular visits to the cardiac care floor, emergency room, general medicine ward, intensive care unit, and occasionally the OB-Gyn floor and psychiatry wing. For a "sit-down break," I got to read the electroencephalograms (EEGs).

As each day was something of a whirlwind, I thought it might be interesting to look at the most frequent diagnoses of the patients I saw.

Here is the graph (Figure 1).

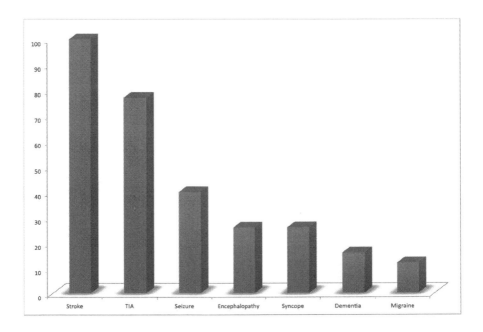

Since the legend may be too small to read, can you guess which was the number one diagnosis? Number two? Number three? These numbers are an estimate, as they are based on claims data, but I think they provide a fairly good picture of the kind of work a neurohospitalist is expected to do (at least in my hospital), and which diagnoses to brush up on! The results held no real surprises, but I didn't realize the magnitude of #1 and #2! (The diagnoses are listed below.)

For any neurohospitalists out there, how do these consults compare with your own?

Legend for Figure 1.

1. Stroke

2. TIA

3. Seizure

4. Encephalopathy

5. Syncope

6. Dementia

7. Migraine

References

Annals of Neurology. Neurohospitalists: A subspecialty defining itself. Annals of Neurology 2007;A11-A13.

Barrett KM, Freeman WD. Emerging subspecialties in neurology: Neurohospitalist. Neurology 2010;74(2):e9-10.

Douglas VC. A message from the editor in chief. The Neurohospitalist 2011:1(1):4.

Freeman WD, Gronseth G, Eidelman BH. Invited article: Is it time for neurohospitalists? Neurology 2008;70:1282-1288.

Update May 27, 2013

Neurohospitalist medicine is one of the fastest growing subspecialties in neurology. The American Academy of

Neurology "Neurohospitalist Section" had 476 members in 2012, which increased to 572 in 2013. Neurohospitalists have become an essential component of inpatient care at many hospitals.

Chapter 79

NEUROHOSPITALIST QUALITY INDICATORS

February 8, 2011

In my last blog post (see Chapter 78), I tallied the most common diagnoses I encountered while working as a neurohospitalist in a 300 bed community hospital. In a paper from a new journal, *The Neurohospitalist*, the authors reviewed the frequency of neurology and neurovascular consults at the University of California, San Francisco (UCSF), an academic neurology service (Douglas and Josephson 2011).

Their top three results were identical; cerebrovascular disease (stroke and transient ischemic attack (TIA)), seizures, and encephalopathy. Less common diagnoses included neuromuscular disease, headache, syncope, and multiple sclerosis, similar to my experience.

This information provides a "heads up" to anyone considering becoming a neurohospitalist, whether at a community or academic hospital. It also provides important data regarding the needs for services and resources to care for people suffering from neurologic disease.

Douglas and Josephson go a step further and link the most common inpatient diagnoses with published Class 1/Level A guideline treatment recommendations. These guidelines could be used as a tool to monitor and potentially improve the quality of care in the inpatient setting.

Table 1. Diagnosis and Quality Indicators (modified from Douglas and Josephson, 2011)
Diagnosis-Quality Indicator

Intracerebral Hemorrhage-Antihypertensive
Subarachnoid Hemorrhage-Nimodipine
Pneumococcal Meningitis-Dexamethasone
Cardiac Arrest-Hypothermia
Encephalitis-Acyclovir for Herpes simplex
Guillain Barre-IVIg or plasmapheresis
Multiple Sclerosis-MRI
Benign Paroxysmal Positional Vertigo-Canalith repositioning

The guidelines they cite are certainly appropriate and represent the standard of care. However, the relative rarity and complexity of many neurologic diseases, combined with their diverse presentations in individuals with a variety of comorbidities chaffs against the concept of universal quality indicators. Those that could be agreed upon are so fundamental that all neurologists probably follow them anyway.

For example, the first proposed quality indicator, "prescription of an antihypertensive at discharge" in a patient with intracerebral hemorrhage with the comorbid diagnosis of hypertension would likely be initiated by any first year medical student. Similarly, the recommendation to obtain a brain MRI in patients with multiple sclerosis is superfluous, as such a study has doubtless already been ordered by the physician or physician's assistant in the emergency room...

Efforts to systematize neurologic care may have some value. It is essential that valuable new treatments not be overlooked or ignored (e.g., tPA). Additionally, in a future that may include rationed care, it may be necessary to insist on quality indicators in order to prevent helpful treatments from being withheld because of concerns of excessive cost (e.g., IVIg or plasmapheresis).

However, until there is convincing evidence that neurologists are NOT providing quality care, let's follow the authors' recommendation to study the delivery of care and "determine the degree to which recommended tests and treatments are being used appropriately at the current time" before instituting quality indicators that are likely to prove cumbersome and vulnerable to misinterpretation and misuse by administrators.

Most neurologists spend long days trying their best to provide high quality care to enhance patient outcomes; maybe we should let them do their jobs, not burden them with "quality indicators." What do you think?

Reference

Douglas VC, Josephson SA. A proposed roadmap for inpatient neurology quality indicators. The Neurohospitalist 2011;1:8-15.

Chapter 80

ANTIPLATELET DRUGS-ARE PHYSICIANS "NONRESPONDERS" WHEN IT COMES TO TESTING?

March 17, 2010

Introduction

Imagine if there were tests to determine whether your patient with vascular disease would respond to potentially life saving treatments like aspirin or clopidogrel (Plavix).

Well, there are.

But does anyone use them?

On March 12, 2010, the U.S. Food and Drug Administration (FDA) issued a black box warning for the antiplatelet agent clopidogrel bisulfate (Plavix). Clopidogrel is a pro-drug, widely used to prevent unstable angina, myocardial infarction and stroke. It requires metabolism by the cytochrome P450 liver enzyme CYP 2C19 to become fully active. Approximately 2-14% of people, depending upon race, are poor metabolizers of clopidogrel and do not achieve full benefit from the drug.

Whereas in the "old days," many doctors observed that some patients were more likely to respond or have side effects to certain treatments than other patients, presumably based on the patient's genetic makeup or other unknowable variables, they had no alternative but to prescribe a drug and hope for the best. If the drug didn't work, they could try another.

Genetic Polymorphism

But trial and error isn't the best approach when trying to prevent myocardial infarction and stroke, when error may mean death or severe disability. Pharmacogenomics allows modern physicians to predict nonresponders to clopidogrel based on their cytochrome P450 (CYP) enzyme genotype. For example, in patients with CYP 2C19*1, clopidogrel is fully active. However, those with CYP 2C19*2 or *3 alleles have decreased enzyme activity and are "poor metabolizers." Additional CYP 2C19 variants *4, *5, *6, *7 and *8 may also be associated with reduced or absent clopidogrel metabolism.

Doubling the dose of clopidogrel increases its effectiveness in poor responders. This simple solution may seem appealing, but the best dose in this group has not been identified, and higher doses may result in unpleasant side effects.

Genetic variability may influence adverse reactions in many clinical scenarios, such as the increase in hemolysis from the antimalarial primaquine in patients with genetic deficiency of glucose-6-phosphate dehydrogenase, increased toxicity from isoniazid in "slow acetylators," and an increased risk of severe rash in patients with HLA-B*1502 exposed to carbamazepine. Many more examples of genetic variations that affect drug response are known, and it is likely that even more remain to be discovered.

Testing-Who Me?

The FDA added information about poor metabolizers of clopidogrel to the label in May 2009, but it seems the word did not get out. At my hospital, given the high volume of stroke patients (like most community hospitals in the USA, I suspect), I find myself writing prescriptions for clopidogrel at least once a day. So far, I haven't ordered a test for CYP 2C19 activity. I don't know anyone else who has either. Most of the hospitalists I spoke with didn't even know there was such a test.

There are aspirin nonresponders too, and there's a test available. Does anyone use it? (According to Doug Simpson, President and CEO of Corgenix, Inc., creators of the AspirinWorks test, less than 250,000 tests of aspirin function are performed annually vis-a-vis the approximately 45 million people on aspirin for cardiovascular indications.) The test is offered at most major labs.

Research demonstrating the cost effective value of gene testing in predicting warfarin dose has just been presented at the American College of Cardiology. Hospitalization rates were 30% lower in the group whose warfarin metabolism was predicted by gene testing as opposed to the control group treated empirically. The study was sponsored by Medco.

Alternative Antiplatelet Agents

Prasugrel (Effient) is a new antiplatelet drug approved for people with heart disease and percutaneous coronary intervention. Like clopidogrel, prasugrel is also a prodrug, but its activity does not seem susceptible to variation in CYP 2C19 genetic polymorphism. Prasugrel significantly decreased the risks of recurrent MI and stent thrombosis compared to clopidogrel in a recent clinical trial. But prasugrel, a "stronger" antiplatelet agent than clopidogrel, increased the risk of intracranial bleeding and is contraindicated in patients with transient ischemic attack (TIA) or stroke. Cilostazol has demonstrated effective stroke prevention in Japan and China, but is approved in the USA only for intermittent claudication. Another alternative antiplatelet agent, ticagrelor (Brilinta), which has been tested against clopidogrel, is pending FDA approval.

Unanswered Questions

Where does testing for antiplatelet efficacy fit in the algo-rithm of treatment for angina, myocardial infarction, TIA or stroke? Perhaps the frequency of poor metabolizers is too low to generate much excitement? Is it impractical to test millions of patients with vascular disease? Can we afford to test all these patients? Alternatively, can we afford not to? Stroke or myocardial infarction, which may result from inadequate treatment, generate high direct and indirect costs of hospitalization and rehabilitation, not to mention human suffering. In as much as poor metabolizers are more common in Asians (3-23%) than Caucasians (2-5%), per-haps racial profiling can help us decide whom to test? Will this added complexity regarding clopidogrel prescribing drive physicians and patients to other antiplatelet agents?

Clinical Trials

What is the impact of genetic polymorphism on the results of clinical trials? To what extent would the prasugrel vs. clopidogrel trial results been different if clopidogrel non-responders had been excluded? Should we include genetic screening for different metabolizers in future drug studies?

Conclusion

"One size fits all" is no longer an acceptable approach to medication therapy for patients who suffer from vascular disease. Pharmacogenomics has kept its promise of allowing us to individualize antiplatelet therapy by proactively identifying "nonresponders" to clopidogrel. Aspirin nonresponders can be identified by a urine test. The challenge for physicians is to figure out who should be tested and when, which test to order, and how to interpret the results. These questions lend themselves to analysis in a formal practice parameter, and I hope the American Academy of Neurology or other august body addresses this topic soon.

Update May 28, 2013

The FDA approved ticagrelor (Brilinta) on July 20, 2011, for patients with acute coronary syndromes to prevent heart attacks and cardiovascular death. Oddly enough, ticagrelor works *less* well when combined with standard doses of aspirin.

Since I investigated this topic, I have ordered clopidogrel function tests for hospitalized patients with cerebrovascular disease. Unfortunately, the turn-around time has been several days, meaning the patient is often discharged before the results are filed in the patient's electronic medical record. The time lag creates an opportunity for the results to "fall through the cracks" until the patient's outpatient neurologist catches up with the patient and reviews the chart.

Chapter 81

PHYSICIAN EDUCATION OR INFOMERCIAL?

October 29, 2010

A colleague of mine, Selim Benbadis, MD, recently published a letter in the journal *Epilepsy & Behavior* (Benbadis et al. 2010) addressing pharmaceutical company sponsored dinner programs and "regulations requiring faculty to exclusively show company slides without editing," a situation he calls "untenable."

Dr. Benbadis, Professor of Neurology and Director of the Comprehensive Epilepsy Program, University of South Florida, Tampa General Hospital, Tampa, FL, argues that, "Academic neurologists are educators as well as physicians." He observes that promotional dinner programs provide an additional opportunity for practicing physicians to have "informal and personal interaction with subspecialists," in addition to formal programs such as grand rounds or CME. Physicians, and ultimately their patients, will benefit. However, he, and many other academic physicians, do not wish to be hamstrung to promotional slides without allowing editing.

Frankly, I'm not sure there is a problem here. These programs are clearly promotional and not CME. Pharmaceutical companies are beholden to Food and Drug Administration regulations addressing program content and need to control it. Further, the drug companies are paying the piper, why shouldn't they call the tune?

On the other hand, if academic faculty refuse to participate, then there won't be any programs...

Dr. Benbadis proposed the following solutions:

1. Pharmaceutical companies should sponsor CME rather than promotional programs.

2. Make faculty responsible for the content and allow companies to pre-approve the faculty's slide deck.

3. Create a new type of educational event (not promotional, not CME).

4. Tag team promotional and CME programs at the same event.

What do you think?

Do you attend pharmaceutical company sponsored dinner programs?

Do you think "promotional programs" have any value?

Do you think a "free dinner" has any power to impact a physician's prescribing?

Would you lecture at a promotional program if you were required to show "only the company's slides?"

Please comment. Thanks!

References

Benbadis SR, Faught RE Jr, Hirsch L et al. Open letter (and invitation) to the pharmaceutical industry: "No, we cannot just present your slide deck..." Epilepsy & Behavior, September 10, 2010, Epub ahead of print.

Chapter 82

NEUROENHANCEMENT-PATHWAY TO A BETTER BRAIN?

November 1, 2009

Introduction

For healthy people struggling to succeed in school or careers, optimizing cognitive function is a necessary goal. A healthy diet, exercise, and adequate sleep all increase the likelihood that one's nervous system will perform up to its natural potential. Avoidance of neurotoxins (alcohol and illicit drugs) is a complementary approach. But what happens when these common sense strategies are not enough? Or when the demands of life dictate that an appropriate diet, exercise, and sleep are unachievable luxuries? Is there a pill that can make a difference? If there is, is it wise to take it? And for the neurologist, is it ethical to prescribe it?

A recent article from the Guidance of the Ethics, Law and Humanities Committee of the American Academy of Neurology focuses on the last question and provides some practical advice for neurologists (Larriviere et al. 2009). A Medscape News article includes some quotes from Dr. Larriviere (Jeffrey 2009).

Larriviere et al. address the ethical considerations of neuroenhancement therapy for adults, defined as prescribing prescription drugs to "normal people" for the purpose of enhancing their memory, cognition, or attention span. "Normal people" are those without neurologic disease who seek to improve or "enhance" their neurologic abilities beyond their baseline. In this respect, neuroenhancement parallels cosmetic surgery where one might wish to "enhance" one's appearance by taking a normally functioning body part, e.g., a nose or a breast, and making it larger, smaller, or reshaping it, in the absence of any known disease or physiologic dysfunction.

According to the authors, popular demand for neuroenhancement therapy is increasing, and neurologists should be prepared to deal with these requests. An overview of "cosmetic neurology" regarding movement, mentation, and mood and affect enhancements is provided by Chatterjee (2004). Margaret Talbot, writing in *The New Yorker*, explores the topic of neuroenhancement and profiles several high functioning users. Psychiatrists have confronted this issue in "normal" people who wish to take antidepressants to alter or improve their mood (Kramer 1993). Neurologists who inject botulinum toxin for the treatment of unwelcome skin folds, ridges or creases (wrinkles) already participate in "cosmetic neurology."

The lead author, Dan Larriviere, MD, JD, has addressed other ethical issues in neurology such as terminating food and nutrition in vegetative patients (Larriviere and Bonnie 2006) and conflicts regarding duty hours and professional ethics resulting from new Accreditation Council for Graduate Medical Education (ACGME) guidelines (Larriviere 2004).

Ethical or Not?
The Ethics, Law and Humanities Committee determined that the prescription of neuroenhancement therapy is

legal. It is also ethical, when intended to improve a patient's well-being. However, it is not "ethically obligatory," because it falls outside the core domain of traditional medical practice. Consequently, neurologists who are not comfortable prescribing neuroenhancement therapy are not ethically bound to do so, although they should explain their reservations to the patient and provide alternatives.

Stimulants, such as caffeine, modafinil, and methylphenidate may transiently improve attention and are used for neuroenhancement, although not approved by the U.S. Food and Drug Administration (FDA) in normal adults for this purpose. Currently, there are no FDA approved medications for neuroenhancement. While drugs are the most likely form of neuroenhancement to be requested, one can envision that technology may soon offer prosthetic devices that improve vision, hearing, or other senses beyond one's normal ability. Few would argue the advantages of such devices. For example, an implantable chip to effortlessly expand one's memory is a common request amongst those in medical training and practice! However, the "downside" of such neuroenhancements, besides such obvious considerations as cost and risks associated with brain surgery, remains unknown.

At the moment, most neurologists probably have their hands full diagnosing and treating well-established neurologic disease, as well as weeding out the "worried well" from their clinics. However, if one considers the public's appetite for nutritional supplements as an indication of their probable consumption of neuroenhancement therapy, requests for neuroenhancement may well be considerable as drug and other approaches become available. Direct marketing to consumers will encourage this demand.

Practical Advice

For neurologists who decide to prescribe neuroenhancement therapy, the authors provide some guidance:

1. Consider the request for neuroenhancement similar to any other chief complaint.

2. Consider that a doctor-patient relationship has been established, with all its moral, ethical and professional obligations.

3. Determine by manner of history, physical, and indicated laboratory testing that the "normal person" who is requesting neuroenhancement is, indeed, free of neurologic disease. (It may be that a request for cognitive enhancement stems from the development of mild cognitive impairment or Alzheimer's disease, for example.)

4. Determine whether the patient has psychiatric illness that may require treatment, and how this illness affects the request for neuroenhancement therapy.

5. Discuss the risks and benefits of the proposed "therapy."

6. Inform the patient whether the drug is FDA approved for neuroenhancement or whether this use is off-label.

7. Discuss the desired goals to be achieved.

8. Discuss when it would be appropriate to stop the therapy.

9. Discuss alternatives, such as cognitive-oriented psychotherapy.

10. Refuse to prescribe neuroenhancement if it will do more harm than good.

The FDA will play an important role as this new category of drugs and devices becomes available. One would hope that neuroenhancement therapy will be subjected to burdens of proof regarding efficacy and safety at least as rigorous as those for standard prescription medications. Formal training regarding the prescription of neuroenhancement therapy should be provided in medical school and residency training.

As long as neurologists follow the primary tenet of making the well-being of their patients their first priority, treating patients with neuroenhancement therapy may prove practical and satisfying for both the patient and neurologist. Prospective studies and monitoring of such treatment are necessary, as the long-term consequences of "enhancing" brain function remain unknown.

References

Chatterjee A. Cosmetic neurology. The controversy over enhancing movement, mentation, and mood. Neurology 2004;63:968-974.

Jeffrey S. New guidance document takes on the ethics of "neuroenhancement." www.medscape.com/viewarticle/710289, October 9, 2009.

Kramer P. Listening to Prozac. Penguin, New York, 1993.

Larriviere D, Williams MA, Rizzo M, Bonnie RJ on behalf of the AAN Ethics, Law and Humanities Committee. Responding to requests from adult patients for neuroenhancements. Guidance of the Ethics, Law and Humanities Committee. Neurology 2009;73:1-7.

Larriviere D, Bonnie RJ. Terminating artificial nutrition and hydration in persistent vegetative state patients. Current and proposed state laws. Neurology 2006;66:1624-1628.

Larriviere D. Duty hours vs professional ethics. ACGME rules create conflicts. Neurology 2004;63:E4-E5.

Chapter 83

THE DOCTOR (OR WHOEVER) WILL
SEE YOU NOW...

August 16, 2009

There is a new dermatology group in town. Last week I decided to give them a try rather than make the two hour trek to Boston and wait another hour for my 10 minute dermatology appointment at the "Academic Medical Center."

In fact, six months before, I had been to Boston for the same problem, but I didn't like the doctor's diagnosis (or his attitude). When I showed him the small, rubbery lesion in the corner of my mouth, he looked at it for a microsecond and said, "It's a wart. I'll burn it off."

"Not so fast," was my response. This was my mouth, a sensitive and essential body part. The idea of a bubble of liquid nitrogen leaving a massive crater in the corner of my mouth, a wound that was certain to hurt every time I ate (at least three times a day) or spoke (a lot more often), and might take weeks to heal, was not too appealing. "Any other options?" I asked.

"You can try Retin-A, just apply it there."

"Will it work?" I asked.

"Probably 50% chance, liquid nitrogen is more like 70%. I'll get you a prescription."

I was hoping for a little more discussion, but I figured it could wait until the doctor came back. (I was still trying to comprehend how a wart had grown in my mouth.) After a few minutes, a nurse returned with a prescription.

"Where's the doctor?" I asked innocently.

"He's with another patient. Do you have any more questions?"

At this point, I wasn't really sure. It seemed that the diagnosis and treatment had been dispensed with, along with me. So I went home and tried the Retin-A for a few months. It caused quite a bit of irritation, but the wart, or whatever it was, stubbornly stayed put. I gave up on the Retin-A and waited for it to go away, but it didn't.

So it was not without a little trepidation that I went to the new dermatologist, hoping for a second opinion and a more reasonable approach. I was amazed when the secretary told me there was an opening the next day. (At the medical center, I had to wait six months to get my first appointment.)

I arrived 20 minutes early and filled out the history and physical form. There were several names listed on the office roster. The receptionist had told me on the phone which dermatologist I would see, but I had forgotten his name.

"You have an appointment with Bryan*."

I picked up one of the business cards on her desk. "Bryan" was a Physician's Assistant (PA)! I didn't even know there were dermatology PAs. I was stunned, angry, disappointed, and a little nauseous. It had not been easy for me to confront this problem again and make this appointment. The secretary had *never* told me I was going to see a PA.

I felt betrayed. I had made an appointment at a doctor's office. Didn't that mean I was going to see a doctor?

Apparently not.

After I reigned in my emotions, I said calmly.

"I was expecting to see a dermatologist," I said, "A board certified dermatologist."

"Oh, Bryan is supervised by the doctor," she responded.

I felt a little better. "Will I see the doctor as well?" I asked. I remembered working with PAs in my old neurology practice. The PA would see the patients first, and then we would see them together. That system didn't save me much time, and I didn't use it much, but one of my partners never saw patients without a PA, and he seemed very satisfied.

"The doctor is in the other office today."

"And where is the other office?" I envisioned an adjacent building...

"In Foxboro," she said.

"I see, the other side of the state."

I felt sick again. "So how exactly is Bryan supervised?" I asked. I imagined state of the art telemedicine equipment in the examining room so the PA could transmit a high definition image of my lesion to the doctor for a diagnosis.

"Oh, Bryan will just give him a call if he has any questions."

"I see."

I thought PA stood for "Physician's Assistant," not "Physician's Replacement."

Imagine the scenario. You purchase a plane ticket. You board the aircraft, stow your carry-on in the overhead bin, squeeze into your economy seat and fasten your seat belt. The flight attendant announces, "Today your pilot is Bryan, our Pilot's Assistant (PA). Should any problems occur, Bryan is well supervised by a *bona fide* FAA pilot, Captain Jack, who happens to be flying another plane, a few hundred miles away, but can always be reached by radio. For

413

additional assistance, Bryan has a co-pilot, a PAA (Pilot's Assistant Assistant)."

The flight attendant reads from her preprinted card, "As everyone knows, the airlines have been in dire economic straights, and these measures have been necessary to control costs. Modern jets are on autopilot most of the time anyway, with just the landings and takeoffs requiring special attention, and rare situations like when there are too many birds in the engine or turbulence over Brazil. Consequently, we have found that a PA is adequate for most air travel. Thank you for flying Acme Airlines. Please enjoy your flight."

Would you stay on the plane?

The receptionist was waiting for me to say something. I didn't know what to do. Maybe I should just reschedule to see the doctor? I made a snap decision.

"Look, I'm already here. Why don't I stay and see Bryan, and I'd like to follow up with the dermatologist?" I had already taken the morning off work. I might as well see what the PA had to offer.

Bryan came in right on time. He washed his hands, which I appreciated. He reviewed my medical history. He asked me about the lesion, how it started, did it hurt, had I already treated it? He was very professional and genuinely concerned. I explained it started after I had a crack in the corner of my mouth. When it healed, there was a lump there.

"I think it's tissue hyperplasia. I'll give you some steroid cream, which might decrease the inflammation, and you can come back in a week and see me and the doctor, and we'll see if it goes away."

I liked Bryan. I liked his manner. I liked his approach. He was careful and took the necessary time. And I liked his diagnosis. Tissue hyperplasia sounded a lot better than a wart.

I tried the cream for a week, but nothing happened. I went back for my follow up.

The dermatologist breezed in with Bryan at his coattails. The doctor didn't stop to wash his hands and briefly said hello on his way to the corner of my mouth. I looked up expectantly.

"It's a wart. I'll burn it off."

Yikes! So here I was, back where I started 6 months before. Bryan had gone through all the proper motions, but he didn't have the experience, the training, to make the correct diagnosis. (A PA's training usually lasts two years, after two years of college, although it may be longer (http://www.bls.gov/oco/ocos081.htm). How does this compare to four years of college, four years of medical school, a year of internship, and three or more years of residency and fellowship of a physician specialist?)

"Not so fast," was my response. But this time, the doctor listened to my concerns. We decided on electro-cautery, after a massive dose of lidocaine to paralyze any pain sensitive neurons anywhere in Eastern Massachusetts. The procedure didn't hurt, but of course it hurts now, but not so much.

I told this story to a few of my friends. They had all had the same experience. An appointment at the "doctor" turned into a visit with a PA or a nurse practitioner (NP).

I think my personal experience would have been a lot more satisfactory if the receptionist had warned me that I would be seeing a PA, so that I didn't arrive in the office with unrealistic expectations. She could have said something like, "Our office is staffed by physicians, physician assistants and nurse practitioners. You may see any one of these when you arrive, depending upon who is available. If you would like to specify a certain provider, please let me know and I will schedule you accordingly."

With respect to PAs and NPs, we are hearing more and more about how important they are to lower health care costs. And maybe they can play a very effective role in those cases that are simple and straightforward. But how does one know ahead of time which cases are "simple and straightforward?" My problem, which was very simple and straightforward to two dermatologists, was not so simple and straightforward to the PA. Of course, this is just one example.

And if PAs and NPs are really "physician-extenders," then what is meant exactly by "supervision?"

In these days of "evidence-based medicine," what is the evidence that PAs and NPs actually save time and money in the long run, and in which clinical environments, while producing equivalent (or superior) results? Before we rush to "physician extenders" who may actually turn out to be "physician replacements," I'd like to see the evidence, if it exists. If it doesn't, maybe we should get some before we jump on the physician-extender bandwagon as a cost saving measure.

In the meantime, next time you go to the doctor, remember, "The healthcare provider will see you now..."

*Bryan is not his real name.

Chapter 84

EEG: A TEST FOR DIAGNOSIS OR MISDIAGNOSIS?

June 22, 2009

Ever since Hans Berger discovered the presence of human brain waves in 1924, the electroencephalogram (EEG) has been an essential part of the investigation of the human nervous system. Despite dramatic advances in brain imaging with computed tomography (CT) and magnetic resonance imaging (MRI), the EEG continues to be an essential tool in the evaluation of altered mental status and seizures. Apart from some technical refinements in data processing (most of us now look at the EEG on a computer screen rather than flipping oversized paper pages), the EEG has remained fundamentally unchanged for decades. Nonetheless, there continue to be reports of EEG misinterpretation.

The following EEG pattern (Figure 1) was submitted by Selim Benbadis, MD, who has taken a great interest in the accurate interpretation of EEG (Benbadis and Lin 2008, Benbadis 2007).

According to Dr. Benbadis, "About 30% of patients seen at epilepsy centers for refractory seizures do not have seizures and have been misdiagnosed...Many of them have histories not in the least suggestive of seizures, and have their diagnosis based largely, and sometimes solely, on an 'abnormal' EEG."

I wonder if other doctors feel that the misinterpretation of EEGs is such a problem. If so, should there be some sort of certification required for neurologists to read EEGs? Do you think it would help? Do you read all of your own EEGs?

Figure 1. EEG

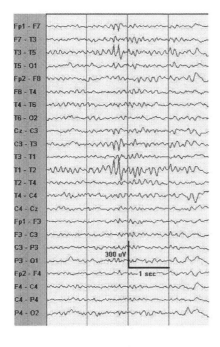

This patient is seen for an episode of LOC (a possible seizure).

No further history is available.

His EEG shows this 8 times.

Your EEG interpretation:

A. Epileptiform
B. Probably epileptiform
C. Of no epileptiform significance

References

Benbadis SR, Lin K. Errors in EEG interpretation and misdiagnosis of epilepsy. Which EEG patterns are overread? European Neurology 2008;59(5):267-271.

Benbadis SR. Errors in EEGs and the misdiagnosis of epilepsy: Importance, causes, consequences, and proposed remedies. Epilepsy & Behavior 2007;11:257-62.

Update May 18, 2013

The poll results for this question indicated that 60% of responders answered correctly, 29% incorrectly, and the remaining 11% do not interpret EEGs.

Chapter 85

COFFEE AND CHOCOLATE-STILL LEGAL IN SEATTLE

May 1, 2009

Yesterday was the last day of the commercial exhibits at this
year's American Academy of Neurology meeting, and I felt
obligated to spend a couple of hours exploring the booths.
After all, the exhibitors are an important part of the annual meeting. If it weren't for all those pharmaceutical companies, we neurologists wouldn't have much to offer our
patients.

I was also curious to see the effect of the new PhRMA
(Pharmaceutical Research and Manufacturers of American)
guidelines regarding promotional items that took effect in
January, 2009 (PhRMA 2008). In short, the new code prohibits promotional items that might potentially influence
a physician's prescribing habits. This rule prohibits items
ranging from World Series tickets to a pen imprinted with
a brand name. Educational items, such as a textbook (<
$100), or patient education materials, such as an anatomi-
cal model of the brain, are allowed. A cup of coffee and a
cookie is also allowed (unless you are from Minnesota or
a New York government employee, which have their own,
stricter guidelines).

My first impression of the exhibit hall was that it was
huge, and relatively quiet. There were no long lines of people with plastic shopping bags waiting to get their names

inscribed on a wooden pen, pick up a free flash drive, Mp3 player, or other sundry, (and dare I say, inconsequential item). There were, however, numerous booths with food, including coffee, chocolate, cookies, donuts, smoothies, and ice cream. When I asked why these items were available, one exhibitor smiled and told me it was because they were "untraceable."

It was the last day of the exhibits, when traffic tends to slow down. But my informal poll of several exhibitors confirmed that attendance in the exhibit hall throughout the meeting was decreased compared to last year. When we speculated on the reasons, we came up with several theories.

1. The weather was great in Seattle, and doctors not attending scientific sessions were making the most of the outdoors. Seattle is a visitor friendly city, with lots of restaurants, shops, and a spectacular waterfront just a few blocks away.

2. The exhibit hall was huge and divided into two large rooms, one behind the other. I didn't even realize there was a second room until I stumbled into it. Probably other attendees didn't either.

3. The poster sessions, usually adjacent to the exhibit hall, are quite effective in encouraging crossover traffic, but this year they were on a different floor.

4. The economy is down. One bookseller told me that people were much more price conscious than in years past, and that the best selling books were the least expensive little handbooks. (My own book,

Epilepsy: 199 Answers, sold at least 2 copies, so at least the economy has not totally collapsed.)

5. According to the AAN press office, meeting attendance is down, but only by a few percentage points. Last year, there were about 12,000 attendees, and this year, there are 11,000+ (final numbers not in yet).

6. Lastly, could it be that the lack of promotional items had decreased traffic somewhat? Hard to say. But it definitely was more peaceful in the exhibit hall, and if you wanted to actually talk to a medical affairs representative or seriously examine a new EEG or EMG machine, it was easier than last year.

The slow traffic was enough of a problem that at least some exhibitors groused about it to the AAN and tried to come up with solutions for a better yield on their advertising dollars next year.

I didn't go home with any promotional items, which is fine since I already have enough pens to last several lifetimes. And, of course, I feel greatly relieved that I will be spared the soul searching regarding the potential influence a flash drive or Mp3 player might have on my prescribing practices. (To be perfectly clear on that point, in my own humble opinion, that was never an issue to begin with.)

However, given the amount of chocolate I ate, including a rather tasty Seattle Space Needle, I may be lugging home an extra pound or two. If everyone else did the same thing, these new PhRMA regulations may unintentionally contribute to an epidemic of obesity among health care providers.

I just hope they don't prohibit coffee as a "performance enhancer" next year, or the economy in Seattle will really take a dive, and I'll never get these blogs done.

References
PhRMA 2008; http://www.phrma.org/sites/default/files/ 369/phrma_marketing_code_2008-1.

Update May 28, 2013

In 2008, Massachusetts passed a law severely restricting the ability of pharmaceutical companies to pay for meals, travel or other perquisites in association with physician medical education, as well as other restrictions (policymed.com 2008). In 2012, after protests from the hospitality industry, Massachusetts relaxed the law to allow for "modest meals and refreshments" for healthcare practitioners (PolicyMed. com 2013).

Additional References
http://www.policymed.com/2008/08/massachusetts-2.html, April 11, 2008.
http://www.policymed.com/massachusetts-code-of-conduct/, March 6, 2013.

Section 12.

Prevention and Treatment Guidelines

Chapter 86

ARE LEVEL "U" GUIDELINES "USELESS"?

September 29, 2010

Introduction

A recent "Special Editorial" in the journal *Neurology* addressed the rating system used by the American Academy of Neurology (AAN) in its evidence-based guidelines (Getchius TSD et al. 2010). Apparently, many readers have expressed frustration with the Level "U" recommendation (see Appendix for explanation of "Levels.") The article states that "U" stands for "insufficient data to support or refute use of a particular treatment or diagnostic test," not "unimportant" or "useless." The authors emphasize, "...a Level U guideline recommendation is not synonymous with a negative recommendation."

Gary Gronseth, MD, Professor and Vice Chair of Neurology, University of Kansas, Kansas City, KA, is one of the coauthors of the article and an evidence-based medicine consultant for the AAN. According to Dr. Gronseth, the AAN has published over 100 guidelines since they began the formal process in 1989. Guideline topics are chosen in three ways; by the AAN Board of Directors, by review of suggestions from members, or are updates of previous topics. A typical budget is $20,000 for a single guideline, which mostly pays for the literature search, articles, and AAN staff time. The expert panel that authors the guideline donates their time. The AAN plans to issue 8 guidelines/year.

AAN Guidelines cover a wide variety of topics and are available free on the AAN website. A number of AAN guidelines have been reviewed in this blog and appear in this collection (i.e., amyotrophic lateral sclerosis, botulinum for spasticity, brain death, microcephaly, nonmotor symptoms for Parkinson's disease, and women with epilepsy, as well as guidelines from other organizations; i.e., intracerebral hemorrhage, traumatic brain injury).

According to the AAN, the purpose of clinical practice guidelines is to "assist its members in clinical decision making related to the prevention, diagnosis, treatment, and prognosis of neurologic disorders. Each guideline makes specific practice recommendations based upon a rigorous and comprehensive evaluation of all scientific data."

The Problem with Level "U"

For clinical neurologists, Level "U" recommendations can be particularly troublesome. For example, a recent Practice Parameter on nonmotor symptoms of Parkinson's disease offered eight Level "U" out of a total of 10 recommendations (Zesiewicz et al. 2010)! There was "insufficient evidence to support or refute treatments" for orthostatic hypotension, urinary incontinence, botulinum toxin for constipation, levodopa for sleep, melatonin for sleep, non-ergot dopamine agonists for periodic limb movements of sleep or restless legs syndrome, REM sleep behavior disorder, or levodopa for anxiety in people with Parkinson's disease.

Similarly, in the Women with Epilepsy Practice Parameter (which I participated in as an author), recommendations for Vitamin K supplementation to reduce the risk of hemorrhagic complications in the newborn were Level "U" (Harden et al. 2009).

Although many epileptologists would recommend Vitamin K for women of childbearing age taking antiepileptic drugs, there is no specific evidence to support these recommendations, resulting in the Level "U" recommendation. Whether one *should* prescribe Vitamin K in the absence of such data is not addressed in these guidelines.

Dr. Gronseth emphasized, "We don't think the guidelines are an appropriate place for expert opinion."

Level "U" recommendations may provide insurance companies an excuse not to pay for certain treatments, which although common practice, may be unsupported by data. The AAN editorial acknowledges that insurance companies take AAN guidelines into account when drafting medical coverage policies, and such fall-out may be possible.

The AAN guidelines perform an important function by engaging a panel of experts to complete a thorough literature review, a Herculean task. The sheer quantity of publications on most topics, numbering in the hundreds if not thousands, have put behind us the days when one could quickly "review the literature" after seeing a patient and return to the examining room minutes later, or even the same day! Subscription services such as Up-to-Date and MD Consult have emerged to assist practicing physicians with this daily struggle.

Conclusions

Personally, I think the AAN's time and money would be better spent to survey a topic for the likelihood of strong recommendations prior to embarking on a full evidence-based guideline. After all, what is the value of an evidence-based guideline if there is no evidence? Consultation with a few experts could rapidly determine whether or not there are sufficient high quality clinical trials to inform physicians about evidence-based practices. If there are few helpful studies, as in the nonmotor symptoms of Parkinson' disease article, another topic should be chosen. If, on the other hand, the purpose of such a Level "U" guideline is to highlight the need for clinical research in a particular discipline, this could be done more expeditiously in another forum.

AAN members who wish to participate in the development of future guidelines may contact the AAN to become reviewers, complete a form to nominate a topic for review, and discuss guidelines on AAN Communities.

References

Getchius TSK, Moses LK, French J et al. AAN guidelines: A benefit to the neurologist. Neurology 2010;75:1126-1127.

Harden CL, Pennell PB, Koppel BS et al. Practice Parameter update: Management issues for women with epilepsy. Focus on pregnancy (an evidence-based review): Vitamin K, folic acid, blood levels, and breastfeeding: Report of the Quality Standards Subcommittee and Therapeutics and Technology Assessment Subcommittee of the American Academy of Neurology and the American Epilepsy Society. Neurology 2009;74:142-149.

Zesiewicz TA, Sullivan KL, Arnulf I et al. Practice Parameter: Treatment of nonmotor symptoms of Parkinson disease. Neurology 2010;74:924-931.

Update June 2, 2013

Guideline development has become a major international endeavor-the Guidelines International Network database features more than 3,700 guidelines from 39 countries (IOM 2011a). In March, 2011, the Institute of Medicine (IOM) of the National Academies published standards for clinical guidelines (IOM 2011a) and systematic reviews (IOM 2011b). The AAN has adopted these standards for future systematic reviews and practice guidelines. According to the AAN, 98% of AAN members are "aware of and use AAN guidelines." The AAN practice section has a blog that accepts comments regarding practice guidelines.

Additional References

Institute of Medicine of the National Academies. Clinical practice guidelines we can trust: standards for developing trustworthy clinical practice guidelines (CPGs). http://www.iom.edu/~/media/Files/Report%20Files/2011/Clinical-Practice-Guidelines-We-Can-Trust/Clinical%20Practice%20Guidelines%202011%20Report%20Brief.pdf. March 23, 2011a.

Institute of Medicine of the National Academies. Finding what works in health care: Standards for systematic reviews. http://iom.edu/~/media/Files/Report%20Files/2011/Finding-What-Works-in-Health-Care-Standards-for-Systematic-Reviews/Standards%20for%20Systematic%20Review%202010%20Report%20Brief.pdf. March 23, 2011b.

Chapter 87

TREATMENT OF CHOREA IN HUNTINGTON DISEASE-NEW AAN GUIDELINE

August 29, 2012

Introduction

Although there are many limitations to evidence-based guidelines, the busier I get, the more I appreciate them. The most recent American Academy of Neurology (AAN) guideline reviews the pharmacologic treatment of chorea in Huntington disease (Armstrong and Miyaski 2012). Uncontrolled chorea results in decreased motor function, falls, and worsens weight loss. Whether patients need treatment for their chorea must be individualized. This AAN guideline does not address other important aspects of Huntington disease such as genetic testing, neuroprotection, or treatment of depression and cognitive decline.

Huntington Disease

Huntington disease is characterized clinically by chorea, cognitive decline and psychiatric impairment. Because of its rarity, most neurologists will have relatively limited experience with the management of Huntington disease. It's prevalence in the US is 4-8/100,000 (Revilla 2011). To put this number in perspective, this prevalence translates to approximately 15,000 cases of Huntington disease compared to more than 2 million for epilepsy. Management is challenging; what the disease lacks in prevalence, it more than makes up for with morbidity and mortality.

AAN Guideline

To prepare the AAN guideline, the authors identified 424 citations from which they selected 33 articles. Studies had to have at least 20 patients, a comparison group, a pharmacologic intervention, and a validated outcome measure. A Unified Huntington's Disease Rating Scale (UHDRS) total motor score decrease of 1 to <2 points was considered "modestly important," a decrease of 2 to <3 "moderately important," and a decrease of >3 "very important."

Recommendations

Three drugs achieved a level B recommendation;* tetrabenazine (up to 100 mg/day), amantadine (300-400 mg/day), and riluzole (200 mg/day). Of these, only tetrabenazine, a vesicular monoamine transporter inhibitor that depletes dopamine and other central monoamines, is approved by the U.S. Food and Drug Administration (FDA) for the treatment of chorea.

Tetrabenazine

In a 12 week, Class I randomized controlled trial of 84 subjects, UHDRS total maximal chorea scores decreased by -5 in the tetrabenazine group vs. -1.5 in the placebo group (p=0.0001). In a Class II study of tetrabenazine withdrawal in 30 subjects, *post hoc* analysis revealed reemergent chorea following tetrabenazine discontinuation (p=0.0486). With respect to adverse events, depression and parkinsonism are two important side effects of tetrabenazine. Depression is of particular importance, as people with Huntington disease are already at increased risks of suicidal ideation and suicide than the general population. Common side effects of tetrabenazine observed in a Class IV continuation study included sedation/somnolence (24%), depressed mood (23%), anxiety (17%) and insomnia (13%). Other less frequent but important side effects are prolonged QT interval and neuroleptic malignant syndrome.

Amantadine

Amantadine, an NMDA receptor antagonist, was examined in two randomized crossover trials (one Class I and one Class II). In the Class I study, 24 subjects took 300 mg/day. Of these, 19 reported improvement on amantadine compared to only 6 taking placebo (p=0.006). However, UHDRS chorea scores were not significantly different. In the Class II study, UHDRS chorea scores decreased by 18% in 24 patients taking amantadine 400 mg/day vs. only 5% for those on placebo (p=0.0007). Adverse events included agitation, anxiety, confusion, diarrhea, exacerbation of morbid thoughts, forgetfulness, hallucinations, nausea, and sleepiness.

Riluzole

Riluzole has antiglutamatergic and antiexcitotoxic properties and is currently FDA approved for the treatment of amyotrophic lateral sclerosis (ALS). Two Class I randomized controlled trials evaluated riluzole for Huntington chorea. In the first study of 63 patients, total maximal chorea decreased at 8 weeks in patients receiving riluzole 200 mg/day vs. placebo (p=0.01). Riluzole 100 mg/day was not effective. The second study of 537 patients did not reveal any difference at 3 years in UHDRS chorea scores in subjects treated with riluzole 50 mg BID vs. placebo. However, more placebo-treated subjects withdrew in order to start anticholinergic medication (14.4%) than those on riluzole (9%) (p<0.0001). Adverse events included elevated liver enzymes, 5 suicides (3 in the riluzole group and 2 in the placebo group), as well as 6 suicide attempts (4 in the riluzole group and 2 in the placebo group).

Nabilone

A Class II randomized, crossover, controlled trial of 22 subjects examined the effects of nabilone (1-2 mg), a synthetic cannabinoid, or placebo for 5 weeks. UHDRS chorea scores decreased by 1.68 in the nabilone group (p=0.009). Adverse effects included sedation, drowsiness and forgetfulness. Nabilone is a Class II controlled substance with high abuse potential, but may be prescribed for "modest decreases" in Huntington chorea (Level C).

Other Drugs

Trials of other agents tended to be negative or inadequate. The data reviewed for ethyl-eicosapentaenoic acid (EPA) and minocycline suggested that these two drugs would not achieve "very important improvements" in chorea (Level B). Similarly, creatine was "possibly ineffective" for "very important" improvements (Level C). Coenzyme Q is "likely ineffective" for moderate improvements in chorea (Level B). There was insufficient data to make recommendations for donepezil, clozapine or other neuroleptics regarding the treatment of Huntington chorea.

Conclusions

This AAN guideline recommends three drugs likely to be helpful in the treatment of chorea in Huntington disease. In addition, it provides negative recommendations of several others. This information should be helpful when discussing treatment options with patients and their families. Physicians without extensive experience in the management of Huntington chorea may not be comfortable selecting and monitoring treatment. Referral to a movement disorder specialist may be helpful. Patients with Huntington disease need close follow-up regarding the possibility of depression, suicidal ideation, and suicide.

N.B. For those who would like to communicate directly with the AAN regarding Guidelines, the AAN has begun a new blog that accepts comments (http://www.aan.com/practice/blog).

*See Appendix for explanation of the American Academy of Neurology Levels of Recommendations

References

Armstrong MJ, Miyasaki JM. Evidence-based guideline: Pharmacologic treatment of chorea in Huntington disease. Neurology 2012;79:597-603.

Revilla FJ. Huntington disease. http://emedicine.medscape.com/article/1150165-overview, August 8, 2011.

Chapter 88

BELL'S PALSY-UPDATED TREATMENT RECOMMENDATIONS FROM THE AAN

November 21, 2012

Introduction

First described in 1821 by Sir Charles Bell, Bell's palsy is an acute, idiopathic, unilateral, peripheral paralysis of the seventh cranial nerve (Gronseth and Paduga 2012). It affects 60,000-90,000 people in the US each year, can occur at any age and affects both sexes equally (Gilden 2004). While most people recover fully, others are left with residual facial weakness that may result in drooling, inability to smile and fully close the eye on the affected side. These limitations in facial expression may adversely impair communication and social relationships (Wysong and Azizzadeh 2011). Long-term sequelae may include involuntary movements of facial muscles (synkinesis). Poor prognostic factors include complete facial weakness, hypertension, impairments of taste, pain other than the ear, and older age (Gilden 2004). Bell's palsy is presumed to be due to reactivation of Herpes simplex virus type 1 in the geniculate ganglion (Gilden 2004). Although evidence is conflicting, a seasonal variation supports an infectious etiology (Narci et al. 2012). Neuroimaging suggests that a narrow labyrinthine segment of the facial nerve canal may increase susceptibility to Bell's palsy when the facial nerve becomes edematous (Murai et al. 2012). Electroneurography can assist prognostication.

On Call at the Montreal General Hospital

I remember one cold winter night during my residency when I agonized over whether to prescribe steroids to an elderly diabetic woman with Bell's palsy. Like many patients with Bell's, she had come to the emergency room fearful of a possible stroke. Her weak facial muscles, asymmetric flattened forehead, and otherwise normal neurologic examination allowed me to offer reassurance that she had not had a stroke. But then I had to decide what to do about the Bell's. Even a short course of steroids was not without potential complications of GI bleed, hyperglycemia, mood swings and others. I knew that treatment was a hotly debated topic, but couldn't recall the bottom line. An American Academy of Neurology (AAN) Evidence-Based Guideline would have come in handy, but AAN Guidelines would not be invented for a couple of more years. I reluctantly telephoned the attending, likely nursing a nightcap while bathed in the warm glow of his fireplace. My esteemed professor didn't know the answer either, and deferred the question back to me, asserting that I was "closer to the recent literature."

Diagnostic Considerations

Bell's palsy and stroke are the two most common causes of sudden facial weakness (Gilden 2004). Part of the importance in accurately diagnosing Bell's palsy is not only to treat the underlying condition, but to recognize that a Bell's palsy is not a stroke. Brainstem lesions and parotid tumors must also be considered in the setting of a seventh nerve paralysis. Additional causes of acute isolated facial nerve weakness include amyloid, diabetes, HIV, sarcoid and others (Gilden 2004). A peripheral facial nerve palsy accompanied by vesicles on the ear (Herpes zoster oticus), known as Ramsay Hunt syndrome, has a viral etiology (Angles et al. 2012).

Tangled Terminology

One can get tangled in a semantic net when discussing the etiology of Bell's palsy because by definition, Bell's palsy is idiopathic (Gronseth and Paduga 2012). Purists will rightly insist that once a specific etiology is determined, e.g., Lyme disease, the problem is no longer a "Bell's palsy," but a "facial palsy due to Lyme disease." This distinction is important because once an etiology is identified, treatment can be directed to the underlying disease. However, in common parlance, Bell's has become synonymous with a seventh nerve mononeuropathy, and many still refer to a "Bell's palsy due to Lyme disease."

Updated Recommendations

The AAN recently updated evidence-based guidelines regarding the use of steroids and antivirals for Bell's palsy (Gronseth and Paduga 2012). Of 340 citations, 9 articles were included. Only controlled trials with prospective data collection including at least 20 patients followed for at least 3 months qualified. Since the last evidence-based guideline on this topic in 2001 (Grogan and Gronseth 2001), two Class I (see Appendix) studies were published that both supported the use of steroids, resulting in the current Level A recommendation. The evidence was much less persuasive for antiviral treatment, resulting in a Level C recommendation, "possibly effective." These conclusions are similar to the AAN's 2001 recommendations, but the endorsement for steroids is now much stronger. Decompressive facial nerve surgery was not addressed in the recent guidelines, perhaps because of the lack of randomized trials.

Antivirals?
Several oral antiviral medications are now available; acyclovir, famciclovir, and valacyclovir. In as much as Bell's palsy is presumed secondary to a viral infection, antiviral medication would seem a logical choice. However, even well-performed studies have failed to show benefit (Engstrom et al. 2008, Sullivan et al. 2007, Gronseth and Paduga 2012). All three of these antiviral drugs target Herpes viruses, which may or may not be responsible for an individual case of Bell's palsy. One could imagine other etiologic mechanisms, such as virus-induced antibody syndromes that preferentially attack the seventh nerve, in which antiviral therapy might not be effective, even if the virus was the inciting agent. There is some suggestion that antivirals offer synergistic effect with steroids, particularly in severely affected patients (Minnerop et al. 2008), but no conclusive evidence to support this contention (Gronseth and Paduga 2012).

Conclusions
This AAN Guideline provides a Level A recommendation for the use of steroids in the treatment of Bell's palsy. This is an impressive conclusion in the face of an illness where approximately 3/4 of patients recover without any treatment. Prompt administration of steroids is likely to be beneficial. Whether an antiviral should be prescribed in addition, and which one, remains an open question and needs further study. There is still more to learn until the day when all cases

of acute peripheral seventh nerve palsy can be ascribed to a known cause and the term "Bell's palsy" becomes obsolete. If these etiologic answers arrive soon, this current AAN Guideline may be the last to address "Bell's palsy."

References

Angles EM, Nelson SW, Higgins GL. A woman with facial weakness: A classic case of Ramsay Hunt syndrome. The Journal of Emergency Medicine 2012, June;dpi:10.1016/j.jemermed.2012.02.061.

Engstrom M, Berg T, Stjernquist-Desatnik A et al. Prednisolone and valaciclovir in Bell's palsy: a randomised, double-blind, placebo-controlled, multicentre trial. Lancet Neurology 2008;7:993-9.

Gilden DH. Bell's palsy. NEJM 2004;351:1323-1331.

Grogan PM, Gronseth GS. Practice parameter: steroids, acyclovir, and surgery for Bell's palsy (an evidence-based review): report of the Quality Standards Subcommittee of the American Academy of Neurology. Neurology 2001;56:830-836.

Gronseth GS, Paduga R. Evidence-based guideline update: Steroids and antivirals for Bell palsy: Report of the Guideline Development Subcommittee of the American Academy of Neurology 2012;79:1-5.

Minnerop M, Herbst M, Fimmers R et al. Bell's palsy. Combined treatment of famciclovir and prednisone is superior to prednisone alone. J Neurol 2008;255:1726-1730.

Murai A, Kariya S, Tamura K et al. The facial nerve canal in patients with Bell's palsy: an investigation by high-resolution computed tomography with multi planar reconstruction. Eur Arch Otorhinolaryngol 2012; Nov 11. Epub ahead of print.

Narci H, Horasanli B, Ugur M. Seasonal effects on Bell's palsy: Four-year study and review of the literature. Iran Red Crescent Med J. 2012;14(8):505-506.

Sullivan FM, Swan IRC, Donnan PT et al. Early treatment with prednisolone or acyclovir in Bell's palsy. NEJM 2007;357:1598-1607.

Wysong P, Azizzadeh B. Facing the truth about Bell palsy. www.medscape.com/viewarticle/739509, March 28, 2011.

Chapter 89

UPDATED GUIDELINES FOR RUPTURED ANEURYSMS FROM THE AMERICAN HEART AND STROKE ASSOCIATIONS

July 3, 2012

Introduction

The American Heart and Stroke Associations have recently updated their 2009 guidelines for the management of aneurysmal subarachnoid hemorrhage (aSAH) (Connolly et al. 2012).

The incidence of aSAH ranges from 2-16/100,000. Management of patients with ruptured cerebral aneurysms is not for the faint of heart. At least 25% of patients die, about half of these before they even get to the hospital, and about 50% suffer persistent neurologic morbidity. In my hospital, "blood in the brain" directs patients to the neurosurgical service. However, these patients fall into the category of "stroke" and may be seen at presentation in the emergency room by neurology consultants or later in their course to address seizures, unexplained altered mental status, and, of course, brain death.

The new guidelines are quite hefty (26 pages) and deserve a detailed review by clinicians who care for this patient population. The update includes 22 Class I recommendations, including 5 new ones since 2009. These

Class I recommendations are summarized below followed by their level of evidence (A, B, C)*.

Class I Recommendations

1. Treatment of high blood pressure with antihypertensive medication is recommended to prevent ischemic stroke, intracerebral hemorrhage, and cardiac, renal, and other end-organ injury (A)

2. Oral nimodipine should be administered (A)

3. Hypertension should be treated, and it may reduce the risk of aSAH (B)

4. Tobacco and alcohol misuse should be avoided to reduce the risk of aSAH (B)

5. Cerebrovascular imaging is indicated immediately after repair to identify remnants that may need re-treatment (B)

6. Clinical validated scales should be used to determine prognosis (B)

7. Urgent evaluation and treatment is recommended due to the risk of early rebleed (B)

8. A high level of suspicion for aSAH should exist in patients with acute onset of severe headache (B)

9. If a noncontrast CT is negative, it should be followed by a lumbar puncture (B)

10. Digital subtraction angiography with 3-dimensional rotational angiography is indicated for aneurysm detection and treatment planning (B)

11. Blood pressure should be controlled with a titratable agent (B)

12. Surgical clipping or endovascular coiling should be performed as early as possible (B)

13. Complete obliteration of the aneurysm is recommended (B)

14. If both coiling and clipping are appropriate, consider coiling first (B)

15. Delayed follow up of vascular imaging is indicated to assess the need of retreatment (B)

16. Low volume hospitals (eg <10 aSAH cases/year) should consider transfer of patients to high volume centers (eg >35 aSAH cases/year) (B)

17. Maintain euvolemia and normal blood volume to prevent delayed cerebral ischemia (B)

18. Hypertension is recommended for delayed cerebral ischemia unless contraindicated (B)

19. Acute symptomatic hydrocephalus requires cerebral or lumbar drainage (B)

20. Heparin-induced thrombocytopenia and deep venous thrombosis need to be identified and treated early (B)

21. Treatment is best determined by a multidisciplinary team (C)

22. Chronic symptomatic hydrocephalus requires a permanent shunt (C)

Conclusions

The diagnosis and management of acute subarachnoid hemorrhage remains challenging. It is interesting that even in these days of very high resolution CT scans, a lumbar puncture is still recommended if the CT is negative to detect possible cases of aSAH. Patients with aSAH tend to be critically ill, require time-intensive management, critical decision making regarding the type and timing of interventions, and rapid response to complications such as acute hydrocephalus, deep venous thrombosis, delayed cerebral ischemia, heparin-induced thrombocytopenia, seizures, and others. Patients are likely to do better when treated by an experienced team of anesthesiologists, cerebrovascular neurosurgeons, endovascular specialists, and neurointensivists. Tertiary care centers are more likely to harbor these resources and should network with smaller hospitals to care for patients with aSAH. Although there may be dissension regarding specific treatment choices in individual cases, there is a consensus that rapid, expert therapy leads to optimal results.

*The classification scheme used in this guideline is different from that used by the American Academy of Neurology (see Appendix). Class I suggests that the procedure/treatment "should be performed/administered." The certainty of the recommendation is then modified by the level of the evidence; A-multiple randomized clinical trials or meta-analysis, B-a single randomized trial or nonrandomized studies, C-consensus opinion of experts, case studies, or standard of care.

References

Connolly ES, Rabinstein AA, Carhuapoma JR et al. Guidelines for the management of aneurysmal subarachnoid hemorrhage. A guideline for healthcare professionals from the American Heart Association/American Stroke Association. Stroke 2012;43:1711-1737.

Chapter 90

ANTIEPILEPTICS AND HIV: AN EVIDENCE-BASED GUIDELINE

June 22, 2012

Introduction

Seizures occur in as many as 11% of people with HIV/AIDS and may require treatment with antiepileptic drugs. Causes of seizures in these patients include drugs, metabolic derangements, neoplasia, opportunistic infections, and the HIV virus (Birbeck et al. 2012, Yacoob et al. 2011). Antiepileptic drugs may also be used to treat HIV/AIDS-related peripheral neuropathy, which occurs in more than one half of HIV-infected patients (Birbeck et al. 2012). Furthermore, psychiatric conditions, refractory headaches, and movement disorders in HIV-infected persons may benefit from antiepileptic drugs (Birbeck et al. 2012, Lee et al. 2012, Okulicz et al. 2011).

Consequently, there is a high likelihood that people with HIV/AIDS will be exposed to a combination of antiretroviral and antiepileptic therapies. For example, in a study of 1,345 patients with HIV/AIDS who were followed at the Southern Alberta Clinic in Canada, 169 (12.6%) were taking antiepileptic drugs (Lee et al. 2012).

Physicians who care for people with HIV/AIDS need to be alert to the possibility of drug/drug interactions between antiepileptic and antiretroviral drugs to avoid loss of efficacy of either drug class or potential toxicities. The

American Academy of Neurology (AAN), in conjunction with the International League Against Epilepsy (ILAE), recently published a guideline addressing this issue (Birbeck et al. 2012). The panel reached its conclusions after a literature search of 4,480 articles and detailed review of 42 articles. The data included class 2, 3, and 4 studies but no class 1 research (randomized, placebo controlled clinical trials with masked outcome assessment).

All of the panel's recommendations are level C, based on relatively "weak" evidence. Level C indicates than an intervention or test is possibly effective, ineffective, or harmful (or possibly useful/predictive or not useful/predictive) for the given condition in the specified population. A rating of level C requires at least one Class 2 study or two consistent Class 3 studies.

Antiepileptic drugs that induce the cytochrome P450 enzyme system, such as carbamazepine, phenobarbital, and phenytoin may increase the metabolism of certain antiretroviral drugs and decrease their efficacy. Antiretroviral drugs that are metabolized by the cytochrome P450 system include protease inhibitors, such as lopinavir and ritonavir, nonnucleoside reverse transcriptase inhibitors, such as efavirenz and nevirapine, and a CCR5 inhibitor, maraviroc (Okulicz et al. 2011). Nucleoside reverse transcriptase inhibitors, such as tenofovir and zidovudine, do not interact with cytochrome P450 enzyme-inducing antiepileptic drugs (Okulicz et al. 2011).

Conversely, certain antiretroviral drugs may reduce serum levels of antiepileptic drugs. For example, the combination of ritonavir and atazanavir may require an increase in lamotrigine dosage. Other drug/drug combinations may also have significant interactions but have not yet been thoroughly studied. Known antiepileptic and antiretroviral drug interactions are summarized below:

- Antiepileptic drugs that affect antiretroviral drugs

Phenytoin reduces lopinavir/ritonavir by 50%
Valproic acid increases zidovudine
- Antiretroviral drugs that affect antiepileptic drugs

Ritonavir/atazanavir decreases lamotrigine by 50%
- Drug/drug combinations that don't change levels
Atazanavir: no change in lamotrigine

Raltegravir: no change in lamotrigine or midazolam

Valproic acid: no change in efavirenz

Antiepileptics to Avoid

A retrospective case-control analysis from the US Military HIV Natural History Study revealed that patients taking enzyme-inducing antiepileptic drugs and antiretroviral therapy were significantly more likely to have virologic treatment failure than those taking non-enzyme-inducing antiepileptic drugs (63% vs. 27%, respectively, p=0.009) (Okulicz et al. 2011). In these patients, enzyme-inducing antiepileptic drugs may have resulted in subtherapeutic levels of highly active antiretroviral therapy (HAART) causing increased viral load. Subtherapeutic treatment may allow development of drug-resistant viral mutations and HIV disease progression (Okulicz et al. 2011).

The authors recommended avoiding enzyme-inducing antiepileptic drugs in patients treated with HAART whenever possible because this combination risks ineffective treatment for both HIV/AIDS and seizures, neuropathy, and other antiepileptic drug indications. Although use of newer non-enzyme-inducing antiepileptic drugs may avoid interactions with antiretroviral drugs, this option may not be available in many clinical settings-including developing nations where cost limits medication choice.

Valproic acid, which is not a cytochrome P450 inducer, increases the level of zidovudine, which may allow a dosage reduction of this antiviral agent and cost savings. In a recent report, valproic acid was successfully used for seizure control in 8 patients treated with HAART (Yacoob et al. 2011). Although there is laboratory evidence that valproate may increase HIV replication *in vitro*, one study did not find any effect on viral load with valproate or other antiepileptic drugs (Lee et al. 2012).

The selection of an antiepileptic drug for patients with HIV/AIDS depends not only on seizure type, comorbidities, hepatic and renal function, adverse event profile, and cost but also on potential drug/drug interactions with antiretroviral therapy. Seizure control and serum levels of antiepileptic drugs should be monitored to insure optimal therapeutic effect. To assess the efficacy of antiretroviral medication, patients should be closely followed for symptoms of opportunistic infections, and viral load should be measured periodically.

Conclusions

Polytherapy risks toxicity and drug/drug interactions, but it is a fact of life for many patients with HIV/AIDS taking combination antiretroviral therapy. Patients with HIV/AIDS and seizures, peripheral neuropathy, psychiatric illness, chronic headache, or movement disorders may have the additional medication burden of 1 or more antiepileptic drugs.

Although the evidence supporting this AAN/ILAE guideline is relatively weak, the guideline highlights drug/drug interactions likely to be clinically significant. The increasing number of antiepileptic and antiretroviral medications will multiply the risk for significant drug/drug interactions. Pharmacists may find that their expertise regarding pharmacokinetic drug interactions is particularly appreciated in HIV/AIDS and epilepsy clinics. Physicians and other healthcare professionals need to stay vigilant for possible drug/drug interactions between antiepileptic drugs and antiretroviral therapy in order to control seizures and other neurologic and psychiatric symptoms, maintain HIV viral load suppression, and prevent drug toxicity.

References

Birbeck GL, French JA, Perucca E et al. Evidence-based guideline: antiepileptic drug selection for people with HIV/AIDS: Report of the Quality Standards Subcommittee of the American Academy of Neurology and the Ad Hoc Task Force of the Commission on Therapeutic Strategies of the International League Against Epilepsy. Neurology 2012;78:139-145.

Yacoob Y, Bhigjee AL, Moodley P, Parboosing R. Sodium valproate and highly active antiretroviral therapy in HIV positive patients who develop new onset seizures. Seizure 2011;20:80-82.

Lee K, Vivithanapom P, Siemieniuk RA et al. Clinical outcomes and immune benefits of anti-epileptic drug therapy in HIV/AIDS. BMC Neurol 2012;10:44.

Okulicz J, Grandits GA, French JA et al. Infectious Disease Clinical Research Program (IDCRP) HIV Working Group. Virologic outcomes of HAART with concurrent use of cytochrome P450 enzyme-inducing antiepileptics: a retrospective case control study. AIDS Res Ther 2011;8:18.

Chapter 91

INFANTILE SPASMS-NEW GUIDELINE FROM THE AMERICAN ACADEMY OF NEUROLOGY

June 19, 2012

Introduction

I still remember my first case of infantile spasms. I was a second year neurology resident and received a page* around 2 am from the Montreal Children's Hospital. When I heard the story from the pediatric resident, I quickly dressed, threw on my winter coat and rushed to the hospital. Our venerable Director of the Division of Pediatric Neurology, Gordon Watters, MD, FRCP, had impressed upon us the urgency to treat infantile spasms as soon as possible in order to minimize brain damage from seizures. I had not reviewed the literature and did not know whether such a recommendation was "evidence-based." Nonetheless, for the possible benefit of the child, and my survival as a resident, I knew there was no time to waste.

When I arrived in the emergency room, the diagnosis was obvious. The infant's mother clutched her close while her daughter's torso jackknifed forward, making her almost impossible to hold. The spasms came in clusters, lasting a few seconds each. I did my best to examine the infant and arranged for ACTH therapy.

Updated Guidelines

Infantile spasms is thankfully a rare disorder, with a prevalence of about 1/5,000 children. When accompanied by psychomotor retardation and a hypsarrhythmic pattern on the electroencephalogram, the triad is known as West syndrome. Treatment goals include stopping the spasms and improving long-term developmental outcomes.

The American Academy of Neurology and the Child Neurology Society have recently updated the 2004 Guideline, which was based on a review of 159 articles. They performed a literature search from 2002-2011 and reviewed an additional 26 articles. Their findings are summarized below:

Recommendations

1. Low dose ACTH is probably as good as high dose (Level B)

2. ACTH may be better than vigabatrin for short-term treatment (Level C)

3. ACTH or prednisolone may be better than vigabatrin for cryptogenic infantile spasms regarding developmental outcome (Level C)

4. Early treatment with ACTH or vigabatrin may result in better developmental outcome (Level C)

5. Insufficient evidence whether any other steroids are as good or better than ACTH (Level U)

6. Insufficient evidence to recommend antiepileptic drugs, the ketogenic diet or therapies other than ACTH or vigabatrin (Level U)

Discussion

Even now, 25 years after I rushed to the hospital that freezing Montreal night, the value of early treatment is still debated. In this updated guideline, six new studies provided Class II, III, and IV evidence for intermediate to long-term outcome. A shorter lag-time to treatment with ACTH or vigabatrin achieved only a Level "C" (possibly effective) recommendation (see Appendix for explanation of "Levels"). While therapeutic nihilists may take comfort in the lack of convincing data, most physicians will still prefer to initiate treatment as soon as possible in the hopes of arresting symptoms and optimizing prognosis.

With respect to treatment choice, if ACTH is used, the best doses, formulation, and treatment duration are still unclear. Adverse effects of hormonal therapy include cerebral atrophy (62%), hypertension (0-37%), infection (14%) and irritability (37-100%).

Vigabatrin received U.S. Food and Drug Administration (FDA) approval in 2009 for infantile spasms as well as adjunctive therapy for partial seizures, despite a black box warning for permanent visual impairment. The clinical significance of MRI abnormalities that may appear during the course of vigabatrin therapy that disappear with the discontinuation of vigabatrin is unknown. There is some evidence to suggest that vigabatrin may be particularly useful when infantile spasms occur in the setting of tuberous sclerosis but this advantage has not been tested in randomized trials.

Future Evidence

A randomized controlled trial of hormonal therapy plus vigabatrin vs. hormonal therapy alone is underway. Results are also pending from a randomized, double blind trial of add-on flunarizine to prevent cognitive decline in children with infantile spasms.

Conclusions

Although there has been progress since the 2004 Guidelines, the 2012 Guidelines still suffer from a lack of high quality evidence-there are no Level A recommendations. However, a Level B recommendation that low dose ACTH is as effective as high dose ACTH supports lower dose treatment and may help reduce the frequency and severity of adverse events. The role of vigabatrin and other therapies is evolving. Physicians faced with the daunting task of treating infantile spasms must still rely heavily on their residency training, personal experience and instincts.

*A pager is an archaic device that could receive a text message but not respond.

References

Go CY, Mackay MT, Weiss SK et al. Evidence-based guideline update: Medical treatment of infantile spasms. Report of the Guideline Development Subcommittee of the American Academy of Neurology and the Practice Committee of the Child Neurology Society. Neurology 2012;78:1974-1980.

Mackay MT, Weiss SK, Adams-Webber T et al. Practice Parameter: Medical treatment of infantile spasms: Report of the American Academy of Neurology and the Child Neurology Society. Neurology 2004;62:1668-1681.

Update June 1, 2013

A recent trial of flunarizine, a neuroprotective agent, did not improve cognition in children with infantile spasms. Current research studies on infantile spasms include genetics, low dose ACTH, pyridoxine and others.

Additional References

Bitton JY, Sauerwein HC, Weiss SK. A randomized controlled trial of flunarizine as add-on therapy and effect on cognitive outcome in children with infantile spasms. Epilepsia 2012;53(9):1570-1576.

Chapter 92

IVIG-NEW AMERICAN ACADEMY OF NEUROLOGY GUIDELINE

April 15, 2012

Introduction

While on rounds seeing critically ill patients with neurologic disease, every now and then another consultant asks, "Should we try IVIg?" Usually, I don't know what to say and have to go look it up. I don't remember learning much about IVIg during residency, and it's not something I prescribe every day. It seems to be used for all kinds of things, from Guillain Barre Syndrome (GBS) to immune rejection prevention in transplant patients. Thankfully, the American Academy of Neurology (AAN) has recently published a new guideline to help clarify the role of IVIg in the treatment of neuromuscular disorders (Patwa et al. 2012).

Indications

The U.S. Food and Drug Administration (FDA) has approved IVIg for two neurologic indications; GBS and Chronic Inflammatory Demyelinating Polyneuropathy (CIDP). IVIg blocks antibodies and can inhibit complement activity, resulting in immunomodulatory and anti-inflammatory effects (Jordan et al. 2006). It may also rarely cause aseptic meningitis, hypercoagulability, renal failure and stroke, as well as many other infrequent adverse events. IVIg is expensive; a 4 dose course for a 70 kg man at 2 gm/kg costs about $25,000, so it's not just another treatment to throw in the mix without a strong indication. A further consideration is that the half-life is only about three weeks, raising the stakes if long-term treatment is required for a chronic disease (Jordan et al. 2006).

Here is a summary of the Guideline's major recommendations:

GBS
Effective in adults (Level A) (see Appendix for explanation of "Levels")
Insufficient evidence in children (Level U)
Don't combine with plasmapheresis (Level B)
Insufficient evidence regarding combining with steroids (Level U)

CIDP
Effective for long-term treatment (Level A)

Myasthenia gravis
Should be considered, especially for moderate or severe cases (Level B)

Multifocal motor neuropathy
Should be considered (Level B)

Lambert-Eaton myasthenic syndrome
May be considered (Level C)

Dermatomyositis

May be considered for nonresponsive dermatomyositis (Level C)

Inclusion body myositis
Insufficient evidence (Level U)

IgM paraprotein neuropathy
Insufficient evidence (Level U)

Postpolio syndrome (see Chapter 18)
Insufficient evidence (Level U)

Lack of Controlled Studies
Diabetic polyradiculoplexoneuropathy, Miller Fisher syndrome, polymyositis

Conclusions
IVIg is a valuable tool for the treatment of immune mediated neurologic diseases like GBS and CIDP. It is usually well tolerated, but serious and mild complications may occur. As is often the case, definitive studies regarding pediatric indications lag behind. Many important questions remain to be answered regarding frequency and duration of IVIg dosing, relative effectiveness compared to plasmapheresis and other therapies, and the possibility of synergies (or incompatibility) with other treatments. More studies are needed to determine whether IVIg will also be useful for diabetic polyradiculoplexoneuropathy, Miller Fisher syndrome, polymyositis, or other challenging immune related diseases such as multiple sclerosis or immune related intractable epilepsy (see Chapter 48).

The AAN Guideline provides a solid reference for clinical decision making, which should be helpful on rounds and in terms of procuring reimbursement.

References

Jordan SC, Vo AA, Peng A et al. Intravenous gammaglobulin (IVIG): A novel approach to improve transplant rates and outcomes in highly HLA-sensitized patients. American Journal of Transplantation 2006;6(3):459-466. http://www.medscape.com/viewarticle/523523, 2/28/2006.

Patwa HS, Chaudhry V, Katzberg H et al. Evidence-based guideline: Intravenous immunoglobulin in the treatment of neuromuscular disorders. Neurology 2012;78:1009-1015.

Chapter 93

DIAGNOSIS AND TREATMENT OF TRANSVERSE MYELITIS-A NEW GUIDELINE

February 29, 2012

Introduction

The incidence of acute transverse myelitis is literally one in a million. Most physicians see relatively few cases, and even neurologists may find it difficult to become comfortable with its diagnosis and treatment. Consequently, the new evidence-based guideline from the American Academy of Neurology (AAN) on clinical evaluation and treatment is particularly welcome. One of the key challenges in treating transverse myelitis is distinguishing idiopathic acute transverse myelitis from all other causes. The guideline references a previous paper from the Transverse Myelitis Consortium Working Group that developed diagnostic criteria for idiopathic acute transverse myelitis (Table 1). The Transverse Myelitis Consortium Working Group paper also provides a useful diagnostic algorithm and detailed suggestions for testing (Neurology 2002).

Table 1. Idiopathic Acute Transverse Myelitis Diagnostic Criteria

- Sensory, motor, or autonomic dysfunction attributable to the spinal cord
- Bilateral signs and/or symptoms

- Clearly defined sensory level
- Exclusion of compressive etiology
- Exclusion of other forms of demyelinating disease (e.g., no cerebral lesions suggestive of multiple sclerosis (MS), no optic neuritis to suggest neuromyelitis optica (NMO), no connective tissue disease, no CNS infection, no history of spinal radiation, no clear arterial distribution to suggest spinal cord infarct)
- Spinal cord inflammation demonstrated by CSF pleocytosis, elevated IgG index or gadolinium-enhanced MRI
- Progression to nadir between 4 hours and 21 days

The most common etiologies to be distinguished from idiopathic acute transverse myelitis are MS, parainfectious myelitis, NMO (Devic's disease), and myelitis related to systemic disease, such as systemic lupus erythematosis (Scott et al. 2011). Up to 36% of patients with transverse myelitis have idiopathic acute transverse myelitis, where a definite etiology cannot be determined (Scott et al. 2011).

Guidelines

The new evidence-based guidelines from the AAN address differential diagnosis, acute symptomatic treatment, and treatment designed to prevent further episodes. After a literature search of English language articles published in 1996-2009, 65 articles met inclusion criteria. The panel's major conclusions are summarized below:

Diagnostic Evaluation

1. Based on two Class III studies, age is "possibly useful" to distinguish spinal cord infarcts from other causes of acute myelopathy, as older patients are more likely to have spinal cord infarcts than acute transverse myelitis. Further, women are more likely to develop inflammatory acute transverse myelitis than spinal cord infarct, indicating that female gender is "possibly useful" as well.

2. Based on two Class III studies, CSF pleocytosis (>10 cells/mm^3) favors an inflammatory myelitis over spinal cord infarct, making CSF evaluation "possibly useful."

MS vs. NMO

Once acute transverse myelitis has been diagnosed and compressive and systemic etiologies ruled out, a major clinical consideration is whether the lesion represents MS (or clinically isolated syndrome) or NMO. Differentiating MS from NMO is clinically important, as the choice of medication for treatment may be dramatically different (e.g., interferon for MS vs. azathioprine for NMO).

Acute transverse myelitis can be complete (acute complete transverse myelitis) (ACTM), which causes symmetric loss of function distal to that level, or partial (acute partial transverse myelitis) (APTM), with incomplete or patchy lesions producing weakness, asymmetric or dissociated sensory symptoms, and occasionally bladder symptoms. Based on multiple Class III studies, those with APTM are more likely to transition to MS than those with ACTM.

Multiple Class III studies suggest that patients with longitudinal extensive spinal cord lesions (≥3 vertebral segments) are more likely to develop NMO than MS, making this criterion "possibly useful."

One Class II and multiple Class III studies suggest that patients with acute transverse myelitis are "possibly" more likely to develop MS (rather than NMO) if there are simultaneous brain lesions on MRI. (However, cerebral lesions may also occur in NMO).

One Class I and several Class III studies endorse aquaporin-4 autoantibodies (NMO-IgG) as "probably" useful in determining the cause of acute transverse myelitis.

Oligoclonal bands are more likely in MS than NMO, but do not appear in parainfectious myelitis or spinal cord infarct based on one Class II and eight Class III studies, making this test "possibly useful."

CSF pleocytosis (>50 cells/mm^3) is more likely in NMO than MS based on one Class III study, making it "possibly useful" as a diagnostic test. (In addition, another Class III study suggested that the etiology was something other than MS if the pleocytosis was > 30 cells/mm^3.)

Relapse

Multiple Class III studies suggest that relapse rates are "possibly" more common in APTM than ACTM. In addition, one Class I study suggests that NMO autoantibodies "probably" predict relapse in patients with acute transverse myelitis.

Treatment

High dose methylprednisolone is usually the initial treatment of acute transverse myelitis (although only Class IV evidence supports this practice, which constitutes "insufficient evidence"). Similarly, "insufficient evidence" supports mitoxantrone. Plasma exchange is "possibly" useful based on one Class II study. Rituximab is "possibly" effective based on two Class III studies. "Insufficient evidence" supports azathioprine, cyclophosphamide, and IVIg to alleviate symptoms or prevent future attacks. Based on the above evidence, the panel made the following recommendations:

Recommendations
Level A-none (see Appendix for explanation of "Levels")

Level B

1. NMO-IgG antibodies are useful to differentiate NMO from MS

2. NMO-IgG antibodies favor recurrence

Level C

1. Age may be useful (older age suggests vascular etiology)

2. Female gender suggests development of MS

3. Brain MRI lesions suggest development of MS

4. Distinction between ACTM and APTM may help determine etiology and relapse risk as those with APTM are more likely to develop MS and recurrences

5. Longer spinal lesions (≥3 vertebral segments) favor NMO over MS

6. CSF cell count and oligoclonal bands may help determine etiology by implicating NMO or other nonMS causes (high cell count) or MS (oligoclonal bands)

Conclusions

An episode of transverse myelitis with rapid loss of spinal cord function requires a prompt diagnostic and therapeutic response. Patients must be immediately assessed for structural lesions that might cause a compressive myelopathy as well as noninflammatory and inflammatory etiologies. This new AAN guideline provides welcome direction for this rare but often disabling disorder. The discovery of aquaporin-4 antibodies and increased understanding of NMO has led to Level B recommendations and highlights the importance of differentiating this newly-defined disease from MS. Physicians should not hesitate to order NMO-IgG antibodies when they suspect NMO. While the evidence supporting steroids as initial treatment of acute transverse myelitis is thin, high dose intravenous (IV) methylprednisolone remains the usual choice. Prospective clinical trials will further elucidate optimal treatments for patients with transverse myelitis of various etiologies.

References

Scott TF, Frohman EM, De Seze J et al. Evidence-based guideline: Clinical evaluation and treatment of transverse myelitis. Neurology 2011;77:2128-2134.

Transverse Myelitis Consortium Working Group. Proposed diagnostic criteria and nosology of acute transverse myelitis. Neurology 2002;59:499-505.

Chapter 94

NEW NICE GUIDELINES TO PREVENT DELIRIUM

November 22, 2011

Introduction

After stroke, transient ischemic attack (TIA), and seizures, the most common neurology consult at my 300 bed community hospital is for delirium, an acute confusional state (see Chapter 78). This diagnosis includes a wide variety of clinical scenarios including encephalitis, hypoxic encephalopathy, intensive care unit (ICU) psychosis, metabolic encephalopathy, nonconvulsive status epilepticus, postictal confusion, postoperative confusion and many others. Often patients have had a "stormy hospital course," and when the dust settled, it became apparent that their mental status had changed. Given proper treatment and time, most patients regain their previous level of intellectual function. But delirium can have a profound effect on prognosis; a prolonged episode of delirium may lead to additional complications such as falls, increased mortality, pressure ulcers, prolonged hospitalization, and the need for long-term care (O'Mahoney et al. 2011).

High Cost of Delirium

Delirium occurs during hospitalization in 6-56% of general hospital populations and 70-87% of those in intensive care (Inouye 2006). Delirium is particularly common in the elderly, complicating the course of at least 20% of the 12.5 million patients 65 years or older hospitalized each year and increasing hospital costs by $2,500 per patient (Inouye 2006). Hospital expenditures attributable to delirium amount to 6.9 billion dollars per year for Medicare (Inouye 2006). The one year mortality of patients with delirium is 35-40% (Inouye 2006).

New Guideline

A recently published clinical guideline developed by the National Institute for Health and Clinical Excellence (NICE) provides suggestions for the prevention of delirium in hospitalized patients (O'Mahony et al. 2011). The guideline is based on eight studies of multicomponent intervention for preventing delirium, only three of which were randomized, controlled trials. The authors estimate that approximately 1/3 cases of delirium could be prevented by multicomponent interventions. The guideline's 13 recommendations for hospitalized patients and adults in long term care are summarized below:

Recommendations

1. Avoid moving patients within and between wards or rooms.

2. Assess all patients for susceptibility to delirium within 24 hours of admission.

3. Implement a multicomponent intervention package to prevent delirium by a trained, multidisciplinary team.

4. Provide clocks, calendars, clear signage, and good lighting in patient rooms. Reorient patients and encourage visits from family and friends.

5. Address dehydration and constipation.

6. Assess for hypoxia.

7. Avoid unnecessary catheterization and identify and treat infections.

8. Address immobility.

9. Address pain.

10. Review medications.

11. Address poor nutrition and make sure that dentures fit.

12. Ensure that visual and hearing aids are available.

13. Promote sleep.

Conclusions

Sometimes it seems that just walking into the hospital, or more commonly, rolling in on a stretcher, triggers the onset of delirium in susceptible patients. The NICE guidelines offer relatively simple interventions that may prevent vulnerable patients from developing delirium. Some of the recommendations represent basic medical care (e.g., assess for pain, avoid unnecessary catheterization, review medications), and others are deceptively simple, such as making sure that patients have their glasses and hearing aids to prevent sensory deprivation and disorientation. (Can you count the times you have tried to interview a hospitalized patient who couldn't find their hearing aid or glasses?) The last recommendation, "Promote good sleep patterns and sleep hygiene," is often overlooked in busy hospitals that function 24/7, but may be very important for patient health.

Any opportunity to decrease the incidence of delirium should be warmly embraced. Hospitals should consider setting up a "delirium prevention committee" in order to integrate these NICE recommendations into routine hospital practice. If these preventive measures achieve anywhere near the projected 30% reduction in cases of delirium, they will not only improve patient outcomes but will be cost effective as well. Patients and neurologists will be grateful for a few less consults for "altered mental status."

References

Inouye SK. Delirium in older persons. NEJM 2006;354:1157-1165.

O'Mahony R, Murth L, Akunne A et al. Synopsis of the National Institute for Health and Clinical Excellence Guideline for Prevention of Delirium. Ann Intern Med 2011;154:746-751.

Chapter 95

PLASMAPHERESIS-AMERICAN ACADEMY OF NEUROLOGY PRACTICE PARAMETER-WHO REALLY BENEFITS?

March 23, 2011

Introduction

Plasmapheresis is expensive, time consuming, and not without risk of significant morbidity (AAN 1996, McLeod et al. 1999). Consequently, this therapy should be reserved for those patients for whom it offers a reasonable chance of benefit. The new evidence-based guideline from the American Academy of Neurology (AAN) updates prior recommendations from 1996 on plasmapheresis (AAN 1996) and provides solid guidance for the practitioner (Table 1). Not only are there Level A (see Appendix) recommendations for the treatment of severe acute demyelinating polyneuropathy (CIDP), but also a Level A recommendation for a disorder that should not be treated with plasmapheresis (chronic or secondary progressive multiple sclerosis).*

Similarly, Level B recommendations suggest that plasmapheresis is helpful for mild Guillain Barre syndrome, steroid resistant exacerbations of relapsing multiple sclerosis, and immunoglobulin A or G, but not M, gammopathies. A lower level of evidence led to a Level C recommendation for fulminating demyelinating central nervous system disease.

Surprisingly, there was insufficient evidence to recommend plasmapheresis for exacerbations of myasthenia gravis, which, at least in my hospital, is the standard of care. There was also insufficient evidence to recommend or refute plasmapheresis for the treatment of pediatric autoimmune neuropsychiatric disorders associated with streptococcus infection (PANDAS), or Sydenham chorea.

The guideline does not advocate specific plasmapheresis treatment protocols regarding the number of treatments or volumes exchanged, which remain a matter of clinical judgment until more evidence accumulates. It also does not weigh the risks and benefits of plasmapheresis versus intravenous immunoglobulin (IVIg). (A prior AAN parameter concluded that plasmapheresis and IVIg were equivalent for acute Guillain Barre syndrome (Hughes et al. 2003). The management of myasthenic crisis, including the use of plasmapheresis and IVIg, is discussed in a recent review (Wendell and Levine 2011)).

This AAN guideline was based on a literature review of 59 articles published with English abstracts from 1995-2009. Articles were ranked regarding the quality of their evidence (Class I-III), which was used to determine the level of recommendation (A, B, C, or U). See Table 1 below:

Table 1. Quality of Evidence for AAN Guidelines (from Cortese et al. 2011)

Disease	Conclusion	Quality
Acute inflammatory demyelinating polyneuropathy/Guillain Barre syndrome	Established effective	Class I
Chronic inflammatory demyelinating polyneuropathy, short-term treatment	Established effective	Class I
Polyneuropathy with monoclonal gammopathies of undetermined significance		
Immunoglobulin A Immunoglobulin G	Probably effective	Class I
Immunoglobulin M	Probably ineffective	Class I
Myasthenia gravis		
Preoperative preparation	Insufficient evidence	Class III
Myasthenic crisis	Insufficient evidence	Class III
Fulminant demyelinating CNS disease	Possibly effective	Class II
Chronic or secondary progressive multiple sclerosis	Established ineffective	Class I
Relapses in multiple sclerosis	Probably effective	Class I
Sydenham chorea	Insufficient evidence	Class III
Acute obsessive compulsive disorder and tics in PANDAS	Insufficient evidence	Class III

Conclusions

These guidelines offer the practitioner an evidence base for decision making regarding the use of plasmapheresis. The presence or absence of evidence may fortify discussions with patients, families, and other interested parties who either request or object to plasmapheresis. From the clinician's point of view, there are no significant changes in the recommendations from the 1996 version. The lack of Class I evidence for some disorders, i.e., myasthenia gravis, fulminant demyelinating central nervous system disease, Sydenham's chorea, and acute obsessive compulsive disorder and tics in PANDAS points to the need for continued research to inform clinical practice.

*The recommendations regarding multiple sclerosis are endorsed by the National Multiple Sclerosis Society.

References

American Academy of Neurology, Report of the Therapeutics and Technology Assessment Committee. Assessment of Plasmapheresis. Neurology 1996;47:840-843.

Cortese J, Chaudhry V, So YT et al. Evidence-based guideline update: Plasmapheresis in neurologic disorders. Report of the Therapeutics and Technology Assessment Subcommittee of the American Academy of Neurology. Neurology 2011;76:294-300.

Hughes RAC, Wijdicks EFM, Barohn R et al. Practice parameter: Immunotherapy for Guillain Barre syndrome. Report of the Quality Standards Subcommittee of the American Academy of Neurology. Neurology 2003;61:736-740.

McLeod BC, Sniecinski I, Ciavarella D et al. Frequency of immediate adverse effects associated with therapeutic apheresis. Transfusion 1999;39:282-288.

Wendell LC and Levine JM. Myasthenic crisis. The Neurohospitalist 2011;1:16-22.

Chapter 96

AHA/ASA GUIDELINES FOR THE MANAGEMENT OF SPONTANEOUS INTRACEREBRAL HEMORRHAGE-2010 UPDATE

August 31, 2010

Introduction

Despite the absence of a specific treatment for spontaneous, nontraumatic, intracerebral hemorrhage, early, aggressive medical management can improve patient outcome. To update physicians on state of the art care, the American Heart Association (AHA) and American Stroke Association (ASA) have published a new evidence-based guideline that covers diagnosis, hemostasis, blood pressure management, inpatient and nursing management, prevention of medical comorbidities, surgical treatment, prognosis, rehabilitation, prevention of recurrence, and other considerations (Morgenstern et al. 2010). All of the recommendations summarized below are Class I* ("conditions for which there is evidence for and/or general agreement that the procedure or treatment is useful and effective").

Early diagnosis is important, as >20% of patients deteriorate from the time they are seen by prehospital emergency medical services and arrival in the emergency room. While many hospitals have critical pathways for acute ischemic stroke, they may be less adept at managing the less frequently seen acute hemorrhagic stroke. Emergency management includes neurosurgery and/or neurology consultation and may necessitate blood pressure management, intubation, hematoma evacuation, external ventricular drainage, intracranial pressure monitoring, and reversal of coagulopathy.

Recommendations

Initial assessment includes prompt neuroimaging with CT or MRI. CT angiography and contrast-enhanced CT may be considered to help identify patients at risk of hematoma expansion. In addition, MRI/angiogram/venogram and CT angiogram/venogram are reasonable to identify underlying causes of hemorrhage such as arteriovenous malformations, cerebral vein thrombosis, moyamoya disease or tumors.

Patients with underlying coagulopathies need to be identified, whether due to oral anticoagulants, acquired or congenital factor deficiencies, or quantitative or qualitative platelet deficiencies. Coagulopathies should be corrected if possible. Patients should be initially managed in the intensive care unit, and should receive elastic stockings and intermittent pneumatic compression to prevent venous thromboembolism. Normoglycemia should be maintained, blood pressure controlled, and clinical epileptic seizures treated with antiepileptic medications. Electrographic seizures should also be treated in patients with altered mental status. Prompt surgical removal of the hemorrhage is indicated for patients with cerebellar hemorrhage with neurological deterioration, brainstem compression, and/or hydrocephalus from ventricular obstruction.

Further details regarding these recommendations can be found in the 22 page guideline.

Conclusions

Predicting prognosis for patients with intracerebral hemorrhage remains imperfect, justifying aggressive initial treatment. These updated recommendations provide a solid framework for a comprehensive clinical approach. Information regarding ongoing clinical trials for intracerebral hemorrhage can be found at: www.strokecenter.org/trials.

References

Morgenstern LB, Hemphill JC, Anderson C et al. Guidelines for the management of spontaneous intracerebral hemorrhage. A guideline for healthcare professionals from the American Heart Association/American Stroke Association. Stroke 2010;41:21-8-2129.

*These guidelines use a different rating system than the American Academy of Neurology.

Chapter 97

BRAIN DEATH CRITERIA REVIVED!

July 21, 2010

Introduction

What could be more essential for a physician than to know whether a patient is dead or alive, particularly if someone is about to harvest the patient's organs. Even a tiny mistake in the determination of brain death changes the donor's charity into a suicide and the harvester's surgery into murder.

So it's nice to have an up-to-date brain death guideline.

In 1995, the American Academy of Neurology published a useful guideline for the determination of brain death (AAN 1995). When I recently examined an unfortunate 44 year old woman who suffered a severe hypoxic-ischemic brain injury due to a drug overdose, I relied on this guideline to arrive at a diagnosis of brain death. I needed to be able to comfort the family prior to her organ donation and convince myself that she was, indeed, brain dead. Although she had no brainstem function, she had tremors of her upper extremities. But the 1995 guideline reassured me, "Spontaneous movements of limbs other than pathologic flexion or extension response...are occasionally seen and should not be misinterpreted as evidence for brainstem function."

I was also reluctant to make the diagnosis because I knew that a new brain death guideline was about to be published, but it was still a week away. Why a new guideline? Would anything change? I breathed easier today when I read, "The criteria for the determination of brain death given in the 1995 AAN practice parameter have not been invalidated by published reports of neurological recovery in patients who fulfill these criteria." Whew!

The new AAN brain death guideline for adults (>18) is endorsed by the American College of Radiology, Child Neurology Society, Neurocritical Care Society, and the Radiological Society of North America.

Clinical Questions
The authors posed five clinical questions:

1. Are there patients who fulfill the clinical criteria of brain death who recover neurologic function?

2. What is an adequate observation period to ensure that cessation of neurologic function is permanent?

3. Are complex motor movements that falsely suggest retained brain function sometimes observed in brain death?

4. What is the comparative safety of techniques for determining apnea?

5. Are there new ancillary tests that accurately identify patients with brain death?

A review of 38 articles that met search criteria arrived at only Level "U" recommendations for 4/5 questions due to a lack of evidence-based research (see Chapter 86). However, question #3 achieved a Level "C" recommendation (requires at least one Class II study or two consistent Class III studies).

Practical Guidance

Consequently, the new guideline is essentially "opinion-based" rather than "evidence-based." Until evidence-based studies become available, the authors offered "Practical Guidance for Determining Brain Death," briefly summarized below:

1. Establish irreversible and proximate cause of coma.

2. Exclude the presence of central nervous system drugs, neuromuscular blockade, or severe electrolyte, acid-base, or endocrine disturbance.

3. Achieve normal core temperature (>36 degrees C).

4. Achieve normal blood pressure (systolic ≥100 mm Hg).

5. Neurologic exam (one exam is sufficient in most states) consistent with brain death includes:

a) coma

b) absence of brainstem reflexes

c) absence of ocular movements using oculocephalic testing (Doll's eyes) and oculovestibular reflex testing (calorics)

d) absence of corneal reflex

e) absence of facial muscle movement to a noxious stimulus

f) absence of pharyngeal and tracheal reflexes

g) apnea

Ancillary tests, such as electroencephalography (EEG), cerebral angiography, nuclear scan, transcranial doppler, CT angiography, and MRI/MRA are not required for the clinical diagnosis of brain death. If, however, the patient doesn't tolerate the apnea test, an ancillary test may be used to support the diagnosis of brain death. The time of death should be documented. The guideline includes a helpful checklist for brain death determination.

Future research recommended by the authors includes examining the safety of the apnea test, alternative methods of apnea testing, audits of documentation, and assessing the competence of examiners.

Conclusions

Compared to the 1995 brain death guideline, the 2010 version has not substantively changed. Although the guideline failed to answer 4/5 of its questions, it serves to establish the "state of the art." The new guideline should help create more consistency in the determination of brain death and alleviate some of the trepidation suffered by physicians regarding this exacting task.

References
Report of the Quality Standards Subcommittee of the American Academy of Neurology Practice Parameters:

Determining brain death in adults. Summary statement. Neurology 1995;45:1012-1014.

Wijdicks EFM, Varelas PN, Gronseth GS, Greer DM. Evidence-based guideline update: Determining brain death in adults: Report of the Quality Standards Subcommittee of the American Academy of Neurology. Neurology 2010;74:1911-1918.

Chapter 98

NONMOTOR SYMPTOMS: THE 5TH CARDINAL FEATURE OF PARKINSON DISEASE

May 15, 2010

Notwithstanding which, it has not yet obtained a place in the clas-sification of nosologists; some have regarded its characteristic symp-toms as distinct and different diseases, and others have given its name to diseases differing essentially from it; whilst the unhappy sufferer has considered it as an evil, from the domination of which he had no prospect of escape.

An Essay on the Shaking Palsy
James Parkinson, 1817

Historical Context
Only two of the four cardinal features of Parkinson dis-ease, tremor and postural instability, were included in James Parkinson's original description of "Paralysis agitans" (Parkinson 1817). Unilateral and progression of tremor, interrupted speech, agraphia, loss of posture, and festinat-ing gait are vividly described, but bradykinesia and rigidity, now considered core features of the disease (Ropper and Samuels 2010) were overlooked. Further, the otherwise per-spicacious Dr. Parkinson inaccurately asserted, "the senses and intellect being uninjured."

However, Dr. Parkinson was aware that these patients could suffer nonmotor symptoms. In his original description of patient #6, "the action of the bowels had been very much retarded," possibly related to autonomic dysfunction. He also noted disturbance of sleep due to "tremulous motion of the limbs," perhaps periodic limb movements of sleep (PLMS).

Practice Parameter on Treatment of Nonmotor Symptoms
A new practice parameter of the American Academy of Neurology (AAN) addressed the nonmotor disorders of Parkinson disease (Zesiewicz et al. 2010). These include symptoms due to autonomic dysfunction (i.e., gastrointestinal disorders, orthostatic hypotension, sexual dysfunction, urinary incontinence), sleep disorders, (i.e., restless legs syndrome (RLS), PLMS, excessive daytime somnolence, insomnia, REM sleep behavior disorder), fatigue, and anxiety. Approaches to cognitive, mood dysfunction, and sialorrhea were addressed in a previous guideline.

The analytic process for this practice parameter began in 2005, and data were sparse. Only 46 articles contributed relevant information, highlighting the need for additional evidence-based studies.

Summary of Recommendations
Level A
Modafinil for subjective (but not objective) excessive daytime sleepiness.

Level B
Levodopa/carbidopa for PLMS

Level C

1. Sildenafil for erectile dysfunction

2. Polyethylene glycol for constipation

3. Methylphenidate for fatigue

The remaining symptoms all received level "U" (insufficient data) recommendations; orthostatic hypotension, urinary incontinence, REM sleep behavior disorder, anxiety, botulinum toxin for constipation, levodopa or melatonin for insomnia, and non-ergot dopamine antagonists for RLS and PLMS.

Prior Parkinson Disease Guidelines

Multiple guidelines have been developed by the AAN over the last 10 years to address different aspects of Parkinson disease. These include Neuroprotective Strategies and Alternative Therapies for Parkinson's Disease (Suchowersky et al. 2006a), Diagnosis and Prognosis of New Onset Parkinson Disease (Suchowersky et al. 2006b), Botulinum Neurotoxin for the Treatment of Movement Disorders (Simpson et al. 2008), Treatment of Parkinson's Disease with Motor Fluctuations and Dyskinesias (Pahwa et al. 2006), Evaluation and Treatment of Depression, Psychosis and Dementia in Parkinson Disease (Miyasaki et al. 2006), and Initiation of Treatment for Parkinson's Disease (Miyasaki et al. 2002).

Current Treatment

Modern day neurologists benefit from nearly 200 years of additional observation since the publication of "An Essay on the Shaking Palsy" (Parkinson 1817). It is now apparent that many patients with Parkinson disease suffer cognitive and other nonmotor symptoms. Recognition of nonmotor symptoms is important, as they may significantly contribute to morbidity. An increased appreciation of nonmotor symptoms associated with Parkinson disease is suggested by the recent establishment of a movement disorders program at a psychiatric hospital in Providence, RI. However, as in Dr. Parkinson's day, nonmotor symptoms of Parkinson disease are still often overlooked in practice.

A new screening tool for physicians not available to James Parkinson is a 30 question self-administered questionnaire developed by the International Parkinson's Disease Non Motor Group. The questionnaire may be time efficient for physicians, as patients can complete it in the waiting room. In recognition of the importance of nonmotor symptoms to overall function, the revised version of the Unified Parkinson's Disease Rating Scale includes a section on nonmotor symptoms.

Conclusion

As treatments for the motor symptoms of Parkinson disease continue to improve, other aspects of the disease, such as nonmotor symptoms, advance to the forefront of the patient's and physician's attention. This new AAN guideline will help physicians address the nonmotor symptoms of Parkinson disease, which will enable sufferers to achieve an improved quality of life and escape some of the symptoms of their affliction.

References

Friedman, J. Letter announcing the establishment of a new Movement Disorders Program at Butler Hospital, Providence, RI, March 15, 2010.

Miyasaki JM, Shannon K, Voon V et al. Practice Parameter: evaluation and treatment of depression, psychosis, and dementia in Parkinson disease (an evidence-based review): report of the Quality Standards Subcommittee of the American Academy of Neurology. Neurology 2006;66:996-1002.

Miyasaki JM, Martin W, Suchowersky O et al. Practice parameter: Initiation of treatment for Parkinson's disease: An evidence-based review. Neurology 2002;58:11-17.

Pahwa R, Factor SA, Lyons KE et al. Practice Parameter: Treatment of Parkinson disease with motor fluctuations and dyskinesia (an evidence-based review). Neurology 2006;66:983-995.

Parkinson, J. An essay on the shaking palsy. J. Neuropsychiatry Clin Neurosci 2002;14(2):223-236 (reprinted from 1817).

Ropper AH, Samuels MA. Adams and Victor's Neurology. Chapter 39. Degenerative Diseases of the Nervous System. Access Medicine. McGraw Hill. http://www.accessmedicine.com.ezp-prod1.hul.harvard.edu/content.aspx?aID=3639184, (accessed 2010).

Simpson DM, Blitzer A, Brashear A et al. Assessment: Botulinum neurotoxin for the treatment of movement disorders (an evidence-based review). Neurology 2008;70:1699-1706.

Suchowersky O, Gronseth G, Perlmutter et al. Practice Parameter: Neuroprotective strategies and alternative therapies for Parkinson disease (an evidence-based review). Neurology 2006a;66:976-982.

Suchowersky O, Reich S, Perlmutter J et al. Practice Parameter: Diagnosis and prognosis of new onset Parkinson disease (an evidence-based review). Neurology 2006b;66:968-975.

Zesiewicz TA, Sullivan KL, Arnulf I et al. Practice Parameter: Treatment of nonmotor symptoms of Parkinson disease. Neurology 2010;74:924-931.

Chapter 99

PRACTICE PARAMETER SUPPORTS BOTULINUM TOXIN A FOR SPASTICITY

February 6, 2010

Botulinum toxin type A effectively reduces localized/segmental spasticity in the limbs of children and adolescents with cerebral palsy, according to a recently published Practice Parameter from the American Academy of Neurology (Delgado et al. 2009). The evidence regarding functional improvement, however, was conflicting. Side effects include pain, weakness, unsteadiness, falls, fatigue, incontinence, and dysphagia.

For generalized spasticity, diazepam was "probably effective," and tizanidine "possibly effective." Insufficient data were available to comment on dantroline and oral or intrathecal baclofen. The recommendations were based on an expert review of the literature from 1966-2008.

The practice parameter concluded that botulinum toxin type A is "generally safe," although there have been isolated cases of generalized weakness (FDA 2009). All botulinum toxin products feature a black box warning and must be administered with a Risk Evaluation and Mitigation Strategy (REMS), which includes a Medication Guide and a Communication Plan. Patients need to be educated regarding the possibility of dysphagia, dysphonia, dyspnea, respiratory distress or weakness. Generalized weakness from botulinum toxin injections may be dose related, as this side effect is not seen when small doses are used for cosmetic treatment of glabellar (frown) lines.

Botulinum toxin type A is not approved by the U.S. Food and Drug Administration (FDA) for the treatment of spasticity in children. However, it is approved for this purpose in children and adults in Canada, among other countries.

More than 10,000 children are born with cerebral palsy in the US each year, most of whom will be affected by spasticity. Reduction of spasticity may reduce pain and muscle spasms, improve posture, facilitate brace use, minimize contractures and deformity, and improve mobility, dexterity, and self-care. However, the treatment must be individualized, as spasticity may help some children compensate for muscle weakness.

This Level "A" (see Appendix) recommendation should reassure physicians who treat spasticity with botulinum toxin type A in children with cerebral palsy. Patients should continue to receive education and close follow-up regarding potential systemic toxicity. More research is needed to clarify the role of other antispasticity agents.

References

Delgado MR, Hirtz D, Aisen M et al. Practice Parameter: Pharmacologic treatment of spasticity in children and adolescents with cerebral palsy (an evidence-based review). Neurology 2010;74:336-343.

FDA Requires Boxed Warning for all Botulinum Products, http//www.fda.gov/News/Events/Newsroom/PressAnnouncements/ucm149574.htm, April 30, 2009.

Chapter 100

MILD TRAUMATIC BRAIN INJURY/ CONCUSSIONS-NEW DEPARTMENT OF DEFENSE GUIDELINES

January 22, 2010

Introduction

Concussions can significantly impact mental, physical, and social well-being. The best evidence on diagnosis and management of mild traumatic brain injury/concussion in adults has been published as a clinical practice guideline by the Veterans Administration and Department of Defense (Working Group 2009). The guideline addresses diagnosis and management of patients who are evaluated for symptoms at least seven days after the initial head injury. The well-organized and comprehensive document includes definitions, classifications, charts, algorithms, and references. Algorithms address initial presentation, management of symptoms, and follow up of persistent symptoms. A useful structured interview for collecting head trauma event characteristics is included in the Appendix. The authors use the terms "concussion" and "mild traumatic brain injury" interchangeably. For those who would like to read more, the entire issue of the journal is devoted to the topic.

Soldiers at Risk

The current military situations in Iraq and Afghanistan with numerous deployments and the nature of modern combat expose soldiers to the risk of repetitive mild traumatic brain injury. Although the new guidelines are based on the battlefield experience of soldiers, the results are applicable to civilian and sports injuries. Emergency room (ER) physicians are well acquainted with the problem-more than 1.1 million people with mild traumatic head injury are seen each year in the ER.

Long-Term Sequelae

The evidence that mild traumatic brain injury, especially repeated concussions, may have severe long-term consequences is becoming increasingly appreciated in the world of sports, particularly boxing, football, and hockey. An ex-Harvard quarterback has founded a company that produces a football helmet design to reduce "dings" and "bell ringers," players' parlance for concussions. The state of Oregon, at the request of the Brain Injury Association of Oregon, has passed a new law effective January 2010, requiring school athletic coaches to take courses to learn to recognize concussions in their athletes and how to seek appropriate medical treatment. Known as Max's Law, the statute is named after an athlete who suffered permanent traumatic brain injury in a high school football game.

Comment

While it is difficult to eliminate traumatic brain injury suffered in combat, sports-related brain injuries are another matter. Efforts are ongoing to improve the design and construction of helmets to protect the brain, which should help ameliorate injury. However, if data continue to accumulate regarding the susceptibility of the brain to injury in these common sports, individuals who box, play football, hockey, and other sports that include repetitive impacts to the head must seriously reconsider the risks and benefits of their participation. Parents have a particular responsibility to guide their children regarding activities that are associated with brain damage and may have deleterious and lifelong consequences.

Treatment?

While various therapies may ameliorate symptoms of traumatic brain injury, there is no medication or other treatment known to reverse underlying brain pathology associated with neurocognitive defects due to mild traumatic brain injury. Consequently the importance of prevention is paramount. Neurologists, pediatricians, family physicians, other informed health care providers, as well as coaches and players, may assist in public education. Even an attorney, Michael Kaplen, Esq., has created an education/marketing site regarding head injury.

This review published by the United States Government acknowledges the public health implications of mild traumatic brain injury and provides comprehensive, state of the art guidance for symptomatic treatment of headaches, dizziness, fatigue, vision problems, and other symptoms.

Future Research

More research is needed to minimize brain damage resulting from head injury related to combat and contact sports, including controlled trials of current therapy, the development of effective, new treatments, as well as improved preventive strategies. Boston University has developed an excellent research program at the Center for Traumatic Encephalopathy with respect to sports-related injuries that includes careful neuropathological examination of the brains of deceased athletes.

More Guidelines on the Way

Evidence-based guidelines for sports related concussions for children age 5 and up are expected from the American Academy of Neurology (AAN) in April 2011.

References

Kaplen, M. braininjury.blogs.com.

Working Group. VA/DoD clinical practice guideline for management of Concussion/mild traumatic brain injury. Journal of Rehabilitation Research and Development 2009;46:CPI-CP68.

Update June 3, 2013

Interest in traumatic brain injury continues to grow with much attention to the diagnosis and management of concussions. An entire section of this collection is devoted to traumatic brain injury (Section 1). The American Academy of Neurology presented its new evidence-based guideline on concussion at a press conference I attended at the AAN meeting last March in San Diego, CA. The new guideline addresses adults and children.

Additional References

Giza CC, Kutcher JS, Ashwal S et al. Evidence-based guideline update: Evaluation and management of concussion in sports. Report of the Guideline Development Subcommittee of the American Academy of Neurology. Neurology Epub 2013 March 18.

Chapter 101

AMYOTROPHIC LATERAL SCLEROSIS AMERICAN ACADEMY OF NEUROLOGY PRACTICE PARAMETER UPDATE

January 7, 2010

Introduction

The American Academy of Neurology (AAN) recently published two evidence-based practice parameters (Miller et al. 1999a, 1999b) on amyotrophic lateral sclerosis (ALS) that update the last guidelines published a decade ago (Miller et al. 1999). The new guidelines recommend that riluzole be offered to slow disease progression (Level A) (see Appendix for explanation of "Levels").

Lower level recommendations include supportive therapy such as supplemental nutrition via percutaneous endoscopic gastrostomy (PEG) (Level B) and noninvasive ventilation (NIV) (Level B). Referral to a multidisciplinary clinic, which may prolong survival, also warranted a Level B recommendation. Specific management approaches include botulinum toxin B (Level B) or low dose radiation therapy (Level C) for refractory sialorrhea, and a combination of dextromethorphan and quinidine (pending U.S. Food and Drug Administration (FDA) approval) for pseudobulbar affect (Level B). Patients should also be screened for cognitive and behavioral impairment (Level B). The new guidelines benefit from the continuity of Dr. Robert Miller's leadership as well as two experts from the 1999 paper.

Not Just a "Pure Motor Neuron Disease"

Contrary to the earlier concept of ALS as a pure motor neuron disease, significant effects on cognition and behavior have been appreciated in many patients with ALS (Flaherty-Craig et al. 2006). The new guidelines highlight these observations with the recommendation that patients be screened for cognitive and behavioral problems. Frontotemporal dysfunction may have significant practical implications, such as impaired decision making as well as diminished compliance with noninvasive ventilation and PEG.

Medication Treatment

Unfortunately, there are no new medications that address the underlying pathophysiology of ALS. Riluzole offers only modest benefit and was recommended in the 1997 AAN Practice Advisory (AAN 1997). Most patients still die within two to five years. The new Practice Parameters focus on supportive care and reinforce pragmatic respiratory and nutritional therapy.

Unproven Therapies

The guidelines may also help practitioners dissuade patients and their families from investing money, time, and emotional resources into unproven therapies. For example, the guidelines recommend that creatine *not* be given as treatment for ALS (Level A), that high dose vitamin E should *not* be considered (Level B), and that evidence for benefit from low dose vitamin E was "equivocal" (Level U).

Future Research

The authors highlight 9 topics that require more research; (1) evaluation of lithium as a disease modifying agent, (2) nutrition, supplements, and vitamins, (3) respiratory management, (4) optimal methods of "breaking the news," (5) the role of the multidisciplinary clinic, (6) evidence-based symptom management (anxiety, constipation, cramps, depression, fatigue, exercise, pain, pseudobulbar affect, sialorrhea, spasticity), (7) cognitive and behavioral impairment, (8) communication methods, and (9) palliative care. If this research proves productive, advances in ALS therapy will merit a new practice parameter before 2019.

References

Flahert-Craig C, Eslinger P, Stephens B, Simmons Z. A rapid screening battery to identify frontal dysfunction in patients with ALS. Neurology 2006;67:2070-2072.

Miller RG, Jackson CE, Kasarskis EJ et al. Practice Parameter update: The care of the patient with amyotrophic lateral sclerosis: Drug, nutritional, and respiratory therapies (an evidence-based review). Neurology 2009a73:1218-1226.

Miller RG, Jackson CE, Kasarskis EJ et al. Practice Parameter update: The care of the patient with amyotrophic lateral sclerosis: Multidisciplinary care, symptom management, and cognitive/behavioral impairment (an evidence-based review). Neurology 2009b;73:1227-1233.

Miller RG, Rosenberg JA, Gelinas DF et al. Practice Parameter: The care of the patient with amyotrophic lateral sclerosis (an evidence-based review). Neurology 1999;52:1311-1323.

Practice advisory on the treatment of amyotrophic lateral sclerosis with riluzole: Report of the Quality Standards Subcommittee of the American Academy of Neurology 1997;49:657-659.

Update June 3, 2013

Nuedexta, a combination of dextromethorphan hydrobromide and quinidine sulfate, received FDA approval for the treatment of pseudobulbar affect on October 29, 2010.

Chapter 102

MICROCEPHALY PRACTICE PARAMETER: INVESTIGATIVE APPROACH AND RECOMMENDATIONS

October 18, 2009

Introduction

A recent practice parameter published by the American Academy of Neurology (AAN) and Child Neurology Society addressed the evaluation of the child with microcephaly (Ashwal et al. 2009). Approximately 25,000 children are diagnosed with microcephaly each year in the United States. These children are more likely to have neurologic problems such as mental retardation (50%), epilepsy (40%), cerebral palsy (20%), and ophthalmologic disorders (20-50%). Diverse etiologies may be responsible. Genetic etiologies are found in 15.5-53.3%. Metabolic disorders are rare (1-5%). The yield of neuroimaging is high (43-80%). Not surprisingly, children with more severe microcephaly are more likely to have severe developmental impairments.

The omnipresent tape measure in every pediatrician's office may be the most "cost effective" neurodiagnostic tool available for determining head circumference and the diagnosis of microcephaly. With respect to neuroimaging, MRI is generally more sensitive than CT.

The article includes a useful table of etiologies of congenital and postnatal onset microcephaly. A second table lists the genetic syndromes associated with microcephaly and severe epilepsy. Algorithms outline the steps for the evaluation of congenital microcephaly and postnatal onset microcephaly.

In addition, there are several useful appendices; a list of resources for evaluating children with microcephaly, an MRI-based classification scheme, and a syndromic classification of primary microcephaly and associated genes. Additional e-appendices are available online; metabolic disorders associated with congenital microcephaly, neurodevelopment in children with microcephaly, microcephalic syndromes with prominent ophthalmologic involvement, and microcephalic syndromes with prominent auditory abnormalities.

A very clear Podcast, introduced by Bob Gross, MD, the new editor of *Neurology*, features an interview with the paper's first and second authors. (The Podcast may be downloaded from the Neurology Web site with iTunes or similar software.)

Conclusions

Pediatricians and others who care for children will find no surprises in the recommendations. This practice parameter confirms the current practice of investigating the etiology of microcephaly with MRI and screening for cerebral palsy, epilepsy, sensory deficits, and developmental delay. Genetic and metabolic testing may also be useful. As one would expect, when microcephaly is particularly severe, developmental impairments are more debilitating.

The primary recommendations from this practice parameter are only Level C, a limitation resulting from the lack of Class I and II studies (see Appendix for explanation of "Levels" and "Class"). It is unclear why the AAN and Child Neurology Society chose to devote the necessary resources to this topic (review of 4,500 titles and abstracts and 150 articles) when there are no critical high level recommendations to be made. Perhaps the intent was to review the "state of the art" and emphasize the need for more research? As it stands, complete with tables, figures, and appendices, this practice parameter is an excellent and concise resource for physicians faced with the challenge of managing children with microcephaly.

References

Ashwal S, Michelson D, Plawner L, Dobyns WB. Practice Parameter: Evaluation of the child with microcephaly (an evidence-based review). Neurology 2009;73:887-897.

Chapter 103

WOMEN WITH EPILEPSY PRACTICE PARAMETERS-THE LAUNCH

April 28, 2009

Introduction

The big highlight today at the American Academy of Neurology (AAN) Annual Meeting was a 10 am press conference for the launch of three new Practice Parameters on Women with Epilepsy (Harden et al. 2009a, b, c). Cynthia Harden, MD, Gary Gronseth, MD, Jennifer Hopp, MD, and a woman with epilepsy, Mary Katherine Albritton, composed a panel that explained the parameters and responded to questions from a large international press contingent. Cynthia Harden, MD, Director of the Epilepsy Division at the University of Miami's Miller School of Medicine, was the lead author and organizer of a large panel of authors who painstakingly reviewed hundreds of abstracts, labored over rating them with a variety of methodologies, (at least one of them brand new), and came up with some conclusions that you can hang your hat on.

(I should pause here for an obligatory conflict of interest disclosure. I was one of the 21 authors on the volunteer panel who composed the guidelines, and this work began more than 2 years ago. (The gestation time of the guidelines was more than double the gestation time of its subject matter.) Secondly, I was the medical writer who wrote the guidelines, so I couldn't get paid until they were published. So I am really glad they are finally done!)

Why are these practice parameters so important? For one thing, there are approximately 1/2 million women with epilepsy in the USA, many of whom are treated by family practitioners, internists, and general neurologists, as well as epilepsy specialists, all of whom need guidance to make the best recommendations for their patients. Second, this is the first update to the original guideline on this topic published in 1998.

What is really exciting about these practice parameters is that we now have good prospective data, extending all the way back to 1997 when the North American Pregnancy Registry began, to answer some of the knotty questions regarding teratogenicity. For example, is it epilepsy or antiepileptic drugs that are responsible for the increase in teratogenicity? If it's the drugs, which ones are the worst? The guidelines address other questions as well. Do pregnant women with epilepsy really have more obstetrical complications such as increased hemorrhage and C-sections, and do their seizures really get worse during pregnancy? We don't have the data to respond to all of these and other important questions, but we have answers to some of them, and it is really satisfying to see this progress. Those who agitated for the creation of the pregnancy registries should be congratulated for their foresight.

Major findings of the three practice parameters:

Obstetrical Complications and Seizure Frequency
a. Premature contractions and premature labor are probably not increased, unless the women smoke.

b. Women with epilepsy who are seizure free for at least 9 months prior to pregnancy are likely to stay seizure free during pregnancy.

Folic acid, Vitamin K, Blood levels, Breastfeeding

a. Folic acid should be taken prenatally at 0.4 mg/day, the same as Centers for Disease Control and Prevention recommendations for women without epilepsy (there wasn't enough evidence to create more specific recommendations).

b. Not clear whether antiepileptic drugs contribute to hemorrhagic disease of the newborn, and consequently not clear whether prenatal Vitamin K is indicated.

c. Monitoring antiepileptic blood levels is important, as they may change dramatically during pregnancy, depending upon the antiepileptic drug.

Antiepileptic drugs may be secreted in breast milk, particularly barbiturates and levetiracetam, but it's not clear if it's bad for the infant (unless there is excessive sedation).

Teratogenesis and Perinatal Outcomes

a. Valproate and polytherapy should be avoided because of increased teratogenicity and impaired cognition.

b. Phenytoin and phenobarbital may also lead to reduced cognitive outcomes.

So, for the first time we can say with confidence that there is a drug to avoid in pregnancy (if the clinical situation permits), and that two drugs are worse than one. There appears to be an increased risk of adverse cognitive outcomes with several antiepileptic drugs. Overall, valproate appears to be the worst offender.

If possible, women should have their epilepsy treatment optimized long before they become pregnant, which means monotherapy if possible, the right drug for their seizure type, prenatal vitamins and folate, switch from valproate if feasible, baseline antiepileptic drug levels, optimized management of any comorbidities, and nutritional and other common sense advice for a healthy baby (stop smoking, exercise, keep weight gain under control, etc.).

Mary Katherine Albritton had two children, an 18 month old girl and a three year old boy. The boy was conceived while she was taking lamotrigine and the girl when she was on a combination of lamotrigine and levetiracetam. Both children are normal. She planned her pregnancies and took folic acid one year before she became pregnant. She stated she had a great neurologist (Page Pennell, MD), obstetrician, and perinatologist. She had five seizures with her first pregnancy and three seizures with the second. More recently, she has been seizure-free for two years. Mary is an example of most women with epilepsy who have healthy children.

Dr. Harden emphasized that although there may be a risk of teratogenicity with all the antiepileptic drugs, a woman should not stop medications without her physician's guidance. Increased seizures and status epilepticus may result. Dr. Harden concluded, "Pregnancy for women with epilepsy is a fairly safe undertaking. There are few obstetrical risks, and if the patient is seizure-free prior to the pregnancy, she will probably stay that way during the pregnancy."

As the various pregnancy registries (North American, UK, Australian, European) collect additional patients, more of our questions regarding the management of women with epilepsy will be answered, and the strength of the answers will increase.

References

Harden CL, Hopp J, Ting TY et al. Practice Parameter update: Management issues for women with epilepsy-focus on pregnancy (an evidence-based review): I. Obstetrical complications and change in seizure frequency. Epilepsia 2009;50(5):1229-1236.

Harden CL, Meador KJ, Pennell PB et al. Practice Parameter update: Management issues for women with epilepsy-focus on pregnancy (an evidence-based review): II. Teratogenesis and perinatal outcomes. Epilepsia 2009;50(5):1237-1246.

Harden CL, Pennell PB, Koppel BS et al. Practice Parameter update: Management issues for women with epilepsy-focus on pregnancy (an evidence-based review): III. Vitamin K, folic acid, blood levels, and breastfeeding. Epilepsia 2009;50(5):1247-1255.

APPENDIX

American Academy of Neurology
Recommendation "Levels"

A=Established as effective, ineffective or harmful (or established as useful/predictive or not useful/predictive) for the given condition in the specified population. (Level A rating requires at least two consistent Class I studies.*)

B=Probably effective, ineffective or harmful (or probably useful/predictive or not useful/predictive) for the given condition in the specified population. (Level B rating requires at least one Class I study or two consistent Class II studies.)

C=Possibly effective, ineffective or harmful (or possibly useful/predictive or not useful/predictive) for the given condition in the specified population. (Level C rating requires at least one Class II study or two consistent Class III studies.)

U=Data inadequate or conflicting; given current knowledge, treatment (test, predictor) is unproven.

*In exceptional cases, one convincing Class I study may suffice for an "A" recommendation if 1) all criteria are met, 2) the magnitude of effect is large (relative rate improved outcome >5 and the lower limit of the confidence interval is >2).

American Academy of Neurology "Class" Categories

Class I
Prospective, randomized, controlled clinical trial with masked outcome assessment, in a representative population. The following are required:
a) Primary outcome is clearly defined.
b) Exclusion/inclusion criteria are clearly defined.
c) Adequate accounting for drop-outs and cross-overs with numbers sufficiently low to have minimal potential for bias.
d) Relevant baseline characteristics are presented and substantially equivalent among treatment groups or there is appropriate statistical adjustment for differences.

Class II
Prospective matched group cohort study in a representative population with masked outcome assessment that meets a-d above OR a randomized controlled trial (RCT) in a representative population that lacks one criteria a-d.

Class III
All other controlled trials (including well-defined natural history controls or patients serving as own controls) in a representative population, where outcome assessment is independent of patient treatment.

Class IV
Evidence from uncontrolled studies, case series, case reports, or expert opinion.

Made in the USA
Charleston, SC
03 November 2013